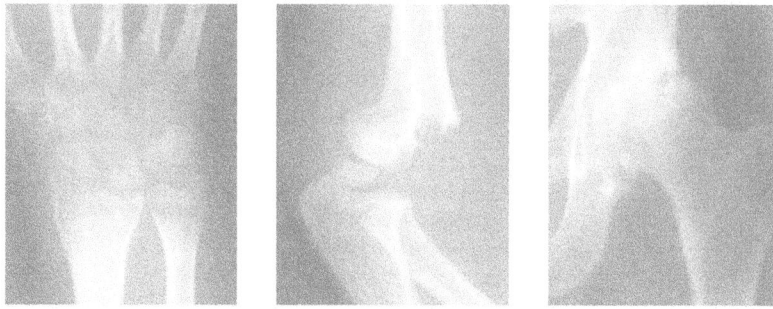

The WHO manual of diagnostic imaging

Radiographic Anatomy and Interpretation
of the Musculoskeletal System

Editors
Harald Ostensen M.D.
Holger Pettersson M.D.

Authors
A. Mark Davies M.D.
Holger Pettersson M.D.

In collaboration with
F. Arredondo M.D., M.R. El Meligi M.D., R. Guenther M.D.,
G.K. Ikundu M.D., L. Leong M.D., P. Palmer M.D., P. Scally M.D.

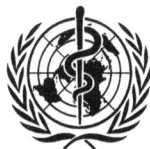

**Published by the World Health Organization
in collaboration with the
International Society of Radiology**

WHO Library Cataloguing-in-Publication Data

Davies, A. Mark

Radiography of the musculoskeletal system / authors : A. Mark Davies, Holger Pettersson; in collaboration with F. Arredondo . . . [et al.]

WHO manuals of diagnostic imaging / editors : Harald Ostensen, Holger Pettersson; vol. 2

Published by the World Health Organization in collaboration with the International Society of Radiology

1.Musculoskeletal system – radiography   2.Musculoskeletal diseases – radiography   3.Musculoskeletal abnormalities – radiography   4.Manuals   I.Pettersson, Holger   II.Arredondo, F.   III.Series editor: Ostensen, Harald

ISBN 92 4 154555 0   (NLM Classification: WE 141)

The World Health Organization welcomes requests for permission to reproduce or translate its publications, in part or in full. Applications and enquiries should be addressed to the Office of Publications, World Health Organization, CH-1211 Geneva 27, Switzerland, which will be glad to provide the latest information on any changes made to the text, plans for new editions, and reprints and translations already available.

Reprinted 2004

Designed in New Zealand
Typeset in Hong Kong
Printed in Malta

Contents

List of editors, authors and collaborators

Editors

Harald Ostensen, M.D., Coordinator, Team for Diagnostic Imaging and Laborabory Technology, WHO, Geneva, Switzerland, co-chairman, The Global Steering Group for Education and Training in Diagnostic Imaging

Holger Pettersson, M.D., Professor of Radiology, Lund University, Sweden, co-chairman, The Global Steering Group for Education and Training in Diagnostic Imaging

Authors

A. Mark Davies, M.D., Consultant Radiologist, Royal Orthopaedic Hospital, Birmingham, UK

Holger Pettersson, M.D., Professor of Radiology, Lund University, Sweden

Collaborators

F. Arredondo, M.D., Professor of Radiology, Universidad Francisco Mairoguin, Guatemala, Guatemala

M.R. El Meligi, M.D., Professor of Radiology, Cairo University, Egypt

R. Guenther, M.D., Professor of Radiology, University Hospital RWTH, Aachen, Germany

G.K. Ikundu, M.D., Lecturer, Department of Radiology, University of Nairobi, Kenya

L. Leong, M.D., Senior Consultant Radiologist, Department of Radiology, Queen Mary Hospital, University of Hong Kong, The Peoples Republic of China

P. Palmer, M.D., Professor Emeritus of Radiology, University of California, Davis, CA, USA

P. Scally, M.D., Consultant Radiologist, Mater Hospital, South Brisbane, Australia

Foreword

Modern diagnostic imaging offers a vast spectrum of modalities and techniques, which enables us to study the function and morphology of the human body in details that approaches science fiction.

However, it should be noticed that even in the most advanced Imaging Department in the economically privileged parts of the world, 70–80% of all clinically relevant questions may be solved by using the two main cornerstones of diagnostic imaging, which are Radiography (X-ray) and Ultrasonography.

It should also be remembered that thousands of hospitals and institutions worldwide do not have the possibilities to perform even these fundamental imaging procedures, for lack of equipment and/ or diagnostic imaging skills.

Therefore, WHO in collaboration with The International Commission for Radiologic Education (ICRE) of the International Society of Radiology (ISR) is creating a series of "WHO Manuals of Diagnostic Imaging", developed under the umbrella of The Global Steering Group for Education and Training in Diagnostic Imaging. Among the members of this group are the major regional and global societies involved in Diagnostic Imaging, including the International Society of Radiology (ISR), The International Society of Radiographers and Radiological Technologists (ISRRT), and the World Federation for Ultrasound in Medicine and Biology (WFUMB).

The full series of manuals will primarily cover the examination techniques and interpretation of Radiography, in a later stage also Ultrasonography. It is meant for health care personnel who in their daily work are responsible for producing and interpreting radiographs, be it radiologists or other medical specialists, general practioners, or radiological technologists working in rural areas.

The manuals are authored by authorities in the specific fields dealt within each manual, supported by a group of collaborators, that together cover the experience, knowledge and needs, which are specific for different regions of the world.

It is our sincere hope that the manuals will prove helpful in the daily routine, facilitating the diagnostic work up and hence the treatment, to the best benefit for the patient.

Geneva, Switzerland and Lund, Sweden, May 2002

Harald Ostensen
Holger Pettersson

Preface

To be asked to author one of the WHO Manuals of Diagnostic Imaging is certainly a great honour, for any radiologist in the world. But to create a manual, that should fit the varying needs in vast areas of the world is certainly also a major challenge.

However, with the excellent support of the group of collaborators referred to us by the International Commission for Radiologic Education (ICRE), we have done our best to fulfil the demands from WHO. Thus we have tried to cover, in a manageable format, the information that is essential for the accurate interpretation of the vast majority of those radiographic musculoskeletal examinations that will appear in a General Radiologic Department.

It is our hope that you, the readers, will find this manual useful in your daily routine work. We sincerely hope that it will facilitate your work, and thereby improve the treatment of your patients.

Birmingham, UK, and Lund, Sweden, January 2002

A. Mark Davies
Holger Pettersson

CHAPTER 1

General Principles

- X-rays are the beam of ionizing radiation emitted from the X-ray tube during the exposure. Although "X-ray" is a term frequently used to refer to the image/film produced, radiograph is the correct term.

- the *radiograph*, irrespective of the projection/view, is a 2-dimensional representation of a 3-dimensional structure. The image produced is therefore made up of multiple overlying structures. Accurate localisation of an abnormality frequently requires two radiographs obtained at right angles to one another e.g. *anteroposterior (AP)* and *lateral projections*. Remember that an object visible on a radiograph may be situated anywhere between the X-ray tube and the film cassette (fig 1.1).

- structures of high density (e.g. bones and metal foreign bodies) will absorb (attenuate) the X-ray beam more than structures of low density (e.g. soft tissues and air).

    — bones will appear white
    — soft tissues will appear grey
    — air/gas will appear black

- remember that *fluoroscopy* (X-ray screening) gives a negative image on the TV-monitor or screen. Therefore, the appearances are reversed with bones black and air/gas white.

- most soft tissue structures have an atomic number (density) approximating to that of water and will attenuate (absorb) the X-ray beam to the same degree. Most soft tissues, irrespective of their nature (e.g. muscle, tendon, blood and pus) will appear with the same grey density on the radiograph.

- fat has a density (atomic number) sufficiently less than that of water for it to be distinguished from the remaining soft tissues provided it is present in an adequate amount. It will appear darker than other soft tissues and lighter (greyer) than air/gas. Fat planes will appear on the radiograph as dark linear strands separating soft tissue structures. Displacement or obliteration of the fat planes may be the only sign on the radiograph of a significant soft tissue abnormality. For example;

Elbow – displacement of the fat pads indicates a joint effusion or haemarthrosis (see Trauma Chapter)

Pelvis – obliteration of the fat plane around the bladder in trauma indicates free fluid or blood within the pelvic cavity.

- *foreign bodies* may be introduced into the body by trauma, ingestion or at the time of surgery. Most will have a density greater than water and will appear whiter than the soft tissues. Metallic foreign bodies will appear white (figs 1.1, 1.2).

- the optimum *exposure* of a radiograph of the skeletal system will demonstrate the bones to show both the cortical and trabecular pattern as well as the soft tissue detail. An overexposed radiograph will appear dark and an underexposed radiograph light/washed-out.

- where possible, radiographs should be examined on a light box with subdued ambient lighting, otherwise important information may be missed.

- *interpretation* of the radiograph(s) requires a careful approach. The individual responsible for interpreting the radiograph should first ensure the following;

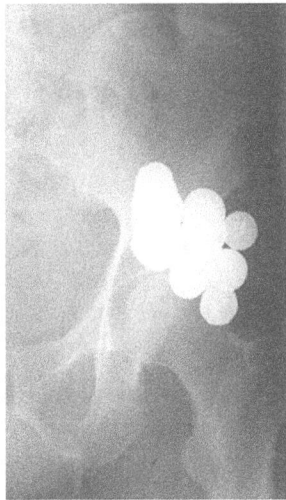

Figure 1.1
AP radiograph of the hip. The multiple rounded white abnormalities are not **in** but **on** the patient, due to at least 10 overlapping coins in the pocket of the trousers that should have been removed prior to the X-ray examination.

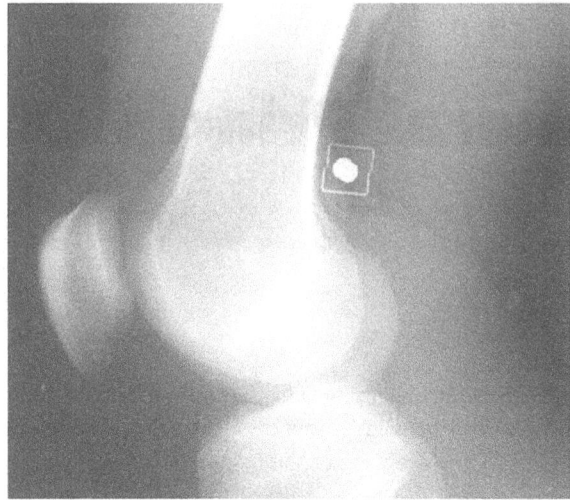

Figure 1.2
Lateral radiograph of the knee of an adult who had been shot with an airgun.

- bones (femur, tibia and patella) = white
- muscles = grey
- air in front and behind knee = black
- rounded white object behind distal femur is a foreign body (airgun pellet)
- the angular objects around the pellet are also foreign bodies. They are metallic staples applied to the skin to show the site of the entry wound
- the black linear shadows adjacent to the pellet represents air introduced at the time of injury.

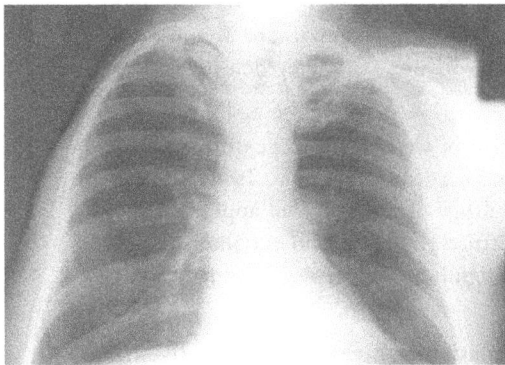

Figure 1.3
Chest radiograph. The abnormality is what is NOT present on the film. The whole right upper limb and shoulder girdle have been surgically removed as treatment for an advanced sarcoma.

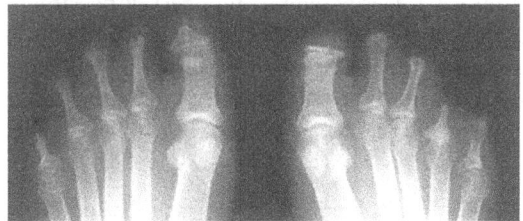

Figure 1.4
Resorption of the phalanges of the toes. The appearances are nonspecific but in this patient from the Indian Subcontinent was the result of longstanding leprosy.

1. Check patient name and side marker (left or right) on film(s) are correct.
2. Check clinical details (age, sex, history etc.)

Then, undertake a systematic review of the radiograph(s). This requires detailed examination of the bones and soft tissue, known areas of complex anatomy and the periphery of the film where pathology may be only partially shown. When necessary, use a bright light (e.g. a bright bulb or angle-poise lamp) to illuminate the radiograph for further inspection of the soft tissues. The assessment should include deciding what is normal from abnormal. Remember that means not just noting new features such as fractures or foreign bodies but also identifying if anything is absent. Is something missing that would normally be seen (fig 1.3)? Review of previous radiographs, if available, is essential to determine whether an abnormality is a new feature and, if not, whether there has been any significant change.

- the interpretation of the radiograph(s) should finish with the production of a report detailing the clinically relevant observations both positive and negative together with a diagnosis, if possible.

- consideration of possible pathologies in a particular case should take into account the life style, country of origin and residence of the patient. Diseases are frequently endemic in certain parts of the world and yet almost unknown in other parts. This will therefore significantly influence the probable causes of an abnormality on a radiograph. For example, figure 1.4 shows the nonspecific appearances of resorption (destruction) of the phalanges of the toes of both feet. If this was a patient from the polar regions then the appearances might be the result of severe frostbite (damage to the bones and soft tissues from prolonged cold). On the other hand, were this a patient from tropical Africa or the Indian subcontinent the possibility of frostbite would be extremely remote. In these areas, leprosy would be a much more likely explanation for the bone destruction.

CHAPTER 2

Terminology

- as with any technical subject, there are numerous terms used to describe the different appearances on a radiograph. Some knowledge of the common terms can be helpful when reading reports. If writing to another colleague, it is important to remember that those reading the report may not understand complex terms. Useful terms include;

sclerotic	— increased bone density
lytic	— bone destruction
cortex	— compact (dense) bone forming the bone surface
medulla	— trabecular bone in the bone marrow
articular	— refers to a joint (an articulation)
demineralization	— decreased bone density (as occurs with osteomalacia/osteopenia/osteoporosis)
ankylosis	— fusion
osteo-	— prefix meaning bony (e.g. osteosarcoma)
chondro-	— prefix meaning cartilaginous (e.g. chondrosarcoma)
fibro-	— prefix meaning fibrous (e.g. fibrosarcoma)
arthro-	— prefix meaning joint (e.g. arthritis)
spondylo-	— prefix meaning spinal (e.g. spondyloarthropathy)
dactyl-	— prefix meaning digit (either finger or toe, e.g. dactylitis)

The figures below show the terminology given to the different portions of a long bone (fig 2.1) and the location of abnormalities in bone (fig 2.2).

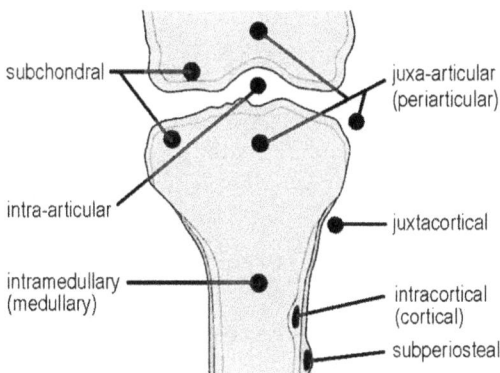

Figure 2.1
Terminology used to describe the different portions of a long bone.
(from Greenspan A, *Orthopedic Radiology* 2nd ed, Raven Press 1992, with permission)

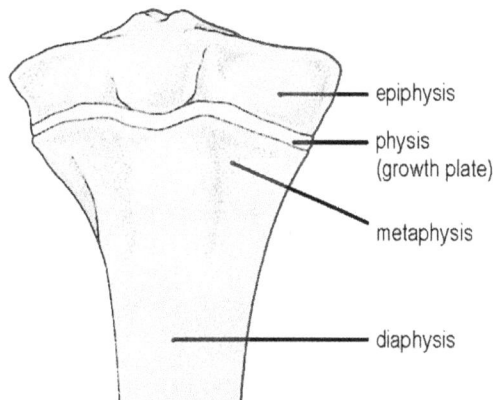

Figure 2.2
Terminology used to identify the location of a lesion in the long bone of the growing skeleton. At maturity (post-skeletal fusion) the physis (growth plate) fuses and is no longer visible.
(from Greenspan A, *Orthopedic Radiology* 2nd ed, Raven Press 1992, with permission)

For description of radiographic projections and positions, the following terms are often helpful:

AP	— anteroposterior
PA	— posteroanterior
lateral	— from the side
oblique	— between lateral and AP (or PA)
decubitus	— lying horizontal
supine	— lying on the back
prone	— lying face down
erect	— standing
axial	— along the axis (of an anatomic structure)
cephalic	— towards the head
caudal	— towards the feet

CHAPTER 3

Normal Anatomy

The anatomical structures that are included in this chapter are those that are radiographically visible on standard radiographs, and that are of clinical importance. The chapter is meant to be used both as a reference on its own, and also as a basis for the understanding of the pathology described in chapters 4–10.

The images in this chapter are all modified, with permission, after Pettersson H, Allison D, *The Encyclopaedia of Medical Imaging*, Vol II, ISIS Medical Media/The NICER Institute, Oslo, 1998.

The projections used are those described in the *"WHO Manual of Diagnostic Imaging, Radiographic Positions and Projections"*. (in print)

3.1 **Skull**

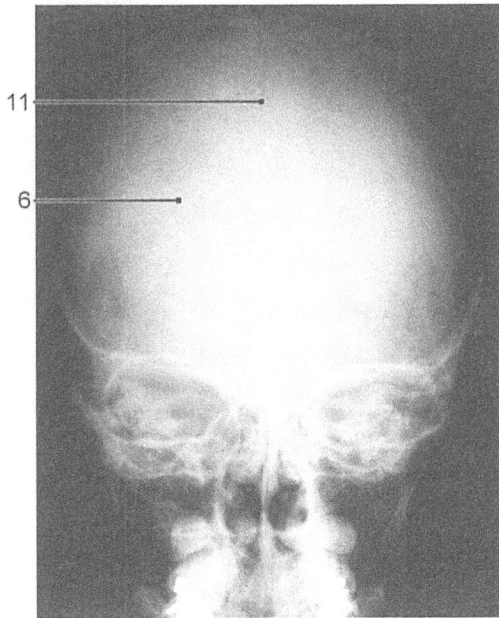

Figure 3.1
Skull, AP projection.

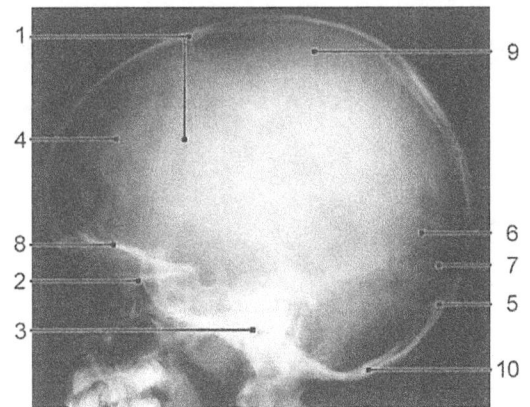

Figure 3.2
Skull, lateral projection.

1. Coronal suture
2. Cribriform plate
3. External acoustic meatus
4. Frontal bone
5. Internal occipital protuberance
6. Lambdoid suture
7. Occipital bone
8. Orbital roof
9. Parietal bone
10. Posterior margin of foramen magnum
11. Sagittal suture

3.2 **Skull Base**

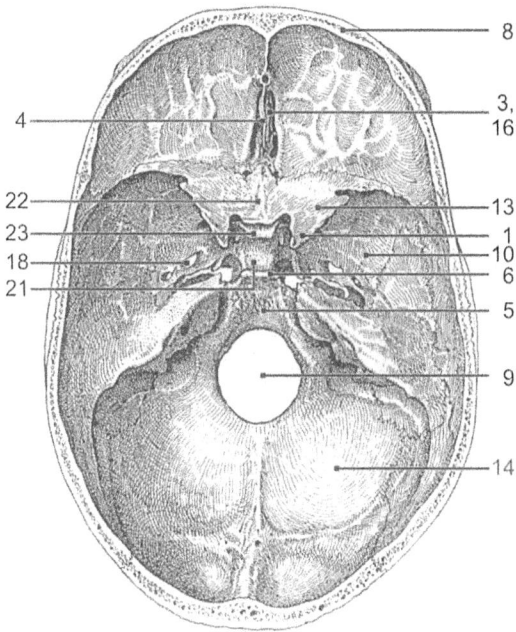

Figure 3.3
Skull base, schematic drawing.

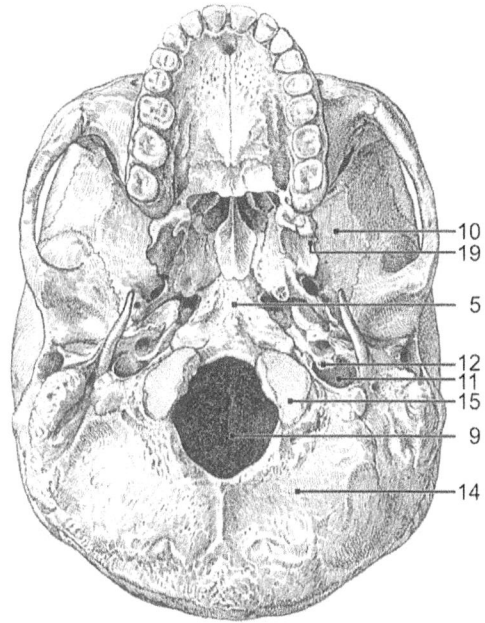

Figure 3.4
Skull base, schematic drawing.

1. Anterior clinoid process
2. Body of sphenoid
3. Cribriform plate
4. Crista galli
5. Clivus
6. Dorsum sellae
7. Ethmoid bone
8. Frontal bone
9. Foramen magnum
10. Greater wing of sphenoid
11. Jugular foramen
12. Jugular tubercle
13. Lesser wing of sphenoid
14. Occipital bone
15. Occipital condyle
16. Olfactory groove
17. Optic canal
18. Oval foramen
19. Pterygoid process
20. Round foramen
21. Sella turcica
22. Sphenoidal plane
23. Tuberculum sellae

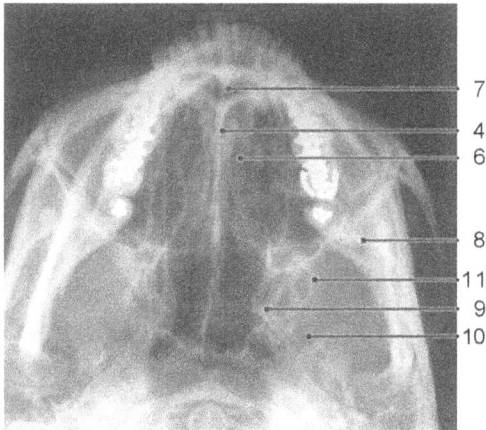

Figure 3.5
Skull base, axial projection.

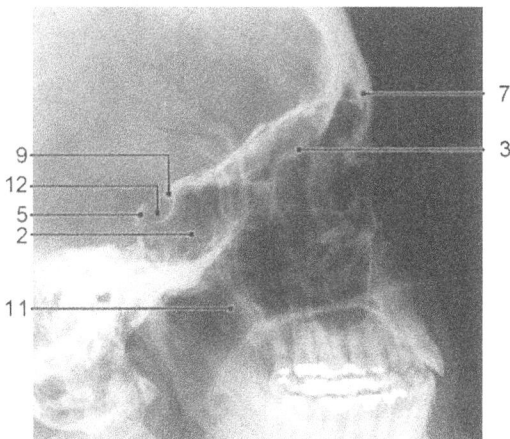

Figure 3.6
Skull base, lateral projection.

3.3 **Face**

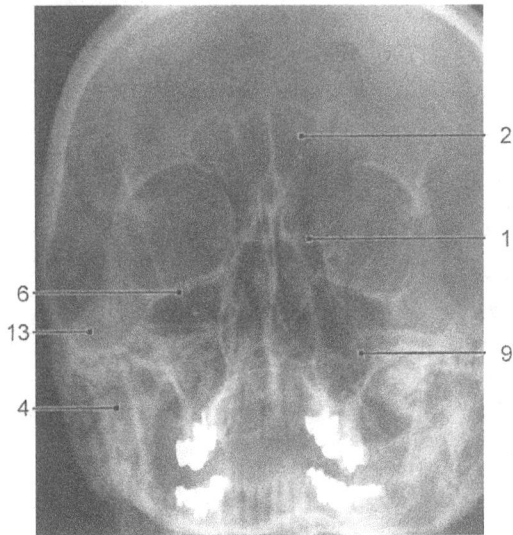

Figure 3.7
Face, PA projection.

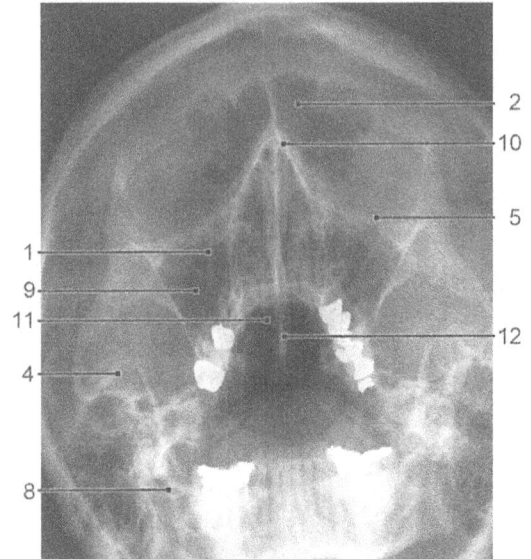

Figure 3.8
Face, PA, semiaxial projection.

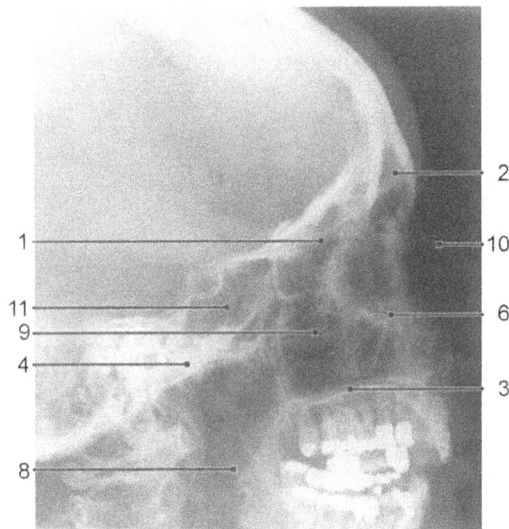

Figure 3.9
Face, lateral projection.

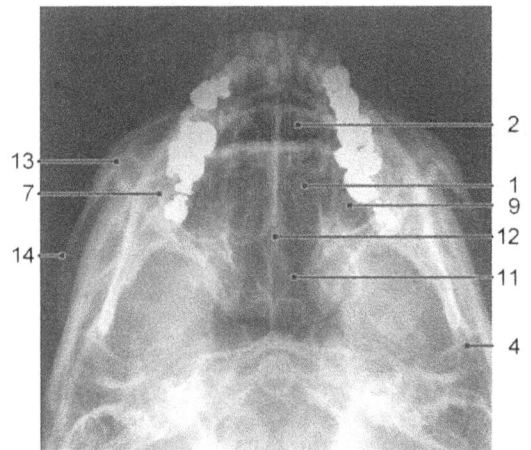

Figure 3.10
Face, axial projection.

1. Ethmoid sinus
2. Frontal sinus
3. Hard palate
4. Head of mandible
5. Inferior concha
6. Infraorbital ridge
7. Mandible
8. Mandibular ramus
9. Maxillary sinus
10. Nasal bone
11. Sphenoid sinus
12. Vomer
13. Zygomatic bone
14. Zygomatic arch

3.4 **Cervical Spine**

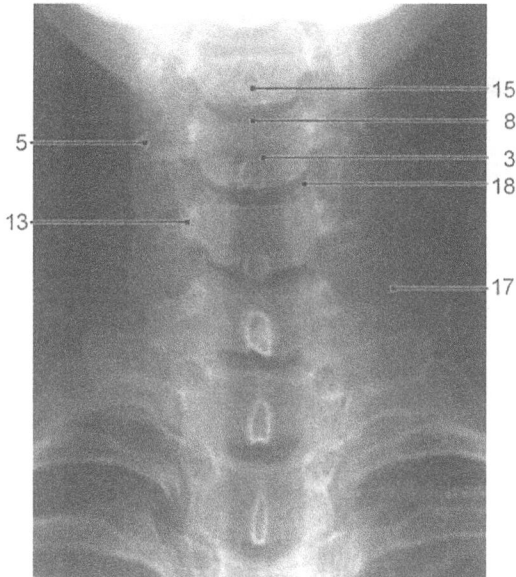

Figure 3.11
Cervical spine, AP projection.

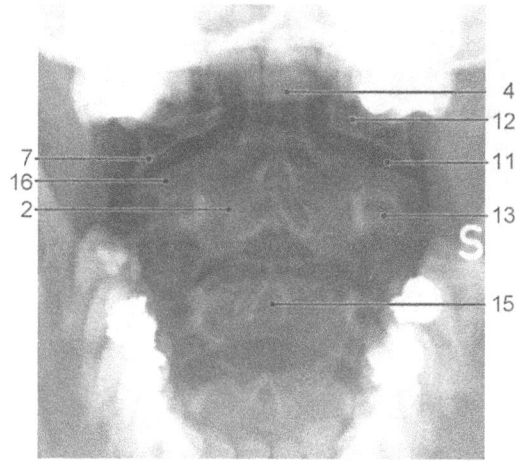

Figure 3.12
Cervical spine, AP projection (open mouth).

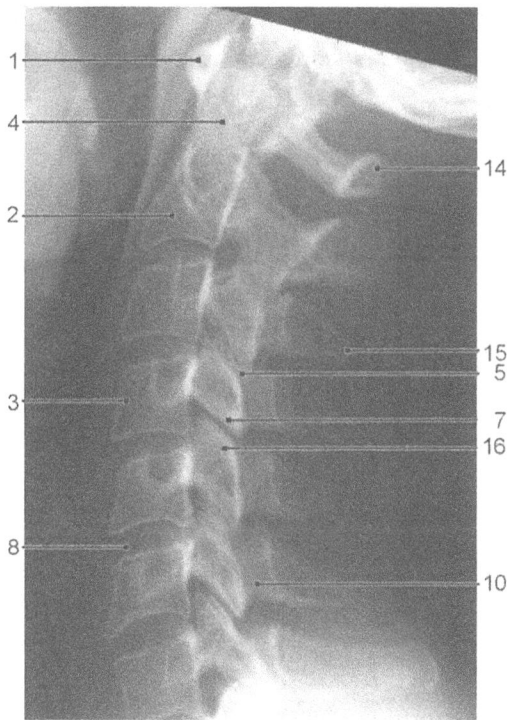

Figure 3.13
Cervical spine, lateral projection.

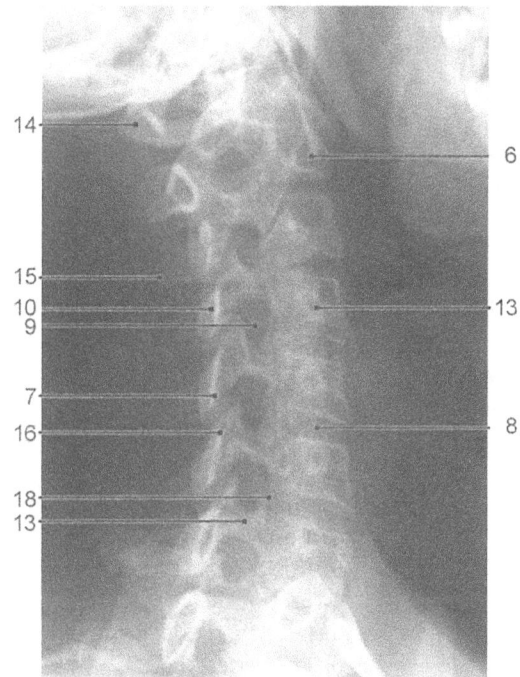

Figure 3.14
Cervical spine, oblique projection.

1. Anterior arch of atlas
2. Axis
3. Body of vertebra
4. Dens of axis
5. Facet joint
6. Transverse foramen
7. Inferior articular process
8. Intervertebral disc
9. Intervertebral foramen
10. Lamina of vertebral arch
11. Lateral atlantoaxial joint
12. Lateral mass of atlas
13. Pedicle
14. Posterior arch of atlas
15. Spinous process
16. Superior articular process
17. Transverse process
18. Uncovertebral joint (joint of Luschka)

3.5 **Thoracic Spine**

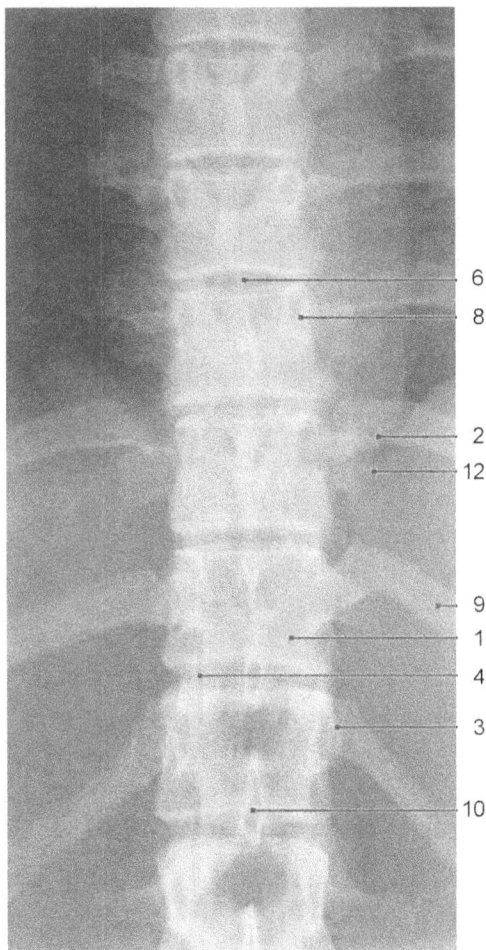

Figure 3.15
Thoracic spine, AP projection.

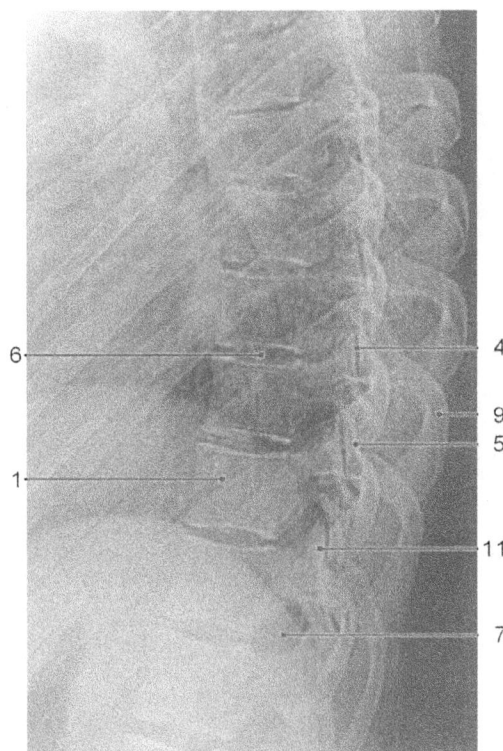

Figure 3.16
Thoracic spine, lateral projection.

1. Body of vertebra
2. Costotransverse joint
3. Costovertebral joint
4. Facet joint
5. Inferior articular process
6. Intervertebral disc
7. Intervertebral foramen
8. Pedicle
9. Rib
10. Spinous process
11. Superior articular process
12. Transverse process

3.6 Lumbar Spine

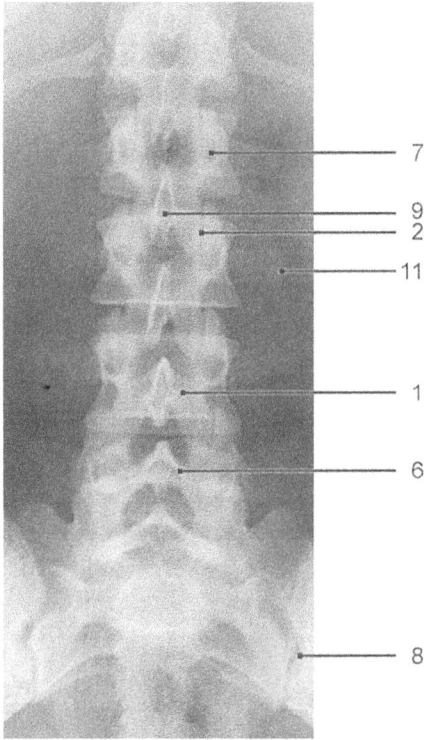

Figure 3.17
Lumbar spine, AP projection.

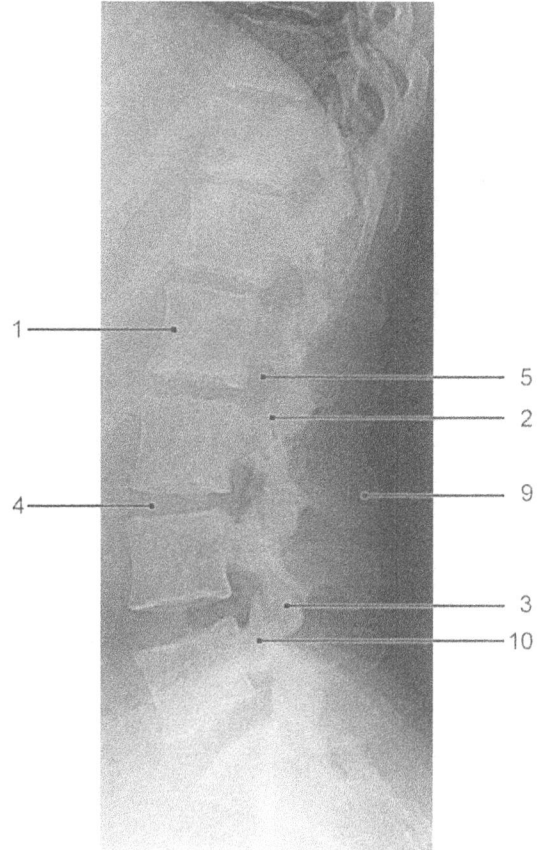

Figure 3.18
Lumbar spine, lateral projection.

1. Body of vertebra
2. Facet joint
3. Inferior articular process
4. Intervertebral disc
5. Intervertebral foramen
6. Lamina of vertebral arch
7. Pedicle
8. Sacroiliac joint
9. Spinous process
10. Superior articular process
11. Transverse process

3.7 **Sacrum**

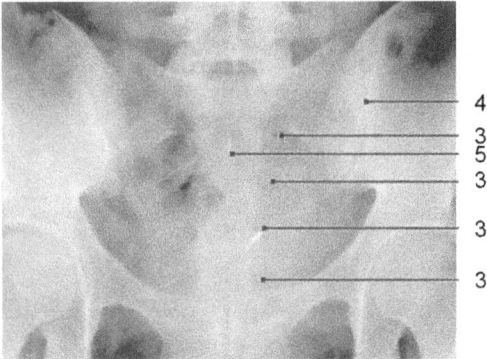

Figure 3.19
Sacrum, AP projection.

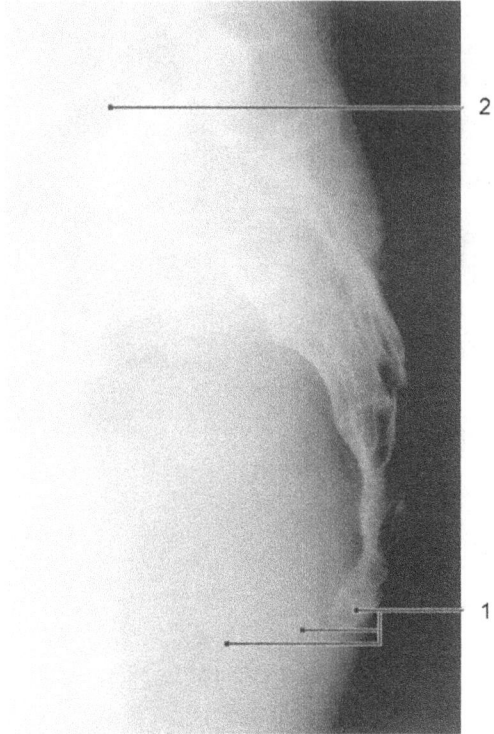

Figure 3.20
Sacrum, lateral projection.

1. Coccyx
2. Intervertebral disc
3. Intervertebral foramen
4. Sacroiliac joint
5. Spinous process

3.8 **Pelvis**

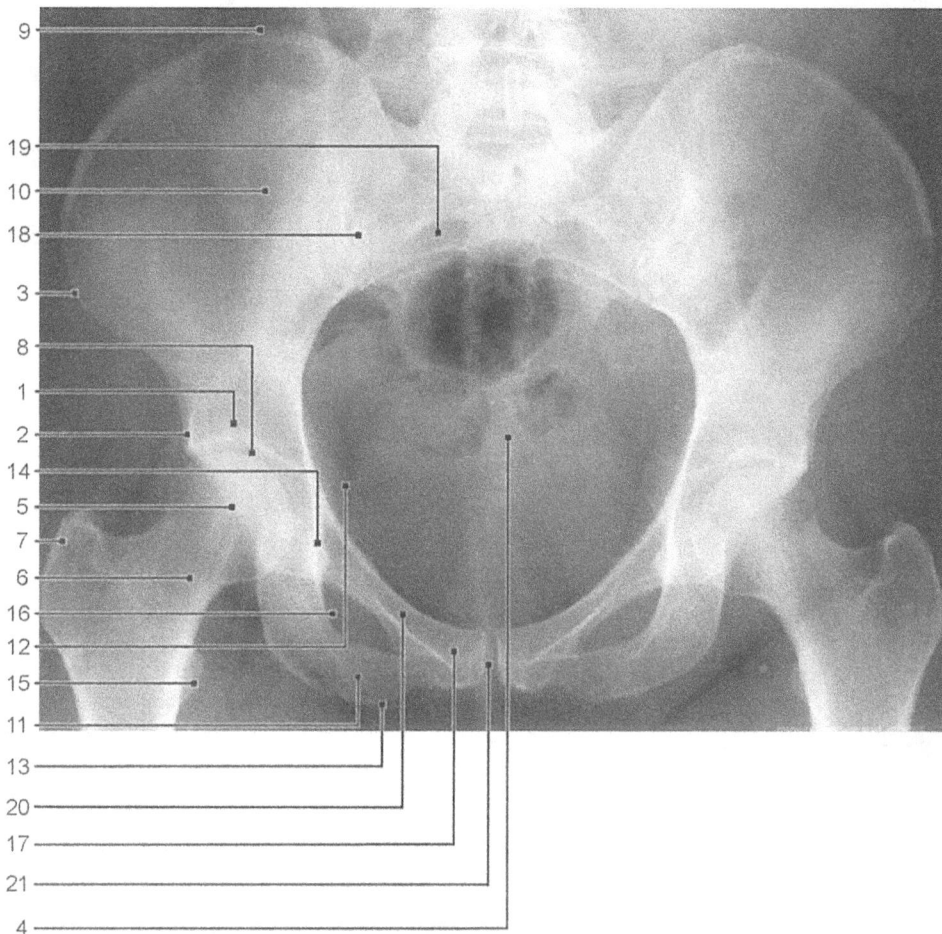

Figure 3.21
Pelvis, AP projection.

1. Acetabulum
2. Anterior inferior iliac spine
3. Anterior superior iliac spine
4. Coccyx
5. Femoral head
6. Femoral neck
7. Greater trochanter
8. Hip joint
9. Iliac crest
10. Ilium
11. Inferior pubic ramus
12. Ischial spine
13. Ischial tuberosity
14. Ischium
15. Lesser trochanter
16. Obturator foramen
17. Pubis
18. Sacroiliac joint
19. Sacrum
20. Superior pubic ramus
21. Symphysis pubis

3.9 **Thoracic Cage**

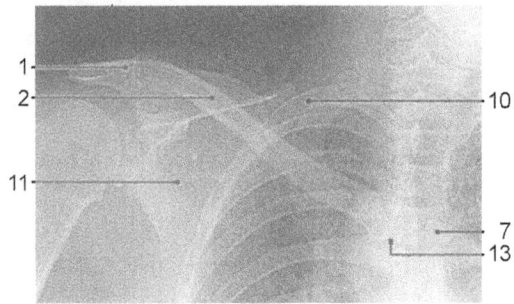

Figure 3.22
Thoracic cage, AP projectionon of upper thoracic cage.

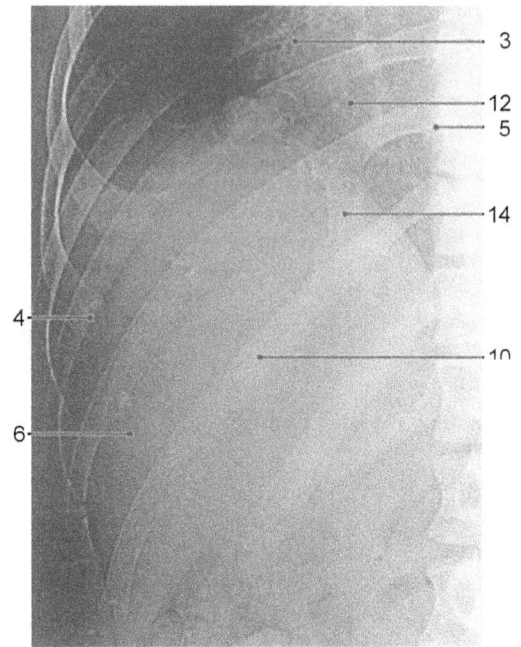

Figure 3.23
Thoracic cage, AP projection of lower thoracic cage.

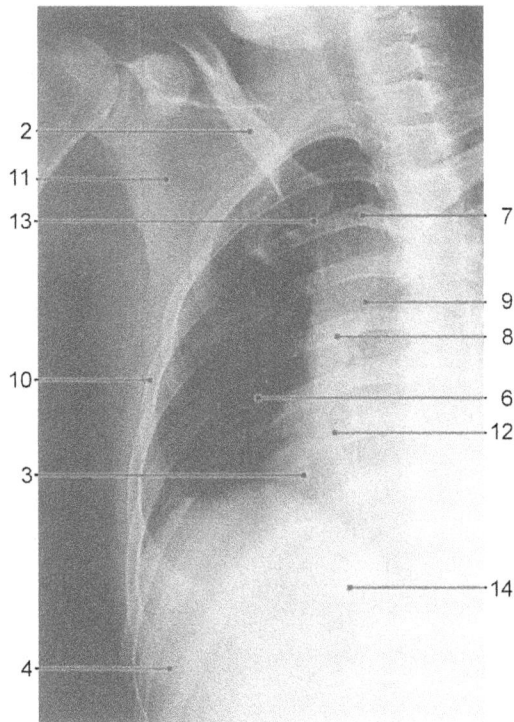

Figure 3.24
Thoracic cage, oblique projection.

1. Acromioclavicular joint
2. Clavicle
3. Costal notch
4. Costochondral junction
5. Costovertebral joint
6. Intercostal space
7. Jugular notch
8. Manubriosternal joint
9. Manubrium sterni
10. Rib
11. Scapula
12. Sternal body
13. Sternoclavicular joint
14. Xiphoid process

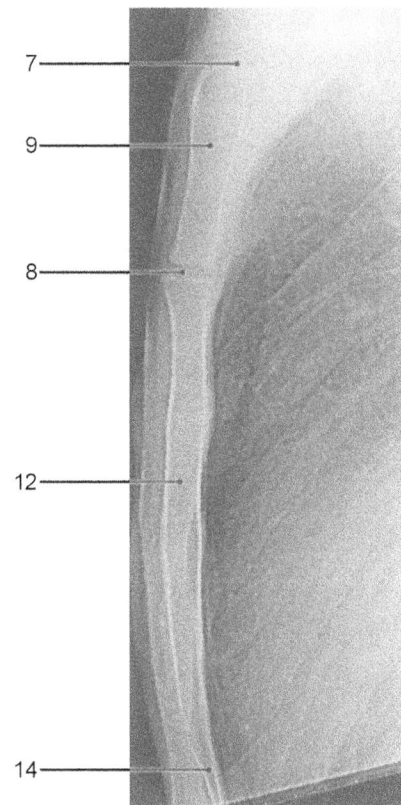

Figure 3.25
Thoracic cage, lateral projection of sternum.

3.10 **Shoulder**

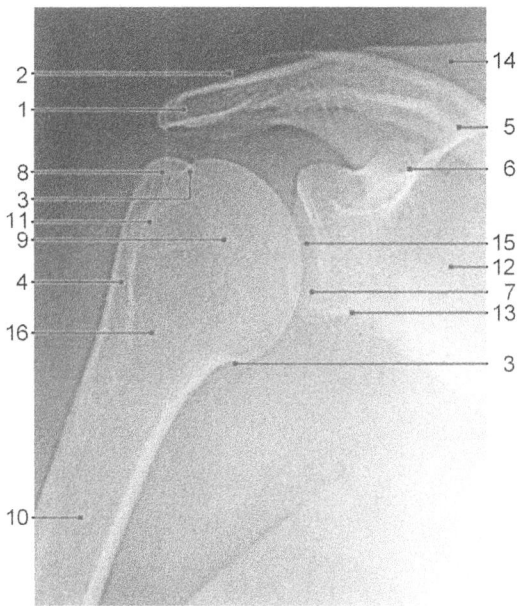

Figure 3.26
Shoulder, AP projection, external rotation.

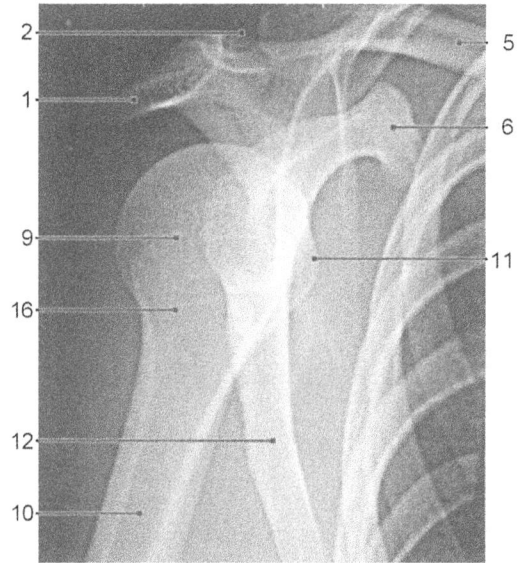

Figure 3.27
Shoulder, axial projection.

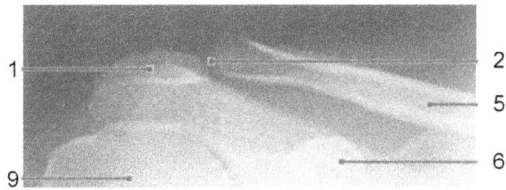

Figure 3.28
Shoulder, AP projection, acromioclavicular joint.

1. Acromion
2. Acromioclavicular joint
3. Anatomical neck of humerus
4. Bicipital groove
5. Clavicle
6. Coracoid process
7. Glenoid cavity
8. Greater tuberosity of humerus
9. Humeral head
10. Humerus
11. Lesser tuberosity of humerus
12. Scapula
13. Scapular neck
14. Scapular spine
15. Shoulder joint
16. Surgical neck of humerus

3.11 **Arm**

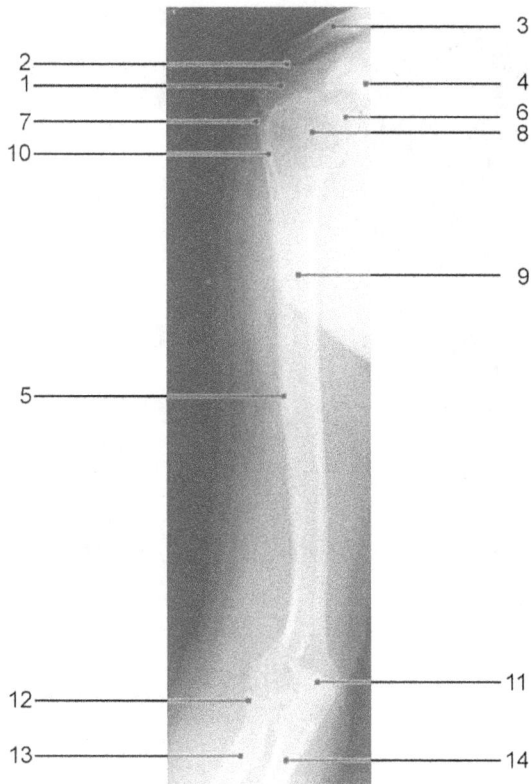

Figure 3.29
Arm, AP projection.

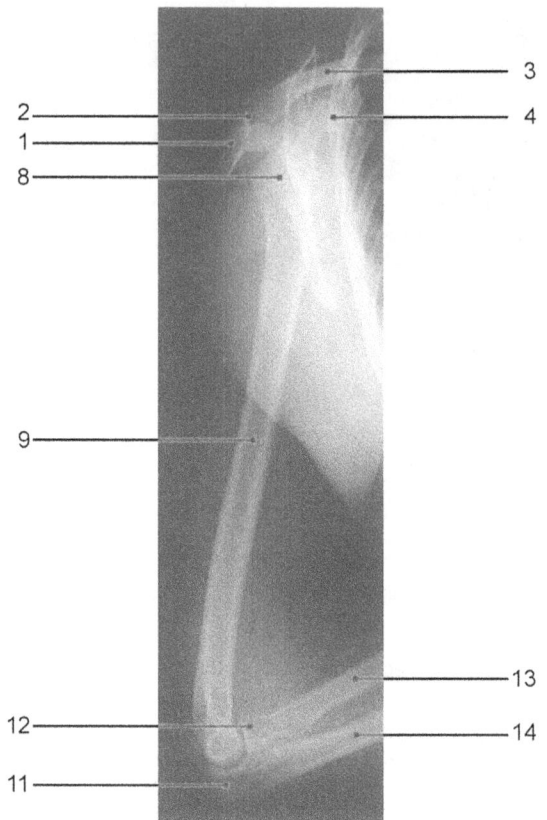

Figure 3.30
Arm, lateral projection.

1. Acromion
2. Acromioclavicular joint
3. Clavicle
4. Coracoid process
5. Deltoid tuberosity of humerus
6. Glenoid cavity
7. Greater tuberosity of humerus
8. Humeral head
9. Humerus
10. Lesser tuberosity of humerus
11. Olecranon
12. Radial head
13. Radius
14. Ulna

3.12 Elbow

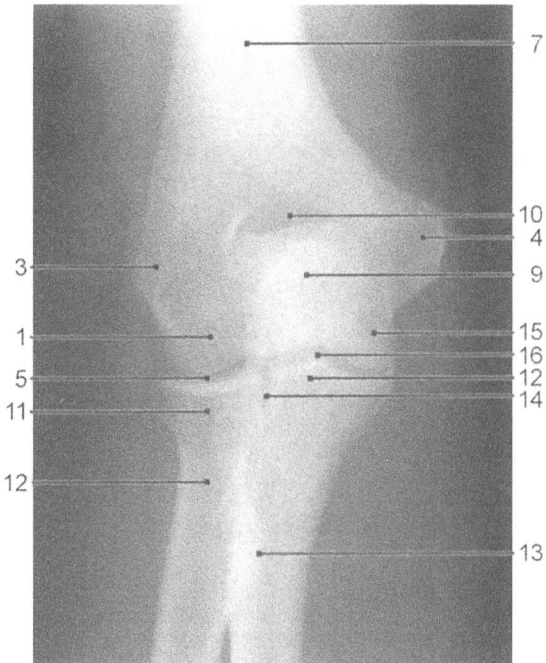

Figure 3.31
Elbow, AP projection.

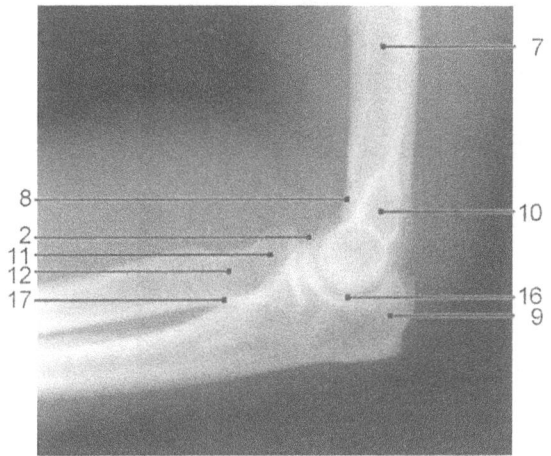

Figure 3.32
Elbow, lateral projection.

1. Capitulum of humerus
2. Coronoid process
3. Epicondyle, radial (lateral)
4. Epicondyle, ulnar (medial)
5. Humeroradial joint
6. Humeroulnar joint
7. Humerus
8. Intercondylar fossa
9. Olecranon
10. Olecranon fossa
11. Radial head
12. Radial neck
13. Radial tuberosity
14. Radioulnar joint, proximal
15. Trochlea of humerus
16. Trochlear notch of ulna
17. Ulnar tuberosity

3.13 **Forearm**

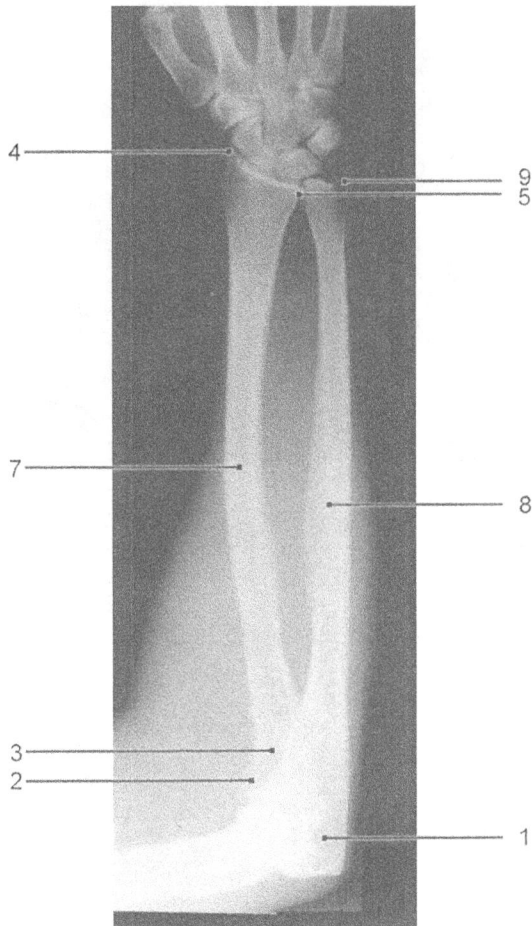

Figure 3.33
Forearm, AP projection.

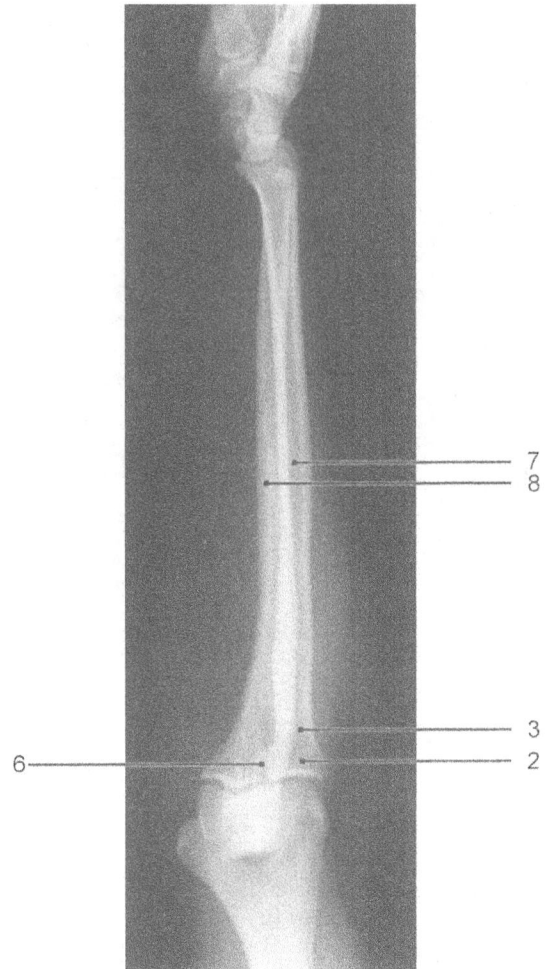

Figure 3.34
Forearm, lateral projection.

1. Olecranon
2. Radial head
3. Radial neck
4. Radial styloid process
5. Radioulnar joint, distal
6. Radioulnar joint, proximal
7. Radius
8. Ulna
9. Ulnar styloid process

3.14 **Wrist**

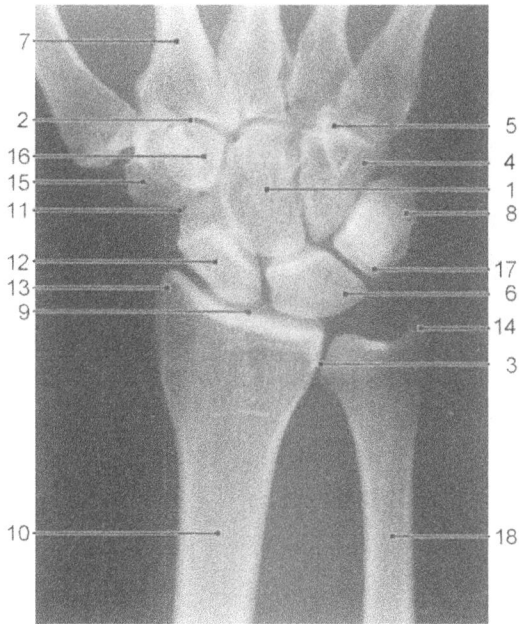

Figure 3.35
Wrist, PA projection.

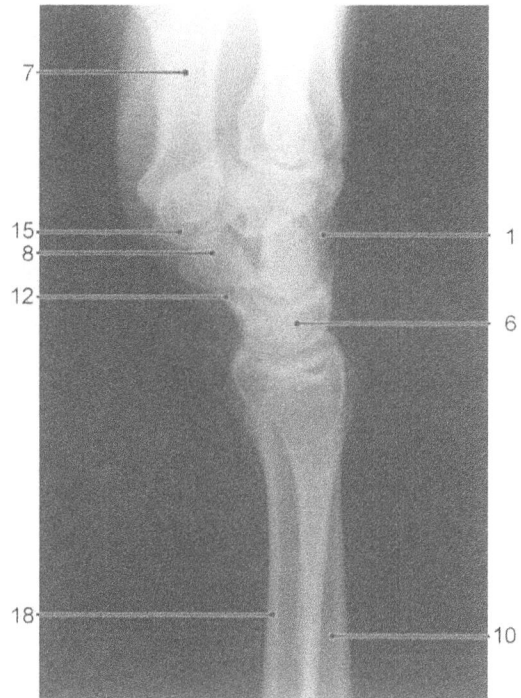

Figure 3.36
Wrist, lateral projection.

1. Capitate
2. Carpometacarpal joints
3. Distal radioulnar joint
4. Hamate
5. Hook of the hamate
6. Lunate
7. Metacarpal bones 1–5
8. Pisiform
9. Radiocarpal joint
10. Radius
11. Scapho-trapezio-trapezoid (STT) joint
12. Scaphoid
13. Styloid process of radius
14. Styloid process of ulna
15. Trapezium
16. Trapezoid
17. Triquetrum
18. Ulna

3.15 **Hand**

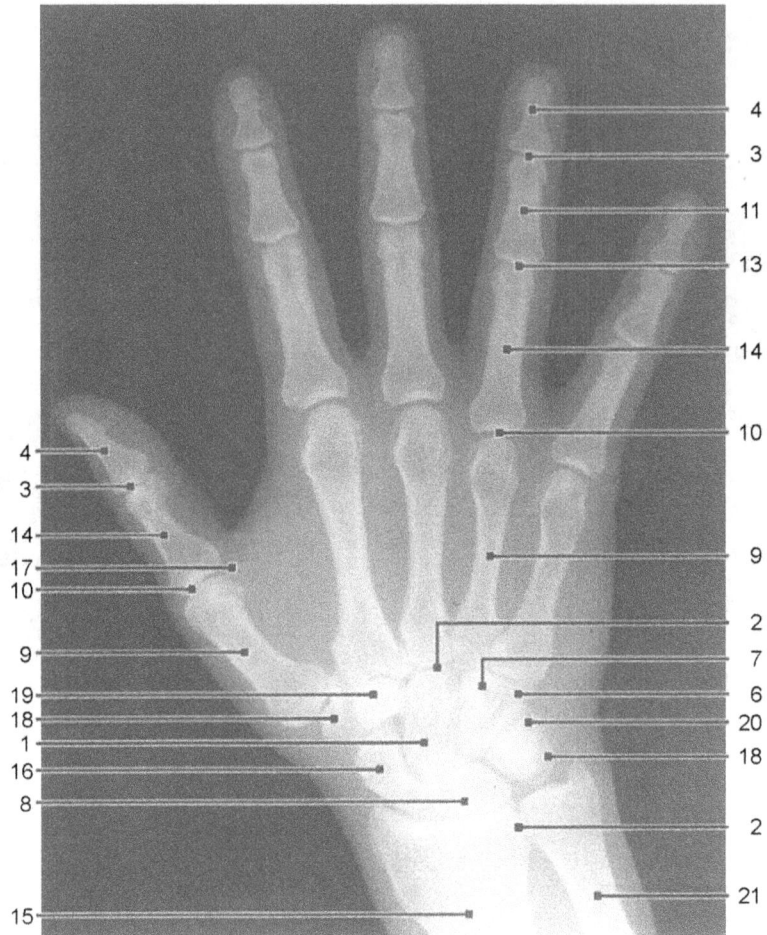

Figure 3.37
Hand, PA projection.

1. Capitate
2. Carpometacarpal joints
3. Distal interphalangeal joints
4. Distal phalanges
5. Distal radioulnar joint
6. Hamate
7. Hook of the hamate
8. Lunate
9. Metacarpal bones 1–5
10. Metacarpo-phalangeal joints
11. Middle phalanges
12. Pisiform
13. Proximal interphalangeal joints
14. Proximal phalanges
15. Radius
16. Scaphoid
17. Sesamoid bones (of thumb)
18. Trapezium
19. Trapezoid
20. Triquetrum
21. Ulna

3.16 **Hip**

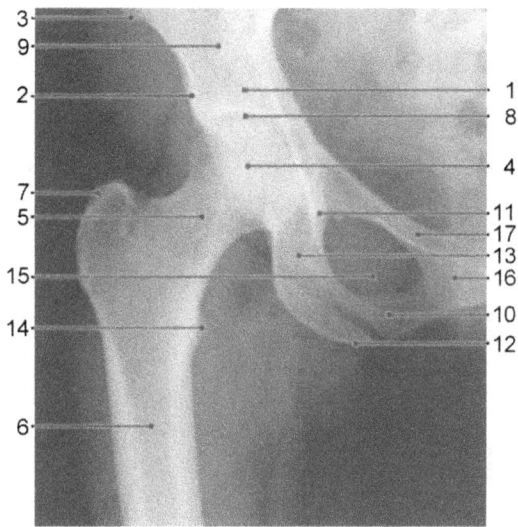

Figure 3.38
Hip, AP projection.

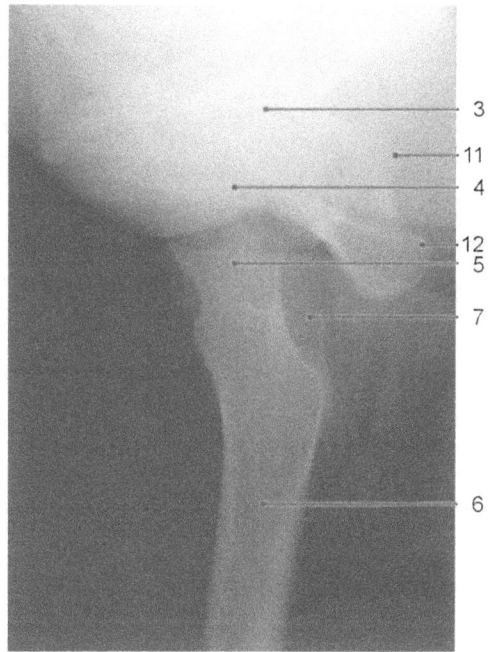

Figure 3.39
Hip, lateral projection

1. Acetabulum
2. Anterior inferior iliac spine
3. Anterior superior iliac spine
4. Femoral head
5. Femoral neck
6. Femur
7. Greater trochanter
8. Hip joint
9. Ilium
10. Inferior pubic ramus
11. Ischial spine
12. Ischial tuberosity
13. Ischium
14. Lesser trochanter
15. Obturator foramen
16. Pubis
17. Superior pubic ramus

3.17 **Thigh**

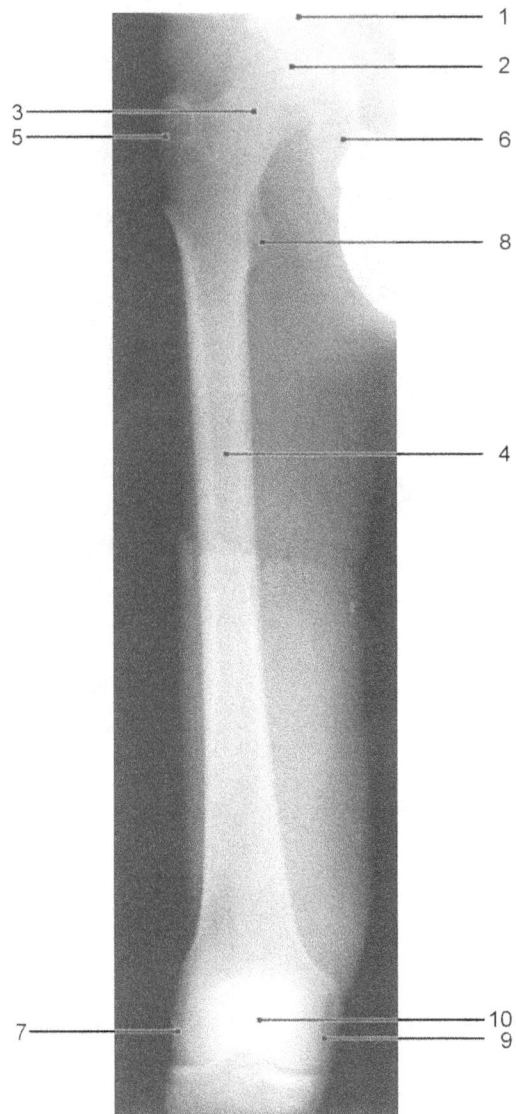

Figure 3.40
Thigh, AP projection.

1. Acetabulum
2. Femoral head
3. Femoral neck
4. Femur
5. Greater trochanter
6. Ischium
7. Lateral femoral condyle
8. Lesser trochanter
9. Medial femoral condyle
10. Patella

3.18 **Knee**

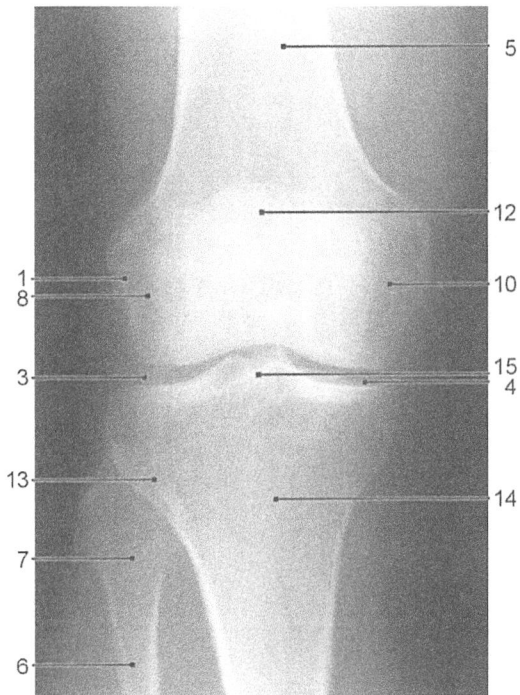

Figure 3.41
Knee, AP projection.

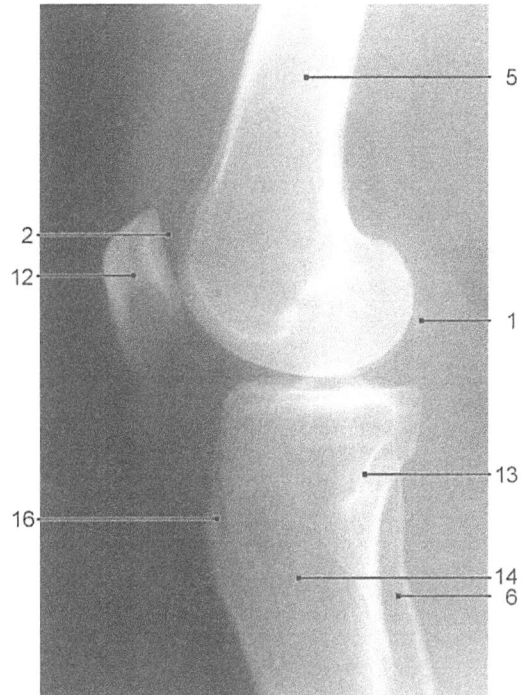

Figure 3.42
Knee, lateral projection.

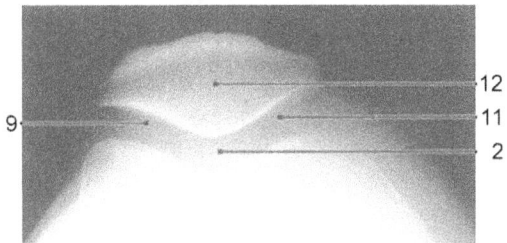

Figure 3.43
Knee, axial view of the patella.

1. Fabella
2. Femoropatellar joint
3. Femorotibial joint, lateral compartment
4. Femorotibial joint, medial compartment
5. Femur
6. Fibula
7. Fibular head
8. Lateral femoral condyle
9. Lateral patellar joint
10. Medial femoral condyle
11. Medial patellar joint
12. Patella
13. Proximal tibiofibular joint
14. Tibia
15. Tibial spine
16. Tibial tuberosity

3.19 Leg

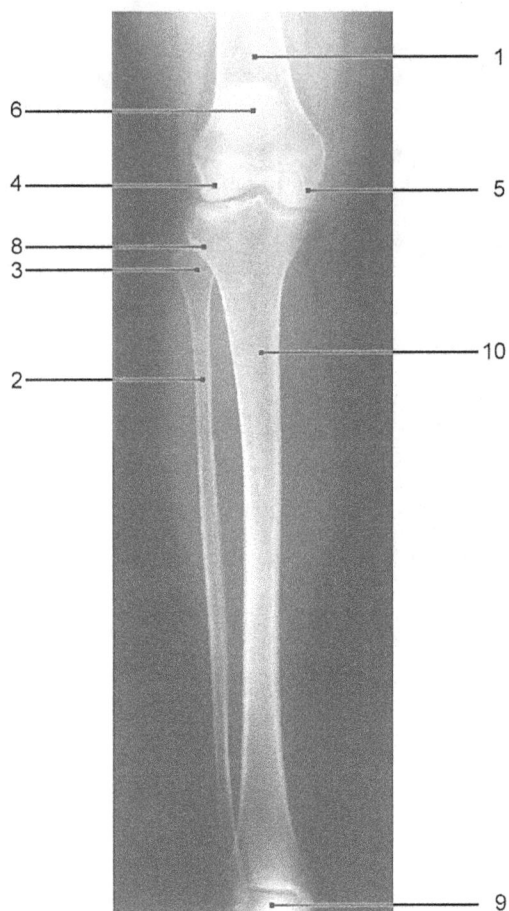

Figure 3.44
Leg, AP projection.

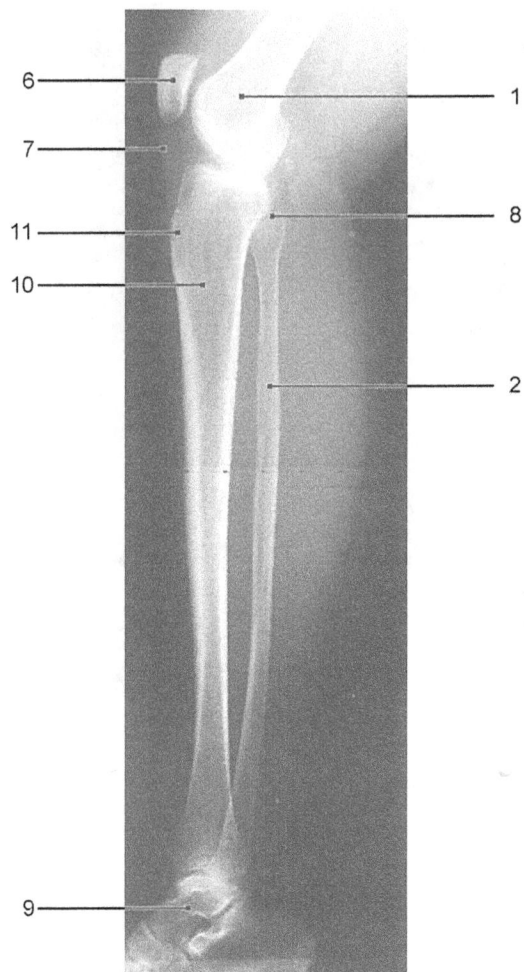

Figure 3.45
Leg, lateral projection.

1. Femur
2. Fibula
3. Fibular head
4. Lateral femoral condyle
5. Medial femoral condyle
6. Patella
7. Patellar tendon
8. Proximal tibiofibular joint
9. Talus
10. Tibia
11. Tibial tuberosity

3.20 **Ankle**

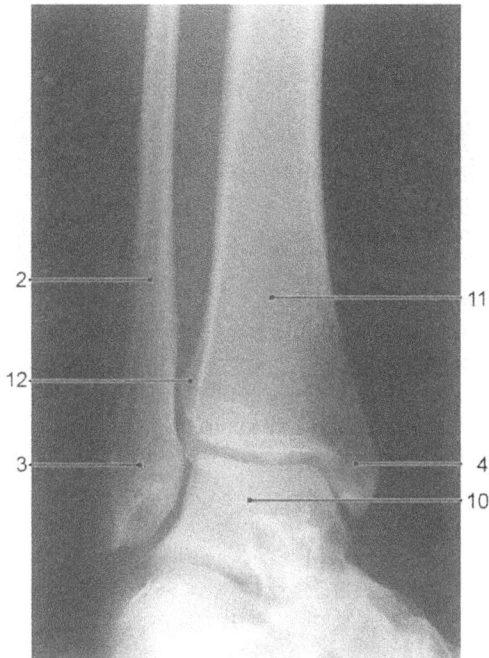

Figure 3.46
Ankle, AP projection.

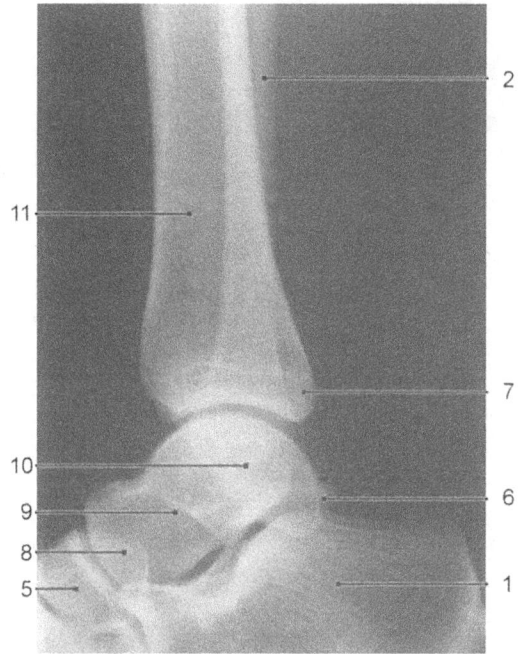

Figure 3.47
Ankle, lateral projection.

1. Calcaneus
2. Fibula
3. Lateral malleolus
4. Medial malleolus
5. Navicular
6. Posterior process of talus
7. Posterior tibial process
8. Talar head
9. Talar neck
10. Talus
11. Tibia
12. Tibiofibular syndesmosis

3.21 **Foot**

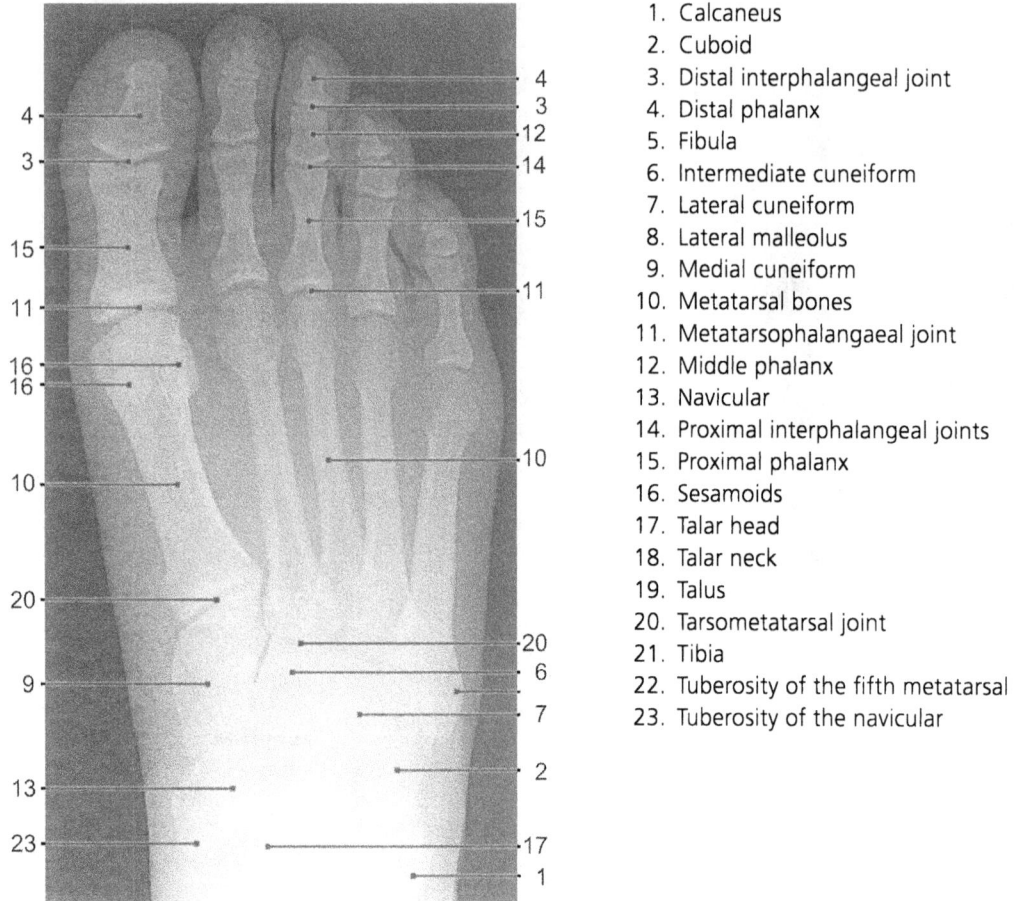

1. Calcaneus
2. Cuboid
3. Distal interphalangeal joint
4. Distal phalanx
5. Fibula
6. Intermediate cuneiform
7. Lateral cuneiform
8. Lateral malleolus
9. Medial cuneiform
10. Metatarsal bones
11. Metatarsophalangaeal joint
12. Middle phalanx
13. Navicular
14. Proximal interphalangeal joints
15. Proximal phalanx
16. Sesamoids
17. Talar head
18. Talar neck
19. Talus
20. Tarsometatarsal joint
21. Tibia
22. Tuberosity of the fifth metatarsal
23. Tuberosity of the navicular

Figure 3.48
Foot, AP projection.

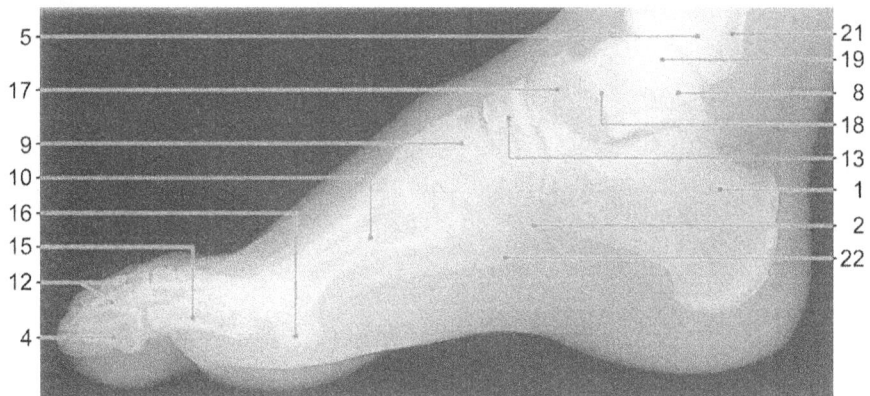

Figure 3.49
Foot, lateral projection.

CHAPTER 4

Trauma

4.1 Classification of fractures and dislocations

4.1.1 General classifications

- a *fracture* is either a complete break in the continuity of a bone or an incomplete break or crack.

- fractures are subdivided according to their cause:

  1. acute traumatic fractures
  2. stress fractures
  3. pathological fractures

- acute traumatic fractures are classified as:

complete	— discontinuity between two or more bone fragments
incomplete	— portion of cortex remains intact
displaced	— space between margins of fracture causing deformity
undisplaced	— bone fragments closely apposed with minimal deformity
closed/simple	— no communication between fracture and skin surface
open/compound	— wound extends from skin surface to fracture

- an open/compound fracture is liable to be contaminated and has a high risk of infection.

- descriptive terms used to indicate the shape or pattern of an acute fracture in the adult are (fig 4.1):

  1. transverse fractures
  2. oblique fractures
  3. spiral fractures
  4. comminuted fractures (2 or more fragments)
  5. compression/crush fractures
  6. depressed (in skull)

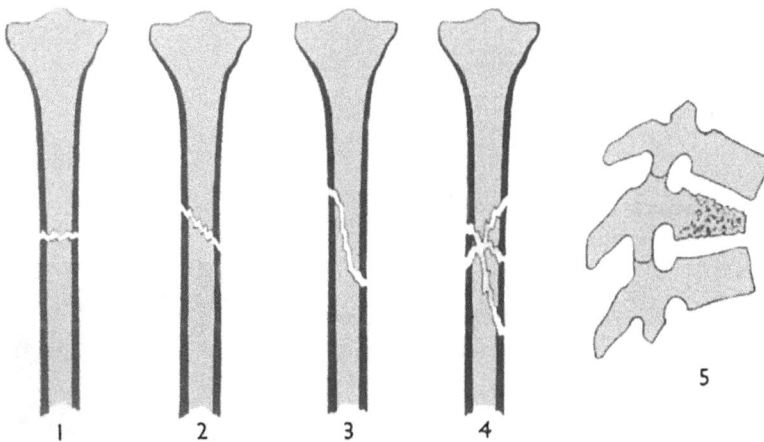

Figure 4.1
Common fracture patterns.

(modified from Adams & Hamblen, *Outline of Fractures* 10th ed, Churchill Livingstone 1992, with permission)

4.1.2 Dislocations

- a joint is *dislocated* (luxated) when its articular surfaces are wholly displaced one from the other, so that apposition between them is lost (fig 4.2).

- *subluxation* exists when the articular surfaces are partly displaced but retain some contact with each other.

- dislocation may occur in isolation or with a fracture (so-called fracture-dislocation) (fig 4.3).

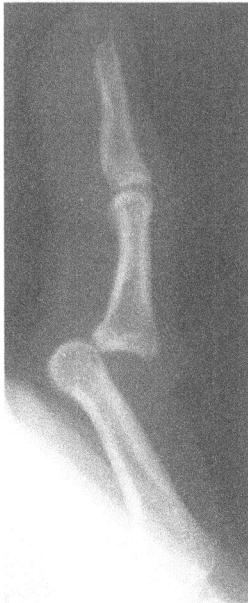

Figure 4.2
Fifth finger showing dorsal
dislocation of the proximal
interphalangeal joint.

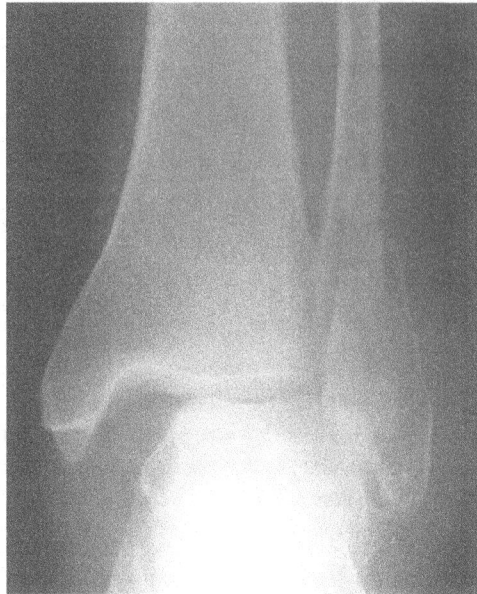

Figure 4.3
AP ankle showing a fracture-dislocation. There is a spiral fracture of the
distal fibula and medial subluxation of the distal tibia with respect to the
top of the talus.

4.1.3 **Fractures in children**

- the pattern of bony injuries in the child are somewhat different to the adult as the skeleton is more elastic and less brittle.

- fractures in children are classified as (fig 4.4);

    — complete
    — greenstick fracture
    — torus (buckle) fracture
    — pipe fracture
    — bowing injury
    — infant's (toddler's) fracture
    — epiphyseal/metaphyseal fractures
    — avulsion injuries

- a *greenstick* fracture is an incomplete fracture. The cortex is broken on one side and buckled on the other with a bending deformity concave to the buckled side (fig 4.4 and 4.5).

FRACTURES IN CHILDREN

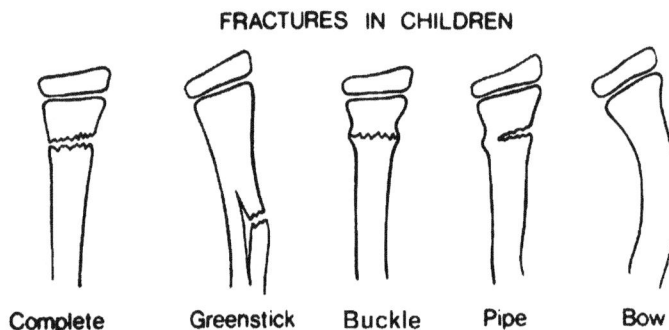

Complete   Greenstick   Buckle   Pipe   Bow

Figure 4.4
Typical fracture patterns in children.

(modified from Lee Rogers *Radiology of Skeletal Trauma* 2nd Ed, Churchill
Livingstone 1992)

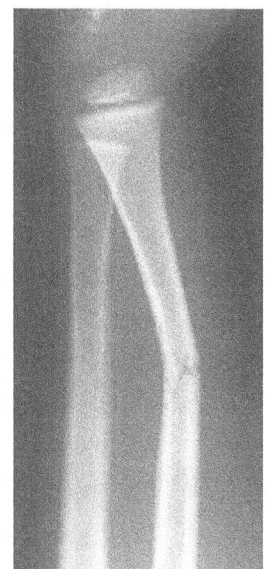

Figure 4.5
Child with a greenstick
fracture of the radius.

- a **buckle** fracture is a buckling of the cortex produced by compression (impaction) forces. Typically seen in the metaphysis of long bones particularly the radius and ulna (fig 4.6).

- a **pipe** fracture is a combination of an incomplete transverse fracture of one cortex and a torus fracture of the opposite side (fig 4.7).

- a **bowing injury** results in the bending of a long bone usually without a fracture, but with an associated fracture of an adjacent bone. Typically affects the radius, ulna and fibula.

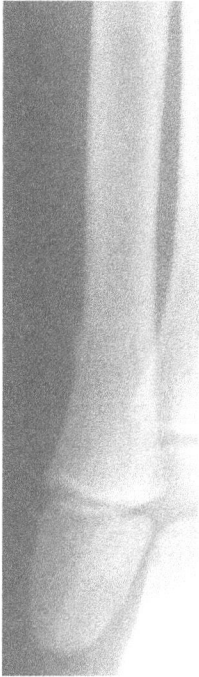

Figure 4.6
Child with a
torus (buckle)
fracture of the
distal fibula.

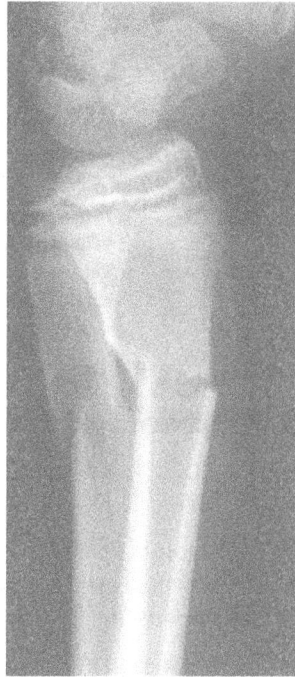

Figure 4.7
Child with a pipe fracture
of the distal radius and
complete fracture of the
adjacent ulna.

- an **infant's (toddler's) fracture** is seen in young children who present with a limp without a clear history of trauma. They are subsequently found to have an occult (unsuspected) undisplaced fracture. Originally described in the distal tibia, it may also be seen in the distal femur and calcaneus.

- a fragment of bone may be avulsed (pulled-off) at the insertion of a ligament or tendon at any age. In adolescents it is the accessory growth centres (the apophyses) which are particularly prone to **avulsion injuries**. These are typically seen in the pelvis (fig 4.8). In the healing phase the hyperplastic callus (new bone formation) may mimic a bone forming tumour.

- in adolescent children the growth plate (physis) is a potentially weak point and is therefore susceptible to trauma. The **Salter-Harris classification of epiphyseal injuries** is illustrated in figure 4.9. The commonest injury (75%) is a Salter-Harris Type 2 with separation of the growth plate and a fracture extending proximally to involve part of the metaphysis (fig 4.10). A complication of a epiphyseal injuries is premature fusion of the growth plate (see Chapter 4.3.2)

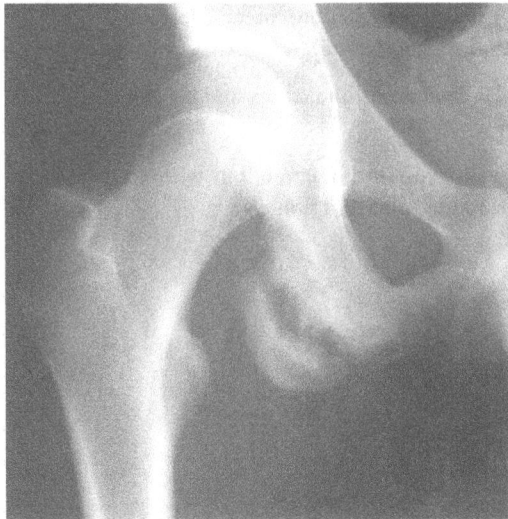

Figure 4.8
Adolescent with a chronic avulsion of the ischial apophysis at the insertion of the hamstrings.

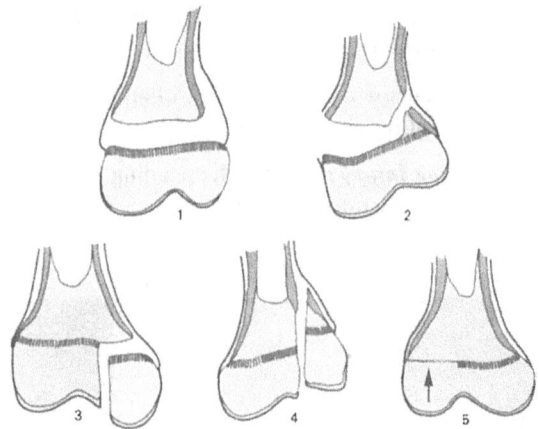

Figure 4.9
Schematic representation of different types of epiphyseal injuries (the Salter-Harris classification).

(from Adams & Hamblen, *Outline of Fractures* 10th ed, Churchill Livingstone 1992, with permission)

4.2 **Radiographic diagnosis of fractures**

- the diagnosis of a fracture on a radiograph depends on identifying the features detailed under the classification in the previous Chapter.

- a fracture is identified by the loss of continuity of the cortex and a dark line traversing the adjacent bone. The fracture line appears dark because the soft tissue (usually haematoma) between the bone ends is of less density than the bone itself.

- a fracture may appear as a dense/sclerotic line if the fracture ends are overlapping. At this site there is therefore twice as much bone attenuating the X-ray beam. The classic example is the depressed skull fracture but it can also be seen with overlapping long bone fractures.

- it is important to obtain two views at right angles for all suspected fractures and dislocations. On occasion a fracture or dislocation may only be visible on one projection (fig 4.10). Two views are also essential to adequately see the degree of deformity at the fracture site.

- it is important that the radiographs always show the joint above and below any suspected long bone fracture, unless it is clinically obvious that the injury is only in the most distal part of the limb. But even then, the nearest joint must always be included on the film.

- in certain circumstances the fracture may not be visible on radiographs at the time of presentation. These include; (a) undisplaced fractures through predominantely cancellous bone such as scaphoid fractures and (b) stress fractures (see Chapter 4.8).

- fracture healing can be assessed with serial radiographs. There are three phases of healing;

    Inflammatory phase: a haematoma (blood clot) forms at the site of the fracture.

    Reparative phase: bone at the fracture margins is deprived of its vascular supply resulting in resorption at the bone ends. On radiographs, fractures which are difficult to see at first, become more easily seen. The cells lining the cortex start to produce immature bone (callus). This is seen as faint calcification around the fracture.

    Remodelling phase: the immature callus is replaced by compact (denser) bone in the cortex and cancellous bone within the medullary cavity.

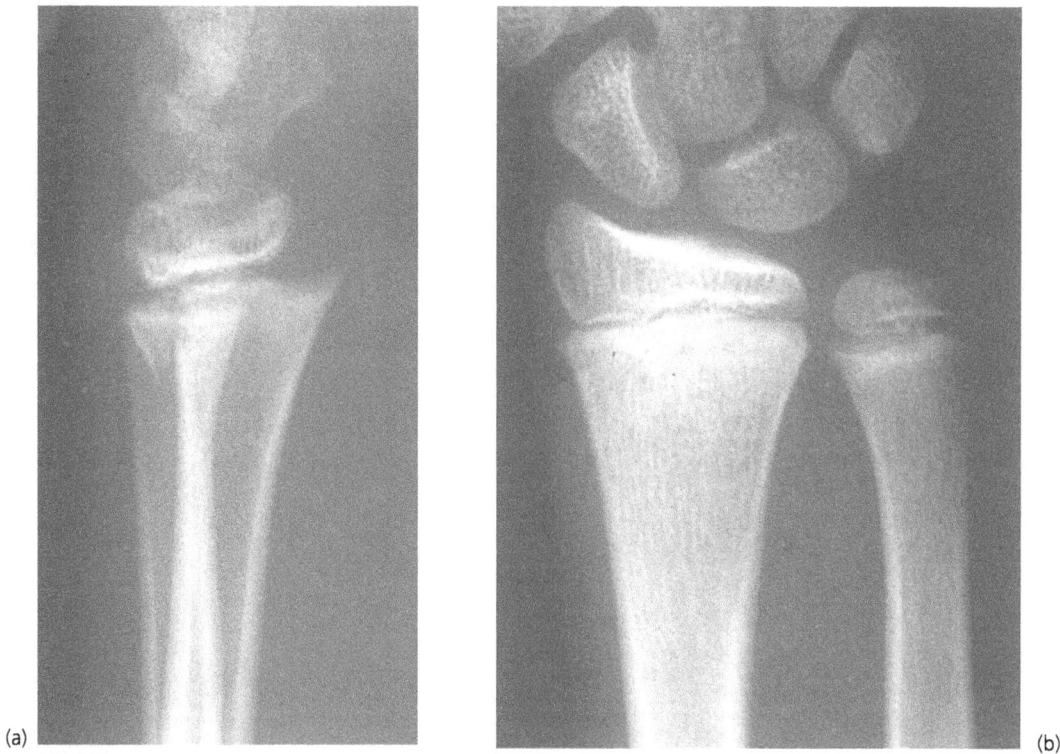

(a)

(b)

Figure 4.10
Lateral (a) and PA (b) radiographs of the wrist in a child with an epiphyseal injury. Note that the injury is
virtually invisible on the PA view.

4.3 Complications of fractures

- complications of fractures may be classified into *intrinsic* (related to the fracture itself) and *extrinsic*
  (the result of associated injury).

- *intrinsic complications* include;

  — delayed union and non-union
  — malunion and shortening
  — avascular necrosis
  — infection
  — degenerative joint disease

- *extrinsic complications* include;

  — injury to adjacent vessels, nerves and tendons
  — injury to viscera
  — fat embolism (*release of marrow fat to the lungs*)
  — reflex sympathetic dystrophy (Sudeck's atrophy)

4.3.1 Delayed union and non-union of fractures

- as a general rule union is considered delayed if the fragments remain freely mobile several months
  after injury but there is nothing in the appearance of the bones to indicate that union will never
  happen.

- if a fracture remains ununited for many months distinctive radiographic features develop which
  indicate that the fracture will fail to heal (i.e. non-union). The bone ends become hypertrophic,
  sclerotic and the fracture line dark and well-defined (fig 4.11). A classic site for non-union is the
  scaphoid fracture.

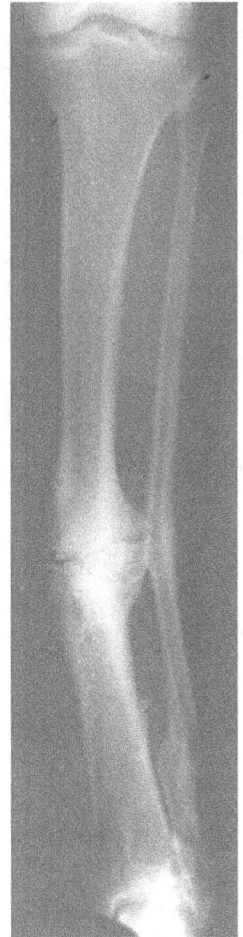

Figure 4.11
Non-union fracture of the tibial diaphysis (shaft). The fibular fractures are soundly united.

4.3.2 **Malunion and shortening**

- mal-union indicates that the fracture has united in an incorrect position. This includes angulation, rotation and overlap at the fracture site (figure 4.12).

- shortening of bone after a fracture may occur due to (figure 4.13);

    1. Malunion with angulation or overlap
    2. Crushing of bone or bone loss
    3. Premature growth plate fusion in children (fig 4.14)

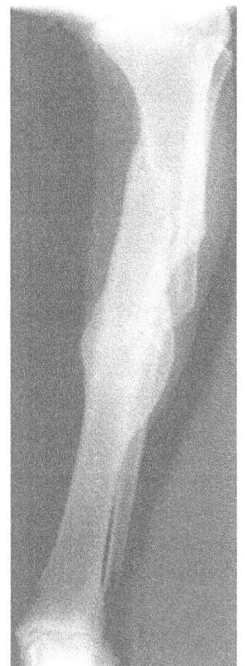

Figure 4.12
Malunion of a fracture of the tibia. The fractures are united but there is marked angulation at the proximal fracture site.

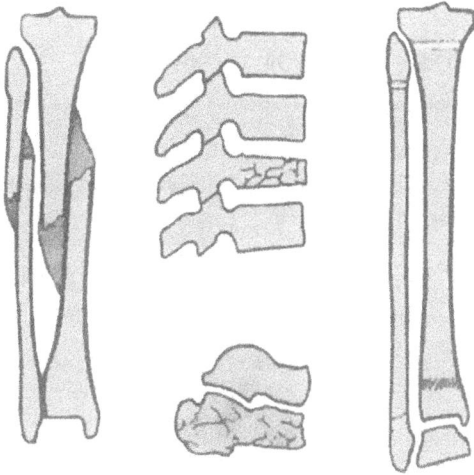

Figure 4.13
Three causes of bone shortening after a fracture. a. Malunion with overlap or angulation. b. Crushing of bone (spine & calcaneum). c. Premature closure of growth plate (tibial) in a child.

(from Adams & Hamblen, *Outline of Fractures* 10th ed, Churchill Livingstone 1992, with permission)

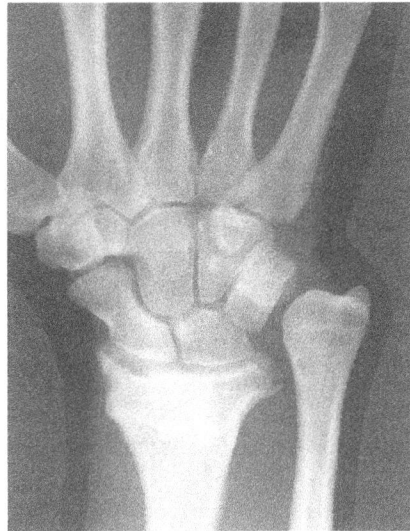

Figure 4.14
Shortening of the radius with relative overgrowth of the ulna due to an old fracture of the distal radial growth plate resulting in premature fusion of the growth plate.

4.3.3 **Avascular necrosis (AVN)**

- avascular necrosis (osteonecrosis) occurs when the blood supply to a bone or part of bone is interrupted. It most commonly occurs as a complication of a fracture, particularly near the articular end of a bone.

- AVN may also occur due to non-traumatic causes (e.g. infection, steroid therapy and sickle cell disease).

- classic sites for AVN after trauma are;

  — femoral head
  — proximal scaphoid (fig 4.15)
  — body of talus

- radiographic appearances of AVN include (fig 4.15);

  — relative increased density of avascular bone
  — fragmentation & collapse
  — late development of premature degenerative joint disease

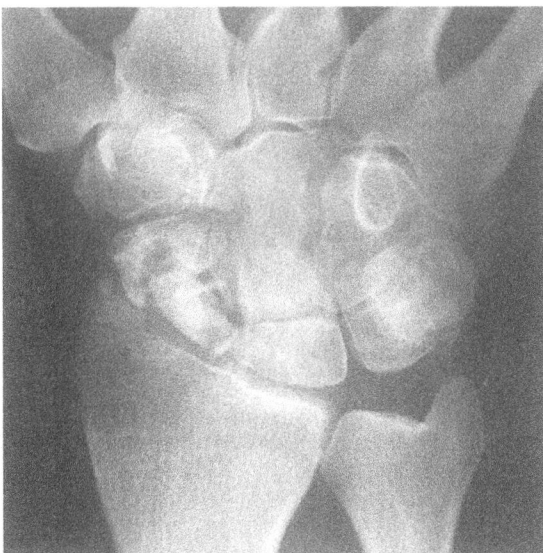

Figure 4.15
Ununited fracture of the waist of scaphoid with avascular necrosis of the proximal pole.

4.3.4 Infection

- infection at a fracture site is most commonly seen in open (compound) fractures.

- infection may be confined to the soft tissues but frequently will involve both the bone (osteomyelitis) and soft tissues (see Chapter 5).

- when there is a dirty open (compound) fracture the possibility of developing gas gangrene due to *Clostridia* or other bowel organisms should be considered.

4.3.5 Degenerative joint disease

- premature degenerative change (osteoarthritis) may develop in the joint adjacent to a fracture due to;

   — extension of fracture to involve articular cortex with loss of joint congruity
   — late sequelae of AVN
   — altered biomechanics of joint due to deformity

- radiographic changes are loss of joint space (indicating cartilage loss), subchondral sclerosis and osteophyte formation (see Chapter 6.1).

4.3.6 Reflex sympathetic dystrophy (RSD)

- RSD, also known as Sudek's atrophy, is a rare cause of prolonged disability after trauma. In many cases the trauma is insufficient to produce a fracture.

- generally attributed to an inappropriate autonomic (neurovascular) response, the patient develops a painful swollen extremity about 2 months after injury. Clinically the extremity is swollen and hyperaemic. The skin has a shiny appearance.

- radiographs show loss of bone density (osteoporosis/osteopenia) which is typically spotty or patchy. It is much more severe than would be expected from mere disuse or immobilization (fig 4.16).

- RSD is usually a self-limiting condition i.e. recovers with time.

- chronic bone or soft tissue infection (fungus, leprosy) must be excluded.

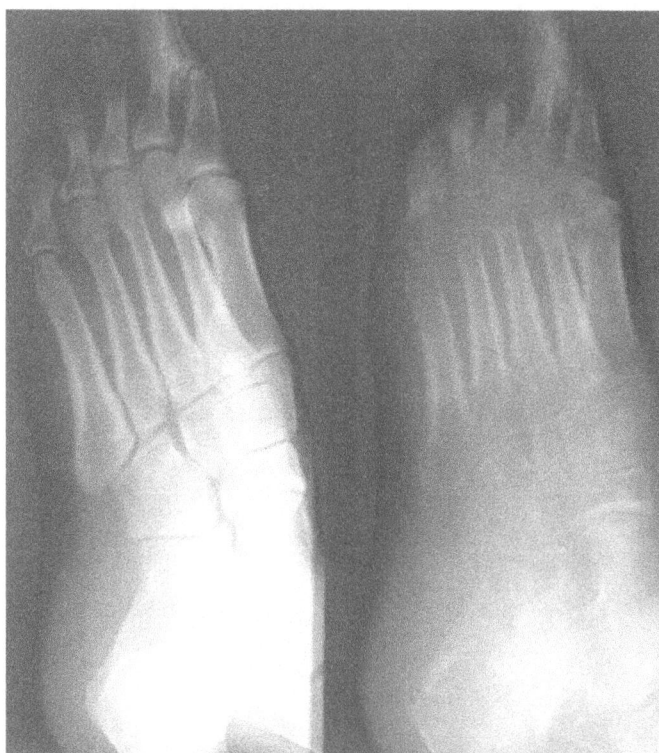

Figure 4.16
Reflex sympathetic dystrophy (RSD). The internal oblique projection of the foot at presentation with trauma is normal. 5 months later the severe loss of bone density (osteopenia) is typical of RSD, but chronic soft tissue or bone infection must be suspected.

4.4 Upper Limb Trauma

4.4.1 Fractures of the shoulder girdle

Fractures of the clavicle

- the clavicle is the most frequent site of fracture in childhood.

- 50% occur in children under 10 years of age. Occasionally it is the result of birth trauma.

- approximately 70% occur in the middle third of the clavicle (fig 4.17). 25% occur in the outer third.

- in children the fracture may be incomplete i.e. greenstick fracture (fig 4.18).

- in adults it is usually a complete transverse fracture.

- if complete, displacement is common due to elevation of medial fragment (from the pull of the neck muscles) and depression of the lateral fragment (due to the weight of the shoulder).

- rarely in severe trauma a midclavicular fracture may be associated with injury of the underlying subclavian artery.

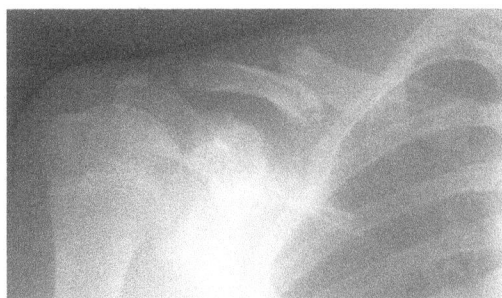

Figure 4.17
Displaced fracture of the midshaft of the clavicle. The ossification centre for the acromion should not be misinterpreted as a fracture (arrow).

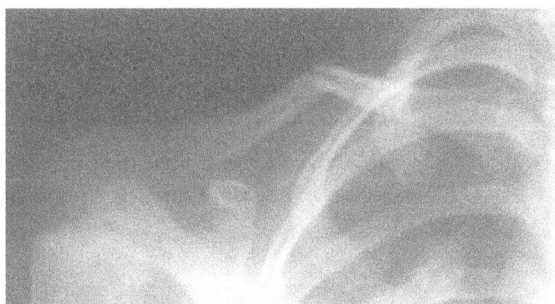

Figure 4.18
Greenstick fracture of the clavicle in a child.

Fractures of the scapula

- scapular fractures usually occur from direct injury, often associated with other injuries to the chest and spine.

- approximately 80% involve the body (fig 4.19) or neck of the scapula. Less common are fractures of the acromion and coracoid.

- fractures of the glenoid may occur in association with shoulder dislocation or from avulsion of the triceps insertion from the inferior glenoid rim.

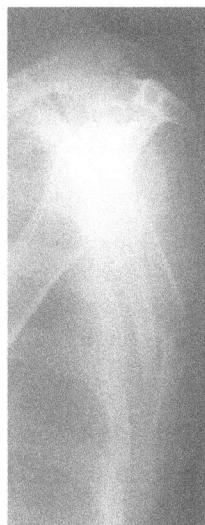

Figure 4.19
Fracture of the blade of the scapula. Lateral projection.

4.4.2 **Injuries of the shoulder and related joints**

Dislocation of the sternoclavicular joint

- an uncommon injury accounting for only 3% dislocations of the shoulder girdle.

- the majority of sternoclavicular joint dislocations are anterior due to an indirect blow to the shoulder levering the medial end of the clavicle forwards.

- the rare posterior dislocation may be associated with injury to the major vessels.

- the dislocation is frequently difficult to identify radiographically. An anteroposterior projection with 40-degree cephalic (towards the head) tilt of the tube may be required. Where available, CT readily confirms/excludes the diagnosis.

Dislocation of the acromioclavicular joint

- a more common injury than sternoclavicular joint dislocation, accounting for 12% of the dislocations of the shoulder girdle.

- indirect trauma causes rupture of the joint capsule and ligaments anchoring the clavicle to the superior aspect of the scapula.

- there is a spectrum of injury from minor subluxation to dislocation with superior displacement of the lateral clavicle (fig 4.20). Weight bearing views (i.e. with the patient erect and holding weights in each hand) may be required to demonstrate the abnormality. The normal width of the acromioclavicular joint in the adult is less than 5 mm.

- pseudodislocation is seen in children and adolescents with a fracture of the lateral end of the clavicle and superior displacement of the medial clavicle.

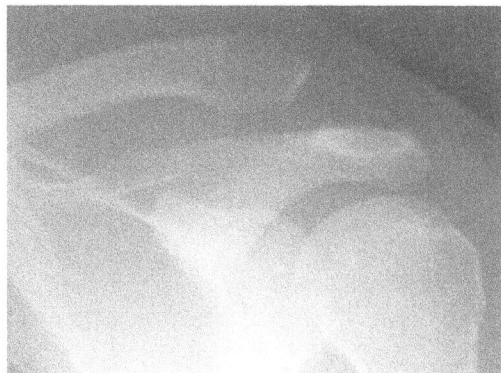

Figure 4.20
Dislocated acromioclavicular joint with superior displacement of the lateral clavicle. (In the uninjured joint, the under surface of the lateral clavicle and the acromion are at the same level, see fig 3.28).

Dislocation of the shoulder

- dislocation of the shoulder occurs at the glenohumeral joint.

- it is the commonest joint dislocated in the body, accounting for 50% of all dislocations. It is however, uncommon in children.

- it can be classified by the direction of the dislocation with respect to the glenoid;

  — anterior (95%)
  — posterior (4%)
  — inferior
  — superior

Anterior dislocation

- commonest form of shoulder dislocation (95%).

- humeral head displaced anteriorly and beneath coracoid (fig 4.21a) or less commonly below the inferior rim of glenoid (fig 4.22).

- 15% associated with fracture of the greater tuberosity (fig 4.21b).

- 8% associated with fracture of anterior glenoid.

- 40% dislocations are recurrent. In chronic cases there is a compression defect on the posterolateral surface of the humeral head.

- bilateral dislocations are seen in association with seizures (epilepsy, electrocution etc.).

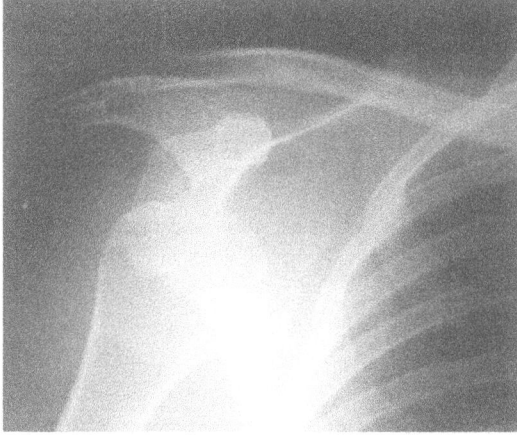

(a)

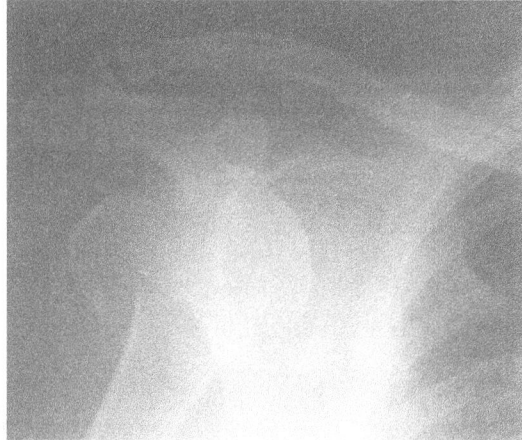

(b)

Figure 4.21
Anterior subcoracoid dislocation of the shoulder. (a) without associated fracture (b) with fracture of the greater tuberosity.

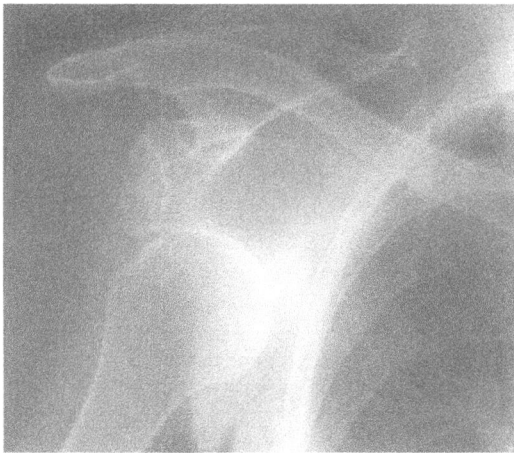

Figure 4.22
Anterior subglenoid dislocation of the shoulder.

Posterior dislocation

- rare form of dislocation but over 50% are missed at time of initial examination.

- convulsive seizures are the commonest cause.

- following dislocation, the humerus is fixed in internal rotation. This gives the so-called "light-bulb" appearance to the humeral head (fig 4.23a). Other signs on the AP projection include loss of congruity of the glenohumeral joint. The posterior displacement is easily seen on a lateral projection (fig 4.23b).

- chronic recurrent posterior dislocation will result in an anterolateral compression defect of the humeral head (fig 4.24b).

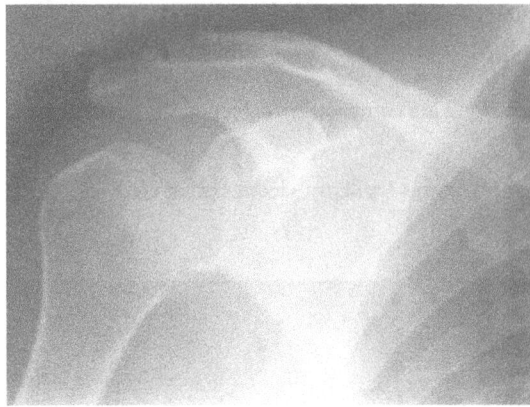
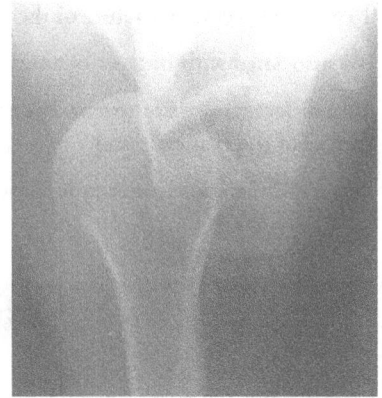

(a)   (b)

Figure 4.23
Posterior dislocation of the shoulder. (a) AP showing loss of congruity of the gleno-humeral joint and a "light-bulb" appearance of the humeral head due to internal rotation. (b) Axial projection showing the posterior dislocation and the compression defect in the anterolateral aspect of the humeral head.

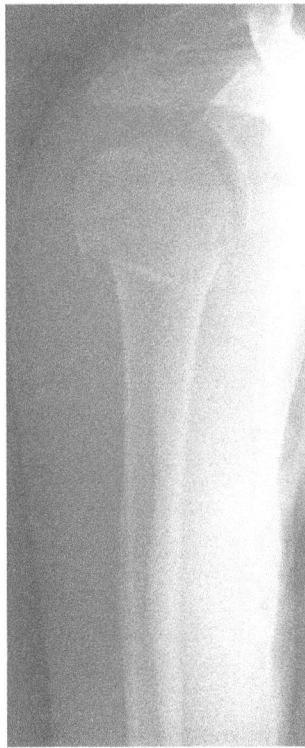
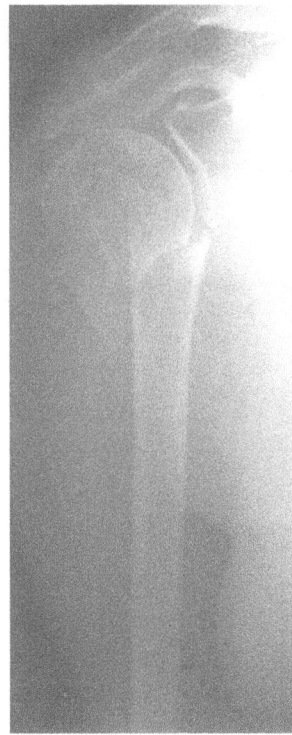

Figure 4.24
Fracture of the neck of humerus.
(a) with minimal displacement.
(b) with moderate displacement.
Note that to completely assess
the deformity and displacement,
lateral projections are also
required.

(a)   (b)

4.4.3 **Fractures of the humerus**

- fractures of the humerus are classified into 6 groups;

  neck of humerus
  greater tuberosity
  shaft
  supracondylar*
  condyle (usually lateral)*
  epicondyle (usually medial)*

  see elbow section below

Fracture of the neck of humerus

- affects the proximal humeral metaphysis (fig 4.24).

- common in elderly women.

- uncommon in children. Usually the fracture separates the proximal humeral growth plate. Do not mistake the normal growth plate in children for a fracture.

Fracture of the shaft of humerus

- usually affects the middle third, either from indirect trauma (resulting in a spiral fracture – fig 4.25a) or a direct blow (resulting in a transverse fracture – fig 4.25b).

- if the fracture is significantly displaced there may be associated radial nerve damage.

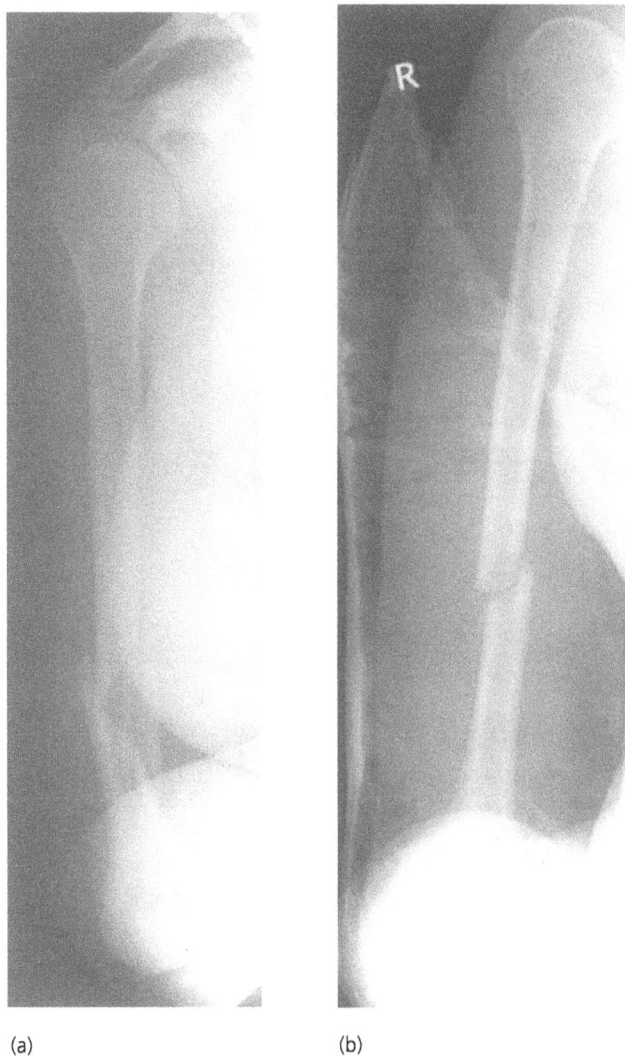

(a)   (b)

Figure 4.25
Fracture of the shaft of humerus (a) spiral fracture from indirect trauma. (b) transverse fracture from a direct blow.

4.4.4 Fractures of the elbow

- the elbow is a common site of injury, particularly in children. Because of the complex anatomy significant injuries may appear subtle on radiographs.

- aids to diagnosing bony trauma on elbow radiographs include;

    — assessment of the ossification centres
    — fat-pad sign

— anterior humeral line
— radio-capitellar line

Ossification centres

• during childhood, six separate ossification centres appear at various intervals up to 12 years. Four of these centres belong to the humerus, one to the radius, and one to the ulna (fig 4.26 and 4.27).

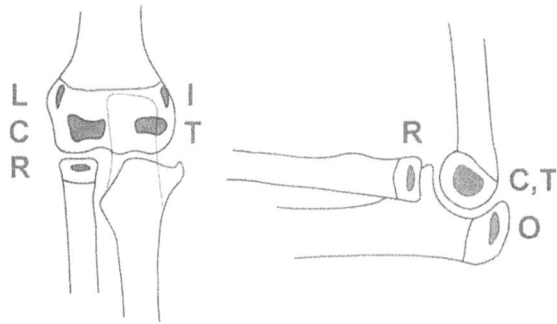

Figure 4.26
Schematic diagram indicating the ossification centres within the cartilaginous ends of the bones of the elbow.

(from Raby, Berman & de Lacey, *Accident & Emergency Radiology: a survival guide*, Saunders, London, 1995, with permission)

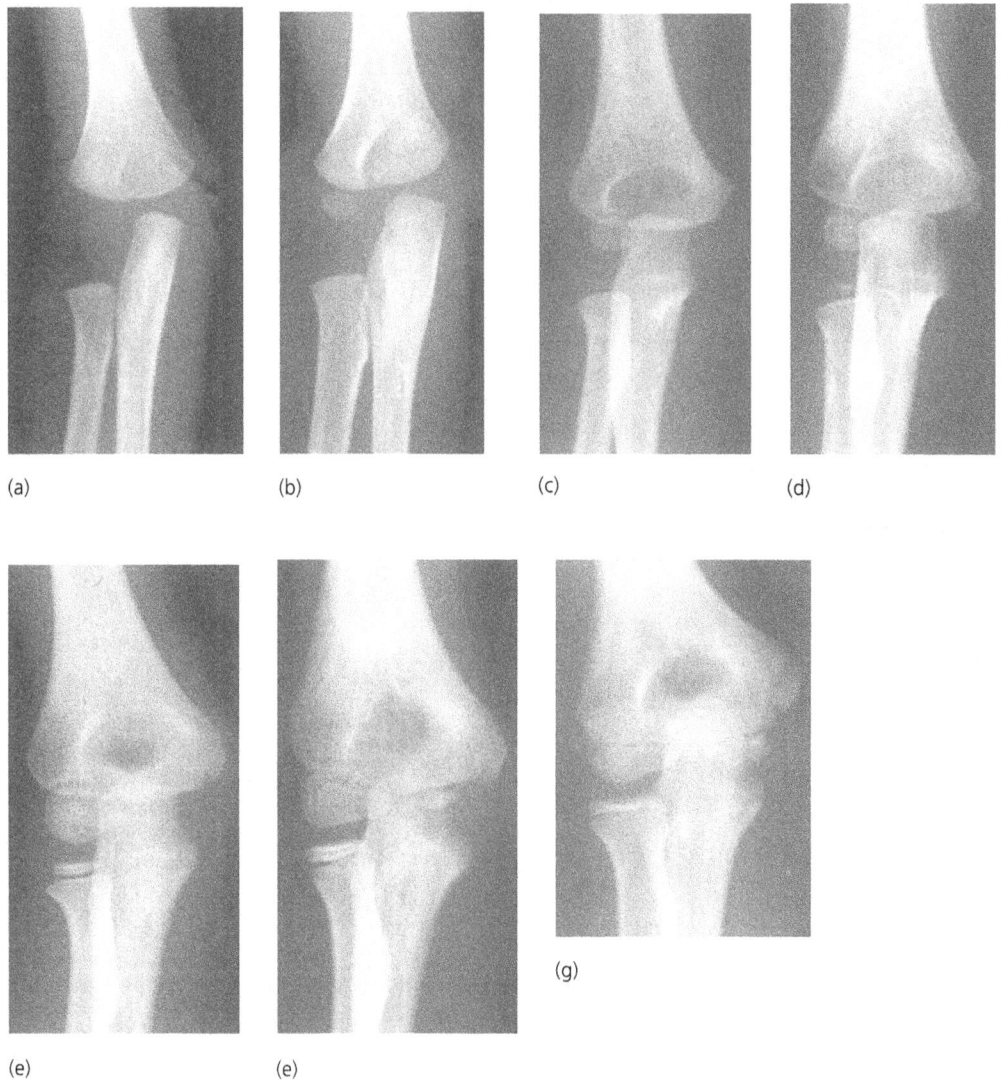

(a)   (b)   (c)   (d)

(e)   (e)   (g)

Figure 4.27
Series of elbow radiographs showing the typical appearances of the ossification centres at different ages. (a) 2 months (b) 4 months (c) 2 years (d) 4 years (e) 6 years (f) 9 years (g) 10 years.

- the age at which each ossification centre appears is NOT important.

- the sequence in which the centres ossify IS important.

- the acronym (aide-memoire) **CRITOL** gives the most common order in which the centres appear.

C	capitellum	3 months
R	radial head	6 months
I	internal (medial) epicondyle	
T	trochlea	
O	olecranon	
L	lateral (external epicondyle)	12 years

- the trochlea always ossifies after the internal epicondyle. If the trochlea is visible the internal epicondyle must be somewhere on the radiograph. An avulsed internal epicondyle may be displaced into the joint space.

Fat pad sign

- there are two pads of fat within the elbow joint capsule which can be seen on lateral radiographs as black streaks in the surrounding grey soft tissues.

- in normal patients the posterior fat pad is hidden within the olecranon fossa. The anterior fat pad may be seen close to the anterior surface of the distal humerus (fig 4.28).

- when there is a joint effusion or haemarthrosis (blood within the joint) the fat pads will be displaced away from the humerus (fig 4.29). A visible posterior fat pad is always abnormal. A visible anterior fat pad is only abnormal if displaced anteriorly.

- when there is a positive fat pad sign (i.e. displacement of the pad), this is strongly suggestive of a fracture. Look carefully for a radial head fracture in adults and a supracondylar fracture in children. However, the fat pad sign may be the only sign of a fracture on the radiograph.

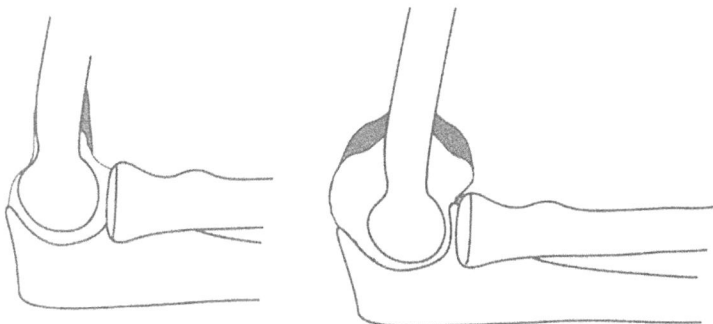

Figure 4.28
Line diagram showing the position of the normal anterior fat pad (left). A joint effusion displaces the anterior and posterior fat pads (black areas) away from the humerus (right).

(from Raby, Berman & de Lacey, *Accident & Emergency Radiology: a survival guide*, Saunders, London, 1995, with permission)

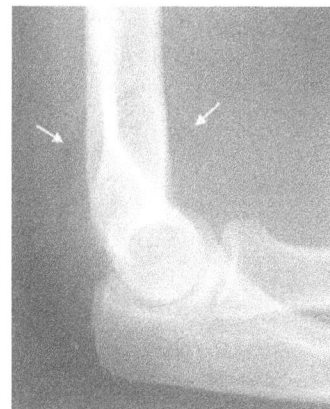

Figure 4.29
Lateral radiograph showing a positive fat pad sign (arrows).

Anterior humeral line

- on a normal lateral radiograph a line traced along the anterior cortex of the humerus will bisect the capitellum between its anterior and middle thirds (fig 4.30).

- if less than one third of the capitellum lies anterior to the line then there may be a supracondylar fracture with posterior displacement of the distal fragment (fig 4.31).

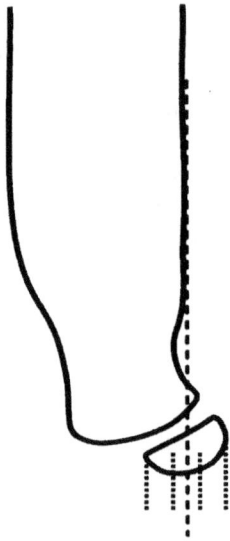

Figure 4.30
Anterior humeral line. The normal line bisects the capitellum at the junction of the anterior and middle thirds.

(modified from Lee Rogers *Radiology of Skeletal Trauma* 2nd Ed, Churchill Livingstone 1992)

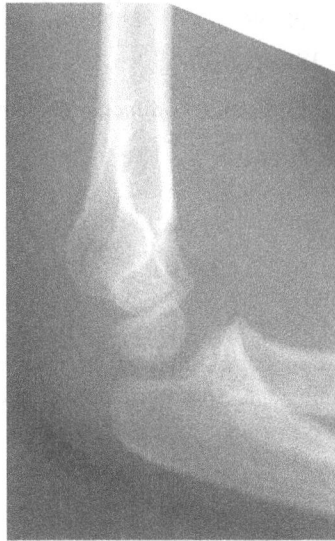

(a)

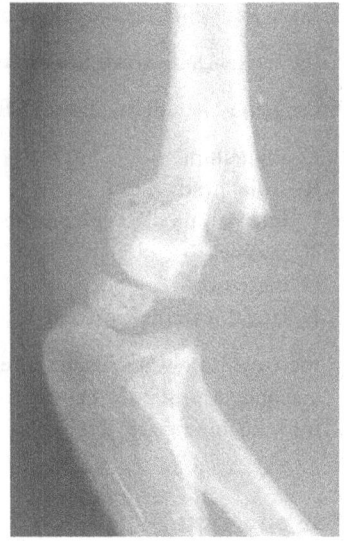

(b)

Figure 4.31
Supracondylar fractures in children. (a) minimal displacement; (b) marked displacement. Note that the anterior humeral line is abnormal in both cases.

Radiocapitellar line

- a line drawn along the centre of the shaft of the proximal radius should pass through the capitellum (fig 4.32).

- if the line does not pass through the capitellum then either the radial head or the capitellum is displaced (fig 4.33).

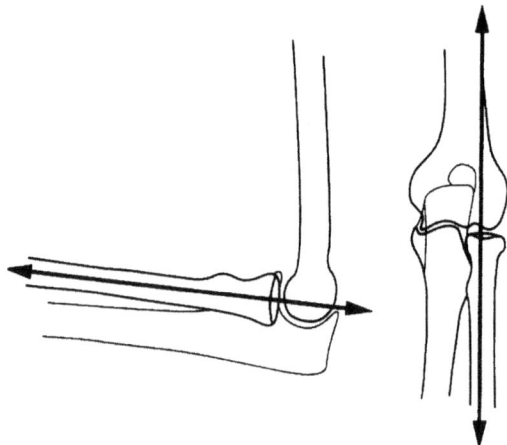

Figure 4.32
Normal radiocapitellar line on the AP and lateral views.

(from Raby, Berman & de Lacey, *Accident & Emergency Radiology: a survival guide*, Saunders, London, 1995, with permission)

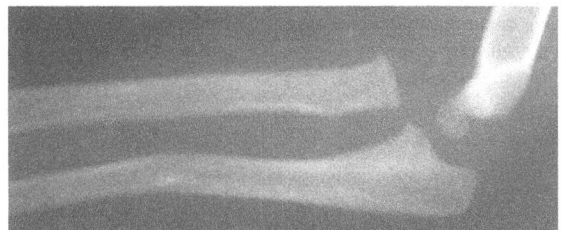

Figure 4.33
There is a fracture of the proximal third of the ulna associated with dislocation of the proximal radius. The radiocapitellar line is disrupted (Monteggia fracture).

Supracondylar fractures

- the commonest fracture of the elbow in children.

- transverse fracture of the distal humeral metaphysis. Approximately 50% are greenstick fractures (fig 4.34).

- posterior displacement of the distal fragment with the anterior humeral line passing through the anterior third or completely anterior to the capitellum (fig 4.31)

- severely displaced fractures may be associated with brachial artery compression.

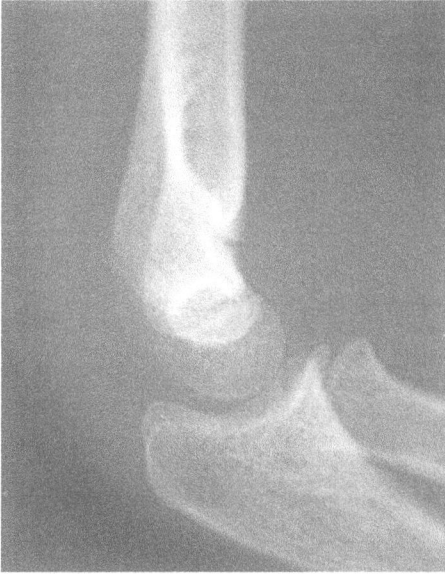

Figure 4.34
Greenstick supracondylar fracture. Note that the anterior humeral line is normal.

Condylar and epicondylar fractures

- there is a spectrum of avulsion injuries of the humeral condyles and epicondyles ranging from those with only minor displacement to those with major displacement (figs 4.35 and 4.36).

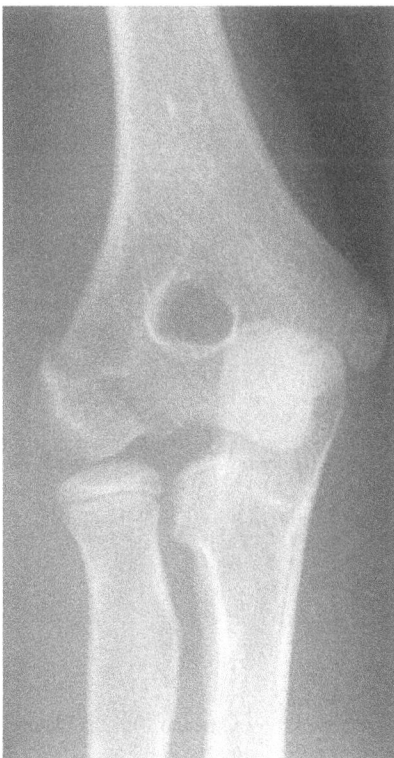

Figure 4.35
Avulsion of the lateral epicondyle in a child with minor displacement.

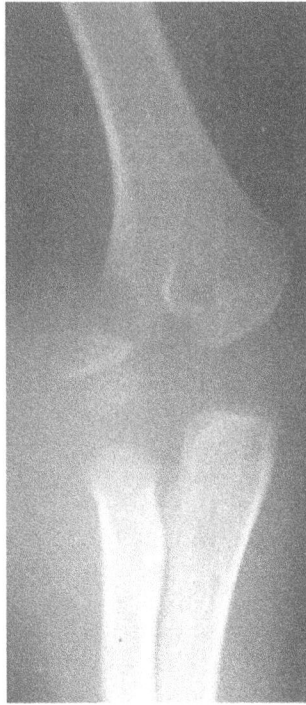

(a)

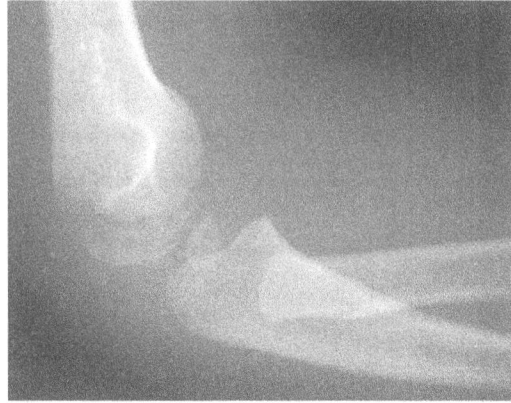

(b)

Figure 4.36
(a) avulsion of the lateral epicondyle in a child with marked displacement.
(b) the lateral projection shows the radiocapitellar line is disrupted indicating that there is a dislocation of the head of radius as well as the avulsion fracture.

- avulsion of the medial epicondyle may be displaced into the joint mimicking the trochlea ossification centre.

Capitellar fractures

- commonest purely intra-articular fracture of the elbow.
- fracture usually identified on lateral projection with fragment rotating anteriorly (fig 4.37).
- AP film may appear normal or show increased density due to the capitellar fragment overlying the lateral epicondyle.

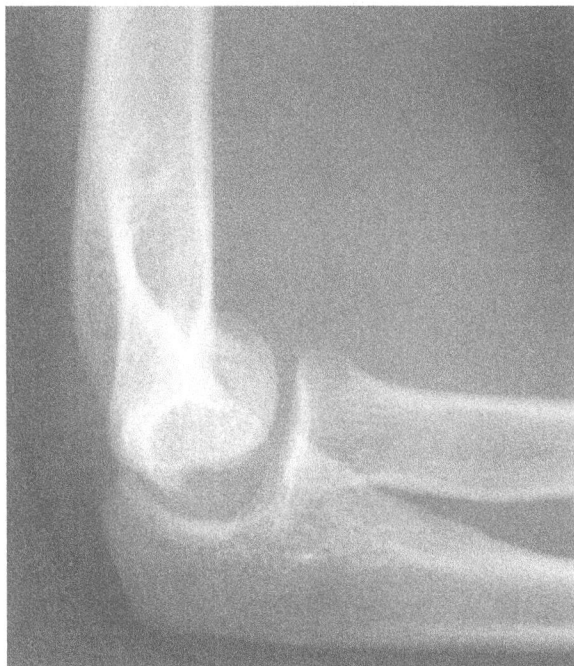

Figure 4.37
Fracture of the capitellum. The capitellum has rotated 90 degrees anteriorly.

Radial head fractures

- account for approximately one third of all elbow fractures.

- commonest in young adults.

- spectrum of injury from minimally displaced to comminuted with displacement (fig 4.38).

- in children tend to appear as a greenstick fracture of the radial neck rather than a fracture of the radial head (fig 4.39).

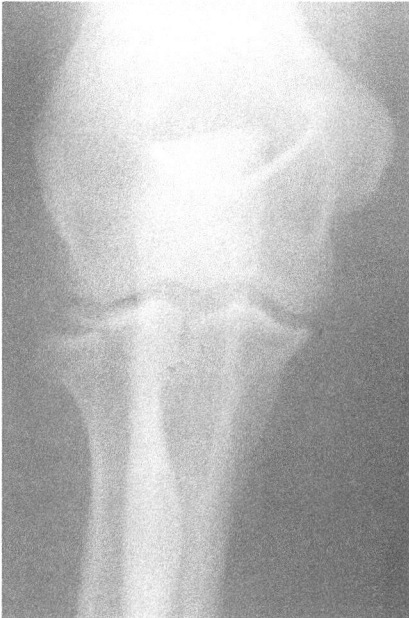

Figure 4.38
Fracture of the radial head with minor displacement.

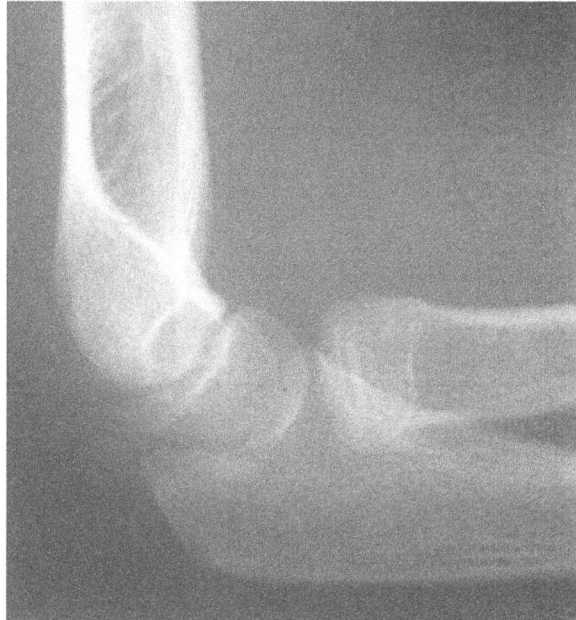

Figure 4.39
Greenstick fracture of the neck of radius in a child.

Olecranon fractures

- result from either a direct blow to the tip of the elbow or avulsion by contraction of the triceps muscle against a fixed flexed elbow.

- the action of the triceps frequently causes marked displacement of the olecranon at the fracture site (fig 4.40).

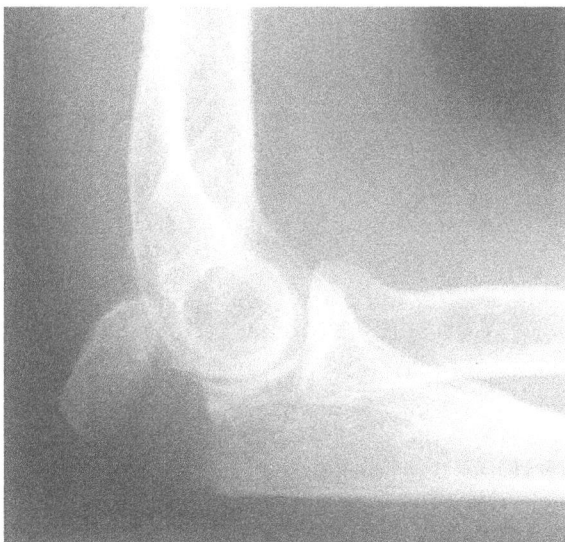

Figure 4.40
Displaced fracture of the olecranon.

Elbow dislocation

- third commonest site of dislocation in the adult after shoulder and fingers.

- commonest site of dislocation in children under 10 years of age.

- 85% posterior or posterolateral in direction (fig 4.41).

- 50% associated with fractures (fig 4.42).

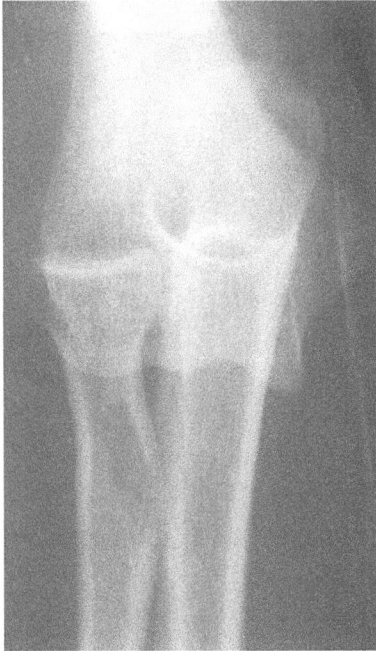
(a)

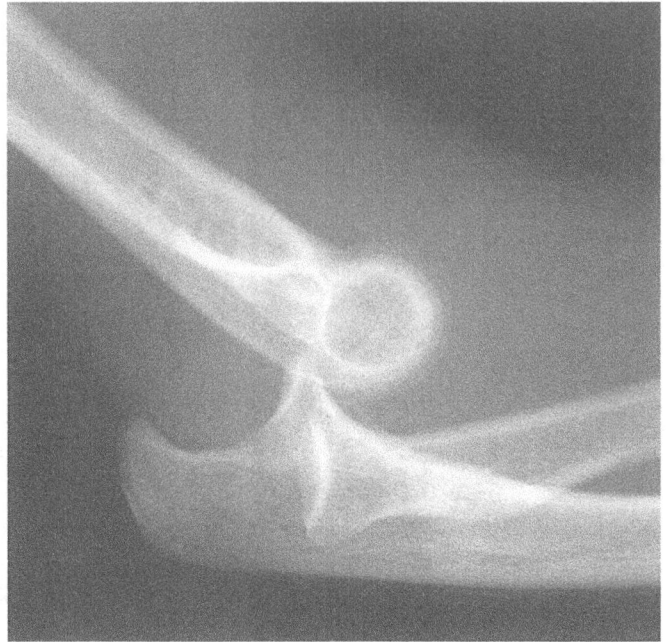
(b)

Figure 4.41
Posterior dislocation of the elbow. (a) AP (b) lateral view.

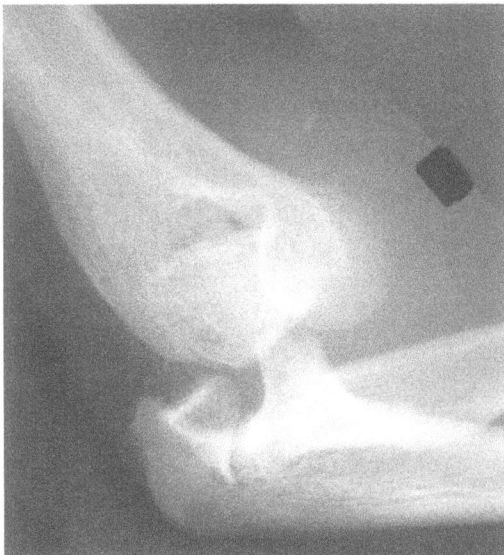
(a)

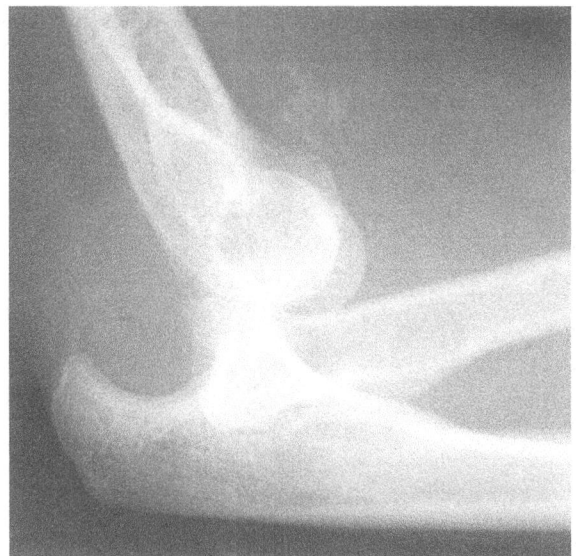
(b)

Figure 4.42
Posterior dislocation of the elbow with a displaced fracture of the radial head. Note that because of the severe trauma it is not always possible to obtain ideal AP (a) and lateral projections (b).

4.4.5 **Fractures of the forearm**

Proximal radio-ulnar fracture-dislocation (Monteggia fracture)

- fracture of the proximal or mid-third ulna, associated with a dislocation of the radial head (figs 4.33 and 4.43).

- the dislocation of the radial head results in disruption of the radio-capitellar line.

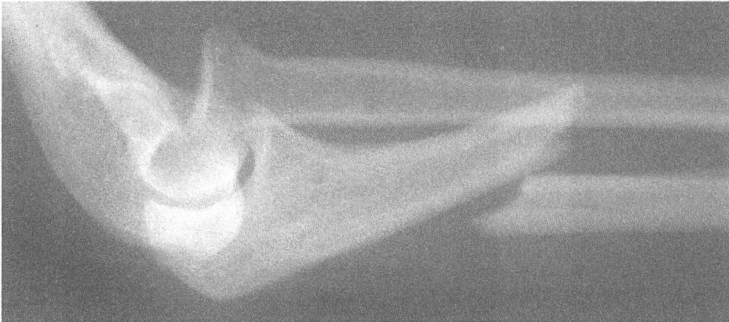

Figure 4.43
Association of a fracture of the proximal third of the ulna and a dislocated radial head (Monteggia fracture). Note the radiocapitellar line is disrupted.

Radius and ulna

- fractures of the shafts of the radius and ulna are most commonly seen in children.

- there is a spectrum of injury from plastic bowing, through greenstick to complete fractures (fig 4.44).

- fractures of the distal forearm are common at all ages. As they typically present with "wrist trauma" they are considered in Chapter 4.4.6 below.

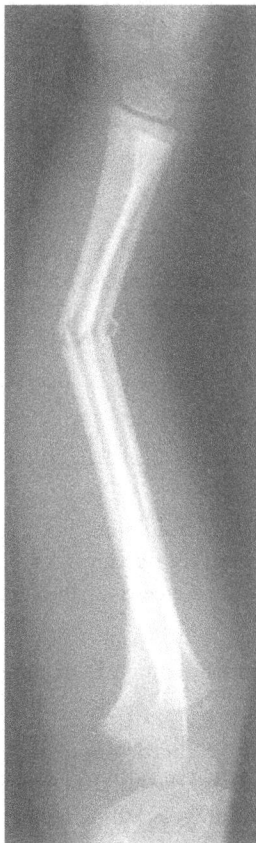

Figure 4.44
Greenstick fractures of the radius and ulna in a child. Note that this is a variant of the Monteggia fracture described above (4.4.5), because the radiocapitellar line is disrupted, indicating that the radial head is also dislocated.

Distal radio-ulnar fracture-dislocation (Galeazzi fracture)

- fracture of the distal third of the radius associated with dorsal dislocation of the distal radio-ulnar joint (fig 4.45). Frequently a distal radio-ulnar joint dislocation can be identified on the lateral projection only (fig 4.45b).

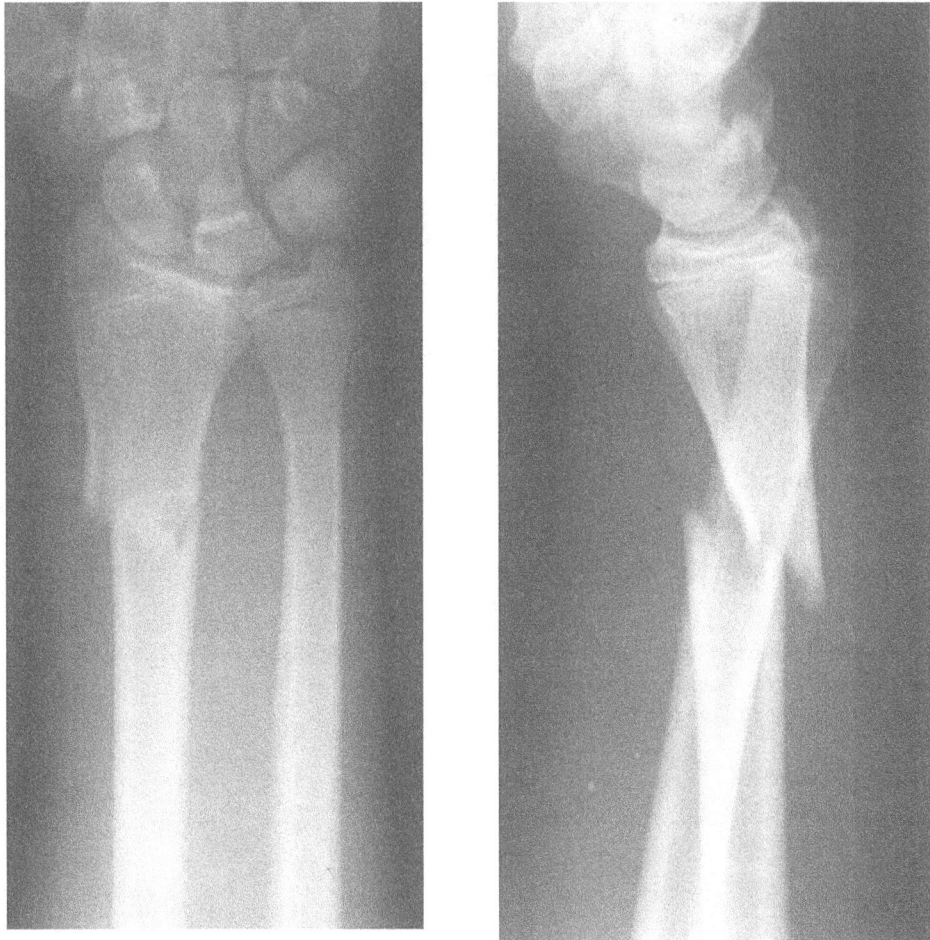

(a)

(b)

Figure 4.45
Association of a fracture of the distal third of the radius with dislocation of the distal ulna (Galeazzi fracture).
(a) PA and (b) lateral projection. Note that the dorsal subluxation of the ulna can only be seen on the lateral projection.

4.4.6 Fractures of the wrist (and distal forearm)

Distal radius and ulna

- fractures of the radius or both radius and ulna are the commonest fractures of childhood. There is a spectrum of injuries from buckle (torus), to greenstick (fig 4.46) to complete fractures (4.47). The commonest combination is a complete fracture of the distal radius with a greenstick fracture of the distal ulna.

- in the adolescent the growth plate is the weakest site. Therefore, the commonest injury is a fracture separation across the distal radial growth plate, (fig 4.48).

- this is also a common site of fracture in the elderly, particularly women with reduced bone density. A fall onto the outstretched hand will result in posterior (dorsal) displacement of the distal fragment (Colle's fracture, fig 4.49). Frequently the distal ulna is also fractured. Anterior (volar) displacement of the distal radial fragment is less common (Smith's fracture, fig 4.50). Posterior or anterior displacement can only be assessed on a lateral projection.

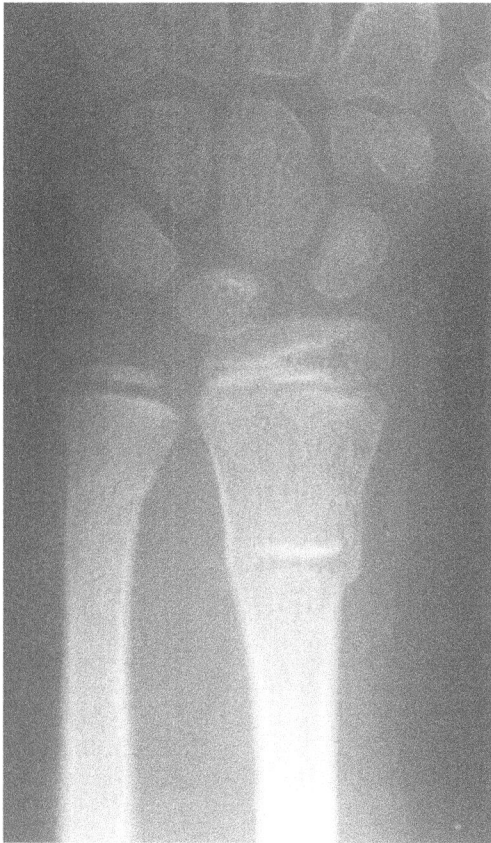
(a)

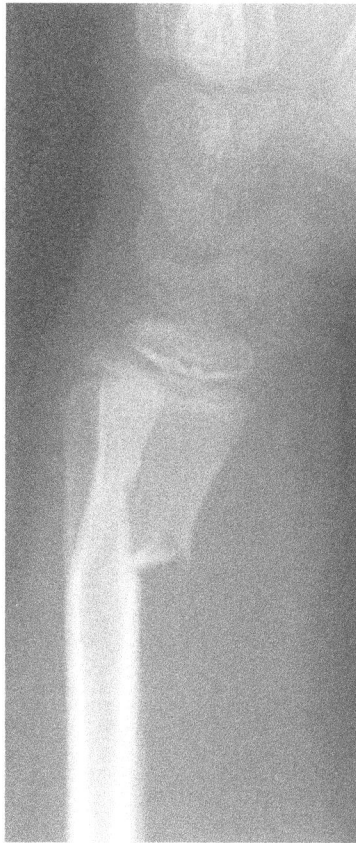
(b)

Figure 4.46
Greenstick fracture of the distal radius with tiny buckle (torus) fracture of the ulna.(a) PA and (b) lateral projection.

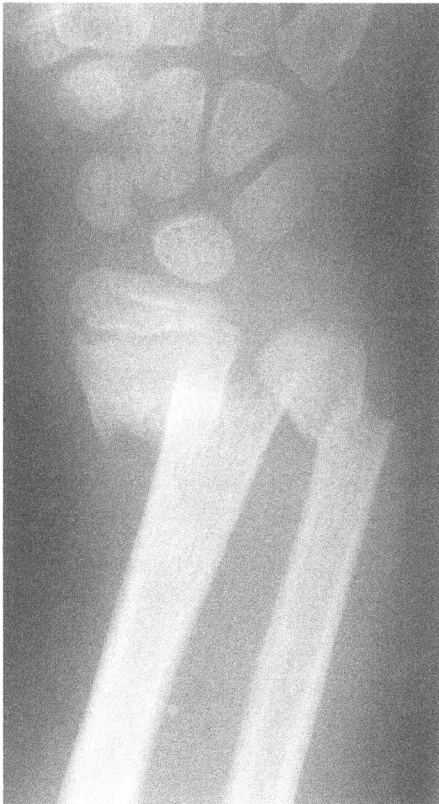
(a)

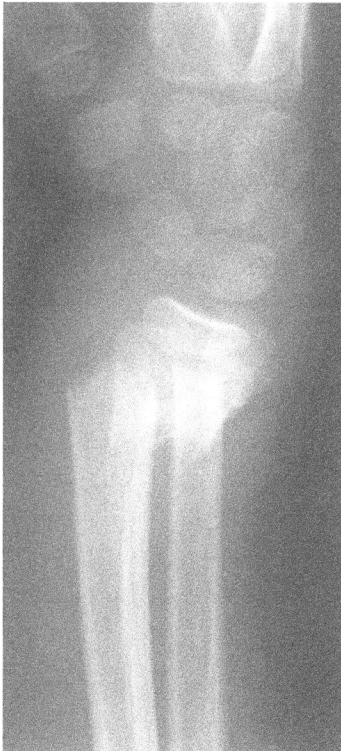
(b)

Figure 4.47
Child with complete fractures of the distal radius and ulna. (a) PA and (b) lateral projection.

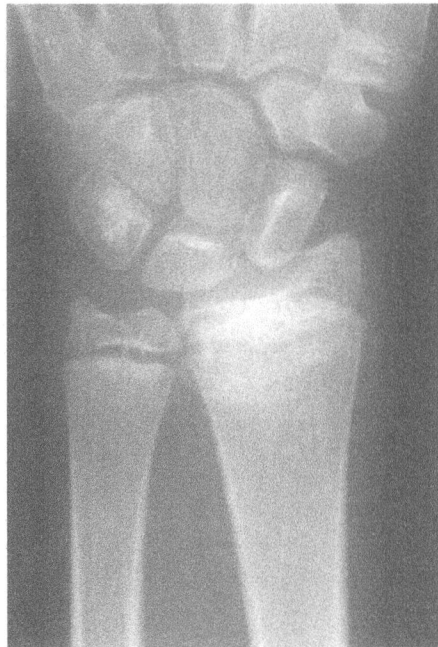

(a)

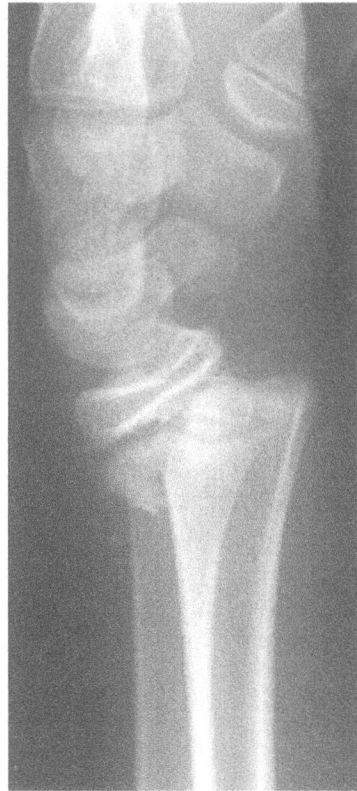

(b)

Figure 4.48
Adolescent with fracture separation of the distal radial growth plate. (a) PA and (b) lateral projection.

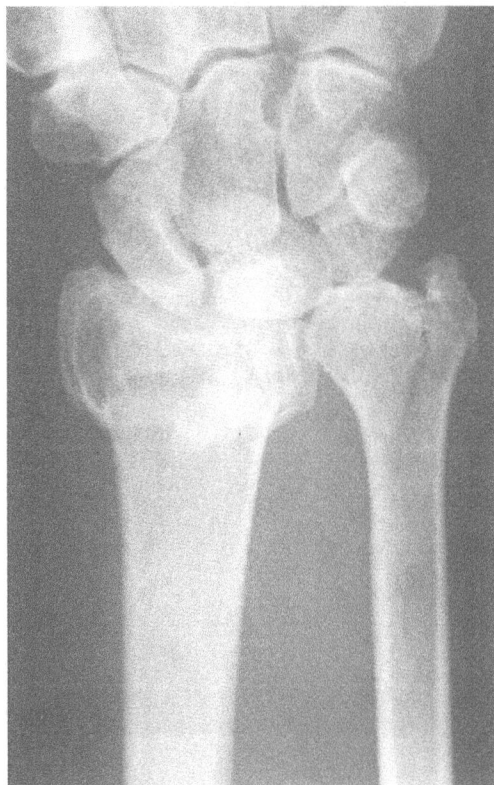

(a)

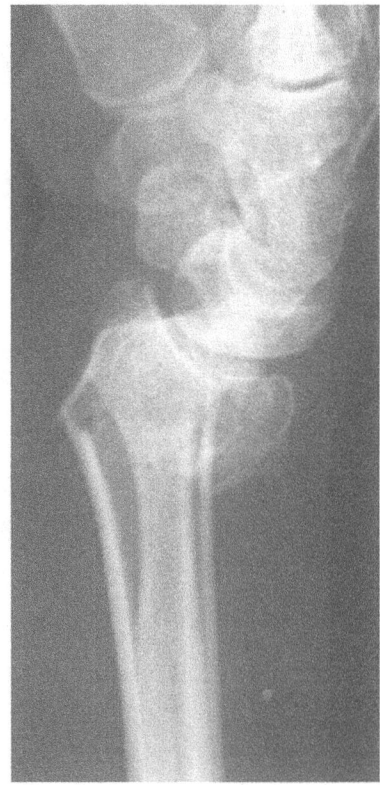

(b)

Figure 4.49
Fractures of the distal radius and ulna with dorsal angulation of the distal fragment (Colle's fracture). (a) PA and (b) lateral projection.

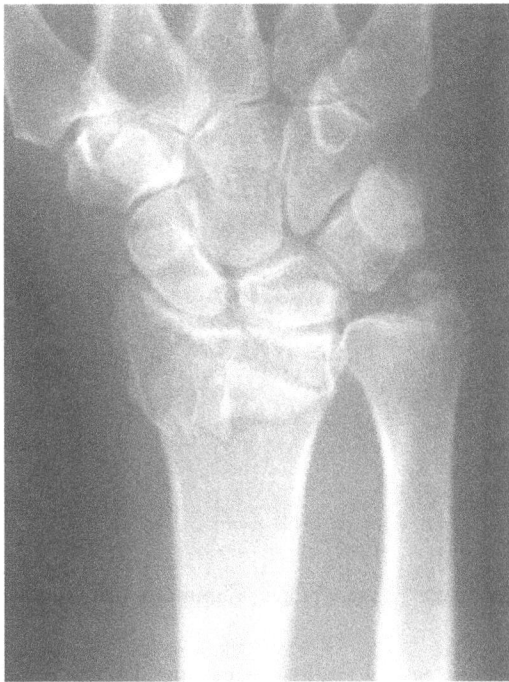
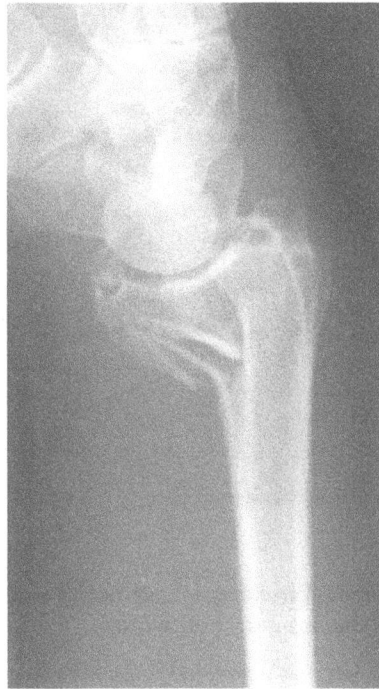

(a)   (b)

Figure 4.50
Fracture of the distal radius and ulna with anterior angulation of the distal fragment (Smith's fracture). (a) PA and (b) lateral projection.

Carpal bones

Scaphoid

- almost all carpal bone fractures are through the scaphoid.

- most are through the waist (midpole) of the scaphoid (fig 4.51), whereas some are through the distal and proximal poles (fig 4.52).

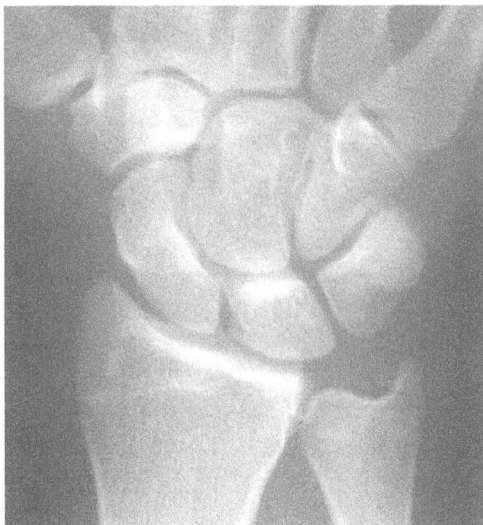
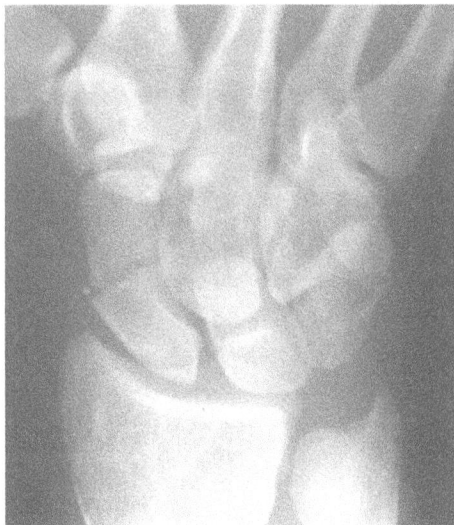

(a)   (b)

Figure 4.51
Fracture of the waist of the scaphoid not visible on the PA film (a) but easily identified on the oblique view (b).

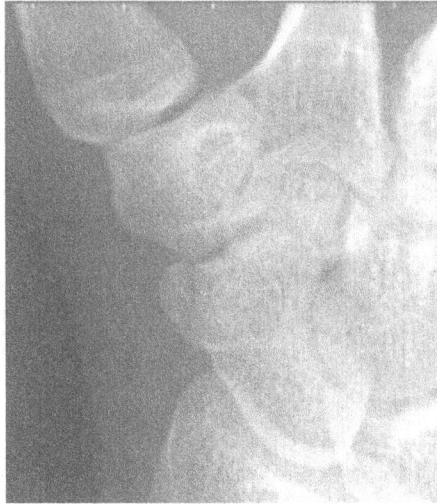

Figure 4.52
Fracture of the distal pole of the scaphoid.

- scaphoid fractures are rare in children, not seen under 10 years of age. Commonest site, unlike adults, is a distal pole avulsion.

- present with pain and localised tenderness over the base of the first metacarpal, known as the anatomical "snuff box".

- soon after the injury the fractures are often subtle or invisible on the radiographs at presentation. For this reason the standard film series should include at least 4 views. Also, in the absence of an obvious fracture on the initial radiographs, when clinical suspicion persists because of pain, it is advisable to repeat the examination after 10 days.

- there is a significant risk of the complications of non-union and avascular necrosis of the proximal pole if the fractures are inadequately treated (fig 4.15). Eventually, this will result in degenerative joint disease of the radio-carpal joints.

Triquetrum

- small flake fractures from the dorsal aspect of the triquetrum, seen on the lateral projection, are the second commonest carpal injury after fracture of the scaphoid (fig 4.53). This injury seldom requires treatment.

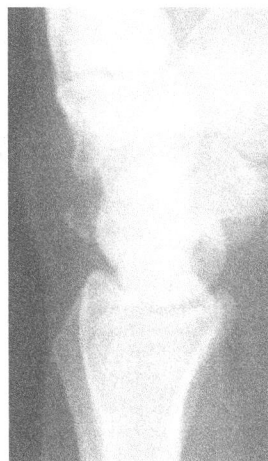

Figure 4.53
Avulsion fracture from the dorsal aspect of the triquetrum.

Lunate

- fractures of the lunate are extremely rare but two types of dislocation are well recognized, lunate dislocation and perilunate dislocation. In the normal position on the lateral projection the capitate sits in the concavity of the lunate. On the PA projection the normal lunate approximates to a rectangle.

Lunate dislocation

- on the PA projection the lunate appears triangular (fig 4.54a).

- on the lateral projection the lunate dislocates anteriorly so that the distal radial concavity is empty (4.54b). The radius and ulna remain in a straight line (fig 4.54c).

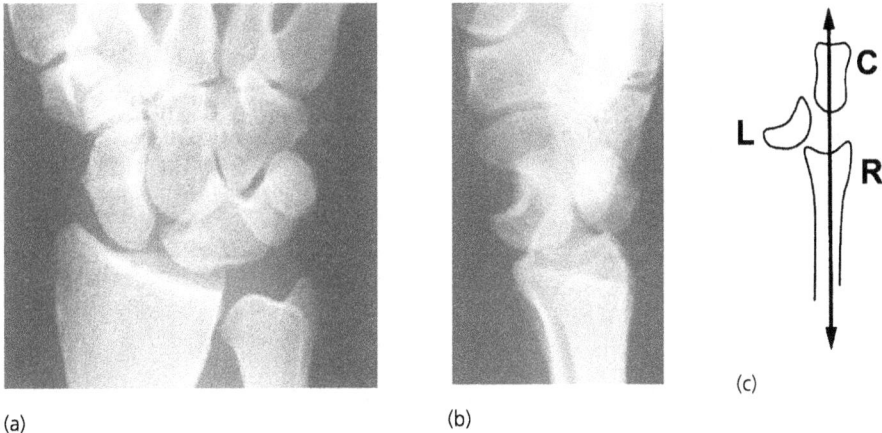

(a)   (b)   (c)

Figure 4.54
Lunate dislocation (a) the PA projection shows a triangular shaped lunate; (b) the lateral shows the lunate displaced anteriorly; (c) line diagram showing the displacement of the dislocated lunate (L) and the normal alignment of the distal radius (R) and capitate (C).

(from Raby, Berman & de Lacey, *Accident & Emergency Radiology: a survival guide*, Saunders, London, 1995, with permission)

Perilunate dislocation

- with this injury, the whole of the carpus (except for the lunate) is displaced posteriorly. The lunate appears triangular on the PA projection (fig 4.55a).

- on the lateral projection the distal concavity of the lunate is empty (fig 4.55b) but the radius and lunate remain in a straight line (fig 4.55c).

- perilunate dislocation is often associated with a scaphoid fracture.

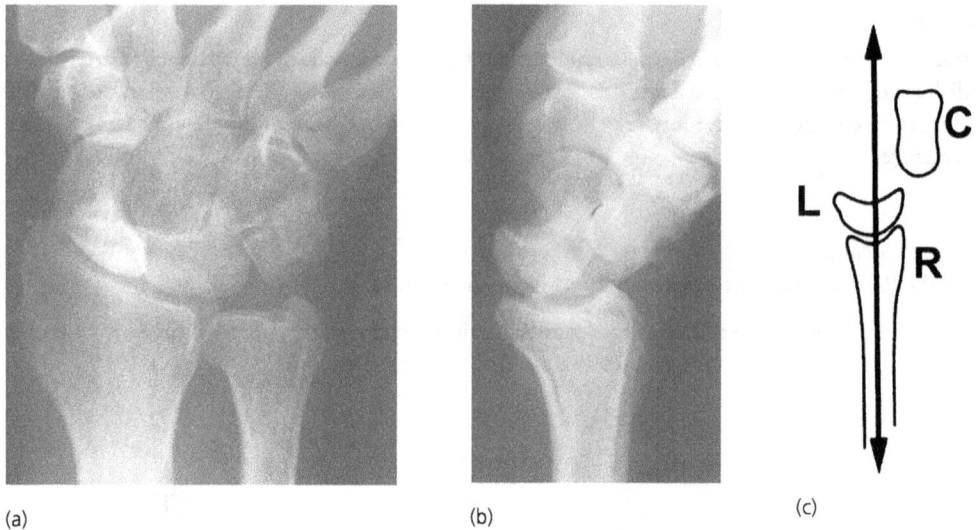

(a)   (b)   (c)

Figure 4.55

Perilunate dislocation. (a) the PA projection shows loss of the normal rectangular shape of the lunate; (b) the lateral projection shows posterior displacement of the capitate; (c) line diagram showing the normal alignment of the distal radius (R) and lunate (L), but the capitate (C) is displaced posteriorly.

(from Raby, Berman & de Lacey, *Accident & Emergency Radiology: a survival guide*, Saunders, London, 1995 with permission)

Carpal subluxation

- a wrist injury may result in damage to one or more of the small intercarpal ligaments. The commonest is rupture of the scapho-lunate ligament. As a result there is widening of the joint between the scaphoid and the lunate (>2 mm) with end-on rotation of the scaphoid (fig 4.56).

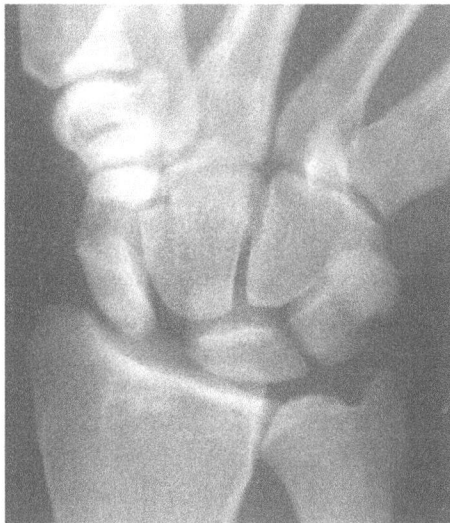

Figure 4.56

Rupture of the scapholunate ligament with widening of the scapholunate joint and rotation of the scaphoid.

4.4.7 **Fractures of the hand**

Metacarpals

- fractures of the metacarpals are fairly common at all ages. Fractures may involve the base, shaft or neck of the metacarpal (figs 4.57–4.59).

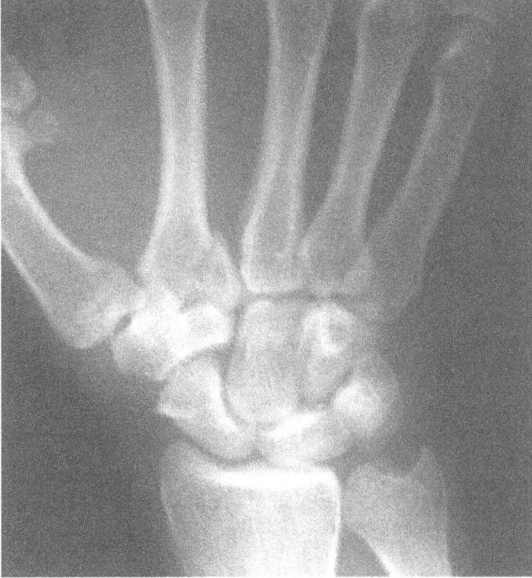

Figure 4.57
Fracture of the base of the second metacarpal extending into the joint.

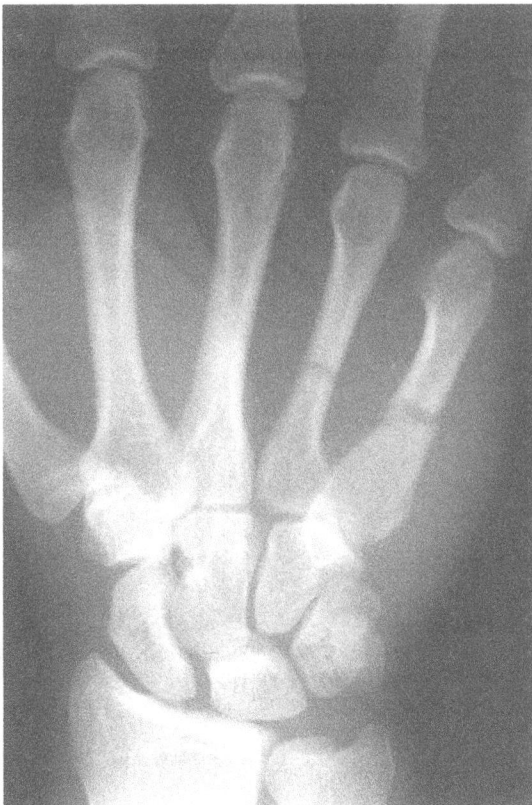

(a)

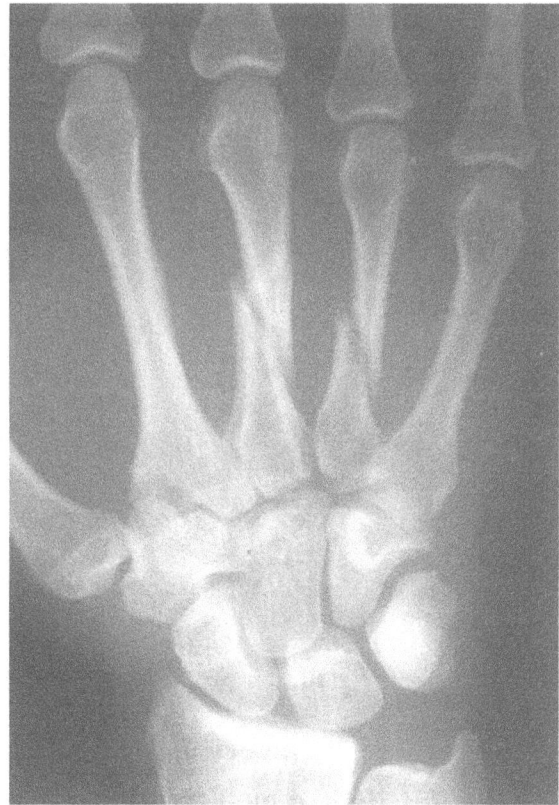

(b)

Figure 4.58
(a) transverse fractures of the shafts of the fourth and fifth metacarpals due to direct trauma; (b) spiral fractures of the shafts of the third and fourth metacarpals due to indirect trauma.

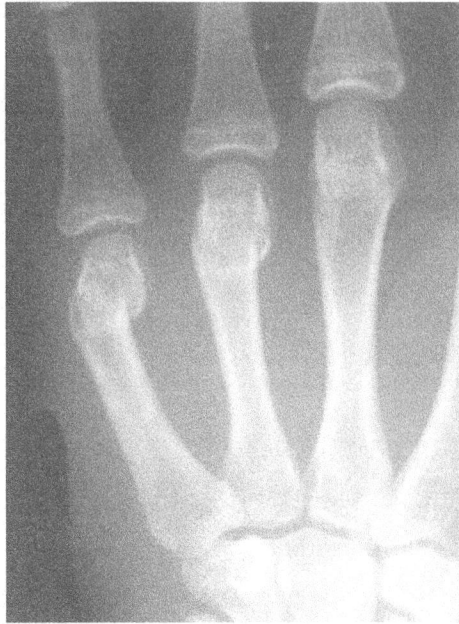
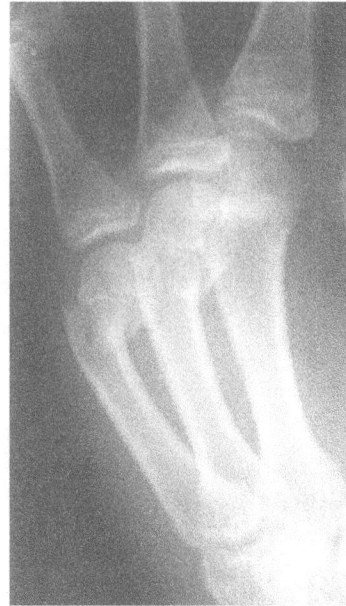

(a)

(b)

Figure 4.59
(a) PA and (b) oblique views of "boxer's" fractures of the necks of the fourth and fifth metacarpals in a child.

Carpo-metacarpal dislocation

- the 4th and 5th joints are the most commonly affected (fig 4.60) and frequently associated with fractures of the bases of the metacarpals. There is a loss of normal joint space at the base of the metacarpal on the PA projection. Dorsal dislocation of the metacarpals is demonstrated on the lateral projection.

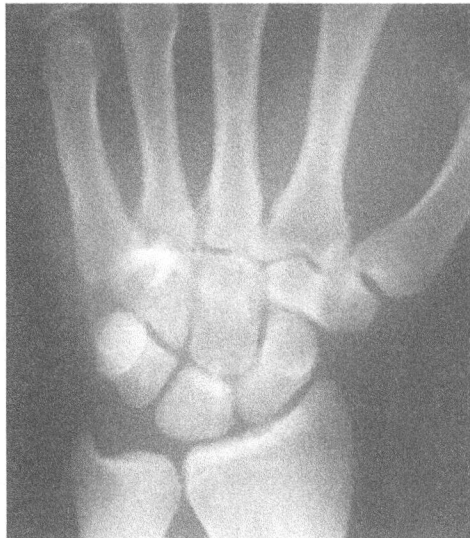

Figure 4.60
Dislocation of the fourth and fifth carpo-metacarpal joints. The joint spaces are obscured on this PA view due to the overlapping bones.

Neck of metacarpal

- fracture of the neck (distal metaphysis) of a metacarpal may be undisplaced; but particularly in the 5th metacarpal there may be marked forward tilting of the distal fragment (fig 4.59) This is known as the "boxer's fracture" as it frequently results from a misplaced blow, as in boxing or fighting.

First metacarpal

- there are two distinct types of fracture of the base of the first metacarpal (fig 4.61a). First, a transverse or short oblique fracture that does not involve the joint (fig 4.61b). This is usually a stable fracture that can be adequately treated conservatively. The second type, is a fracture-dislocation with an oblique fracture through the base of the first metacarpal and extension into the articular surface (Bennett's fracture, fig 4.61c). This type of injury is more serious and, being unstable, frequently requires internal fixation.

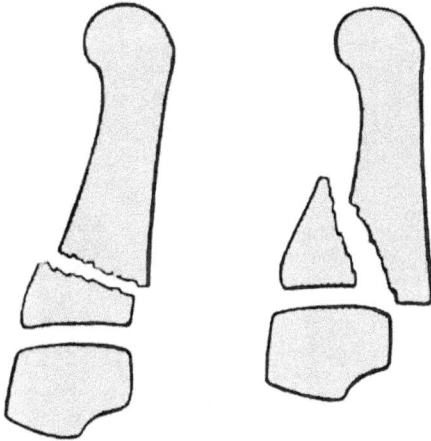

(a)

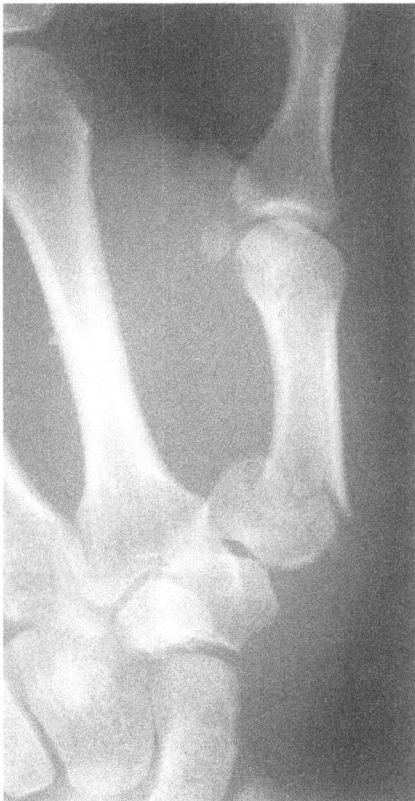

(b)

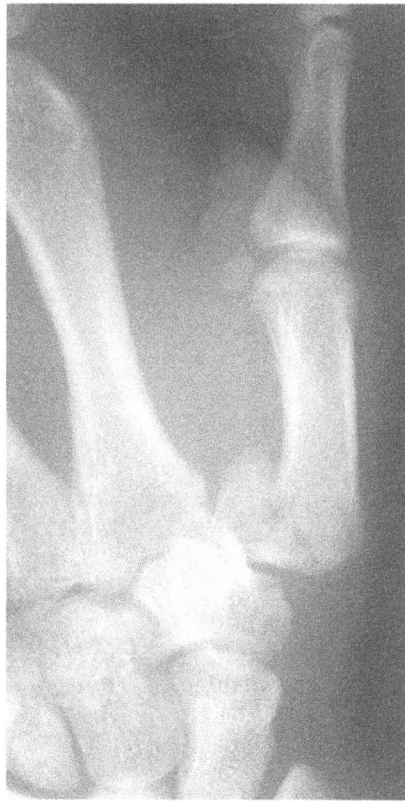

(c)

Figure 4.61
Transverse extra-articular and an oblique fracture dislocation (Bennett's fracture) of the base of the first metacarpal (a) diagram; (b) transverse fracture; (c) Oblique fracture-dislocation (Bennett's fracture).

(from Adams & Hamblen, *Outline of Fractures* 10th ed, Churchill Livingstone 1992, with permission)

Phalanges

- fractures of the phalanges are common. The spectrum of injuries is illustrated in figure 4.62. Further phalangeal injuries are detailed below.

- in children fracture separations of the epiphyses of the bases of the phalanges are fairly often seen (fig 4.63).

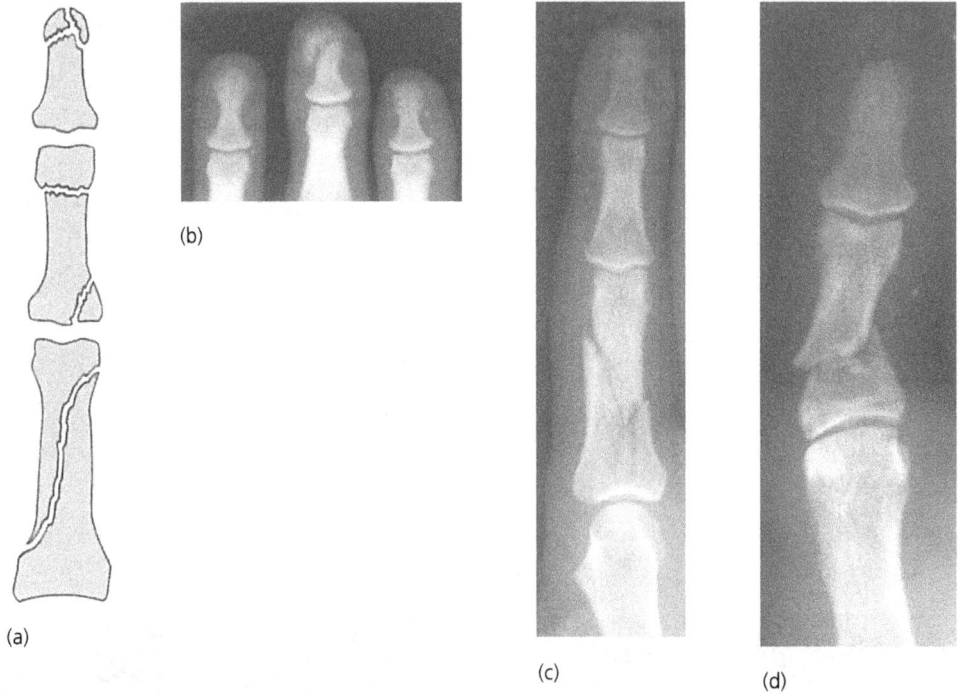

Figure 4.62
Common patterns of phalangeal fractures (a) diagram; (b) fracture of the tip of the terminal phalanx; (c) transverse fracture of the middle phalanx; (d) spiral fracture of the phalanx.

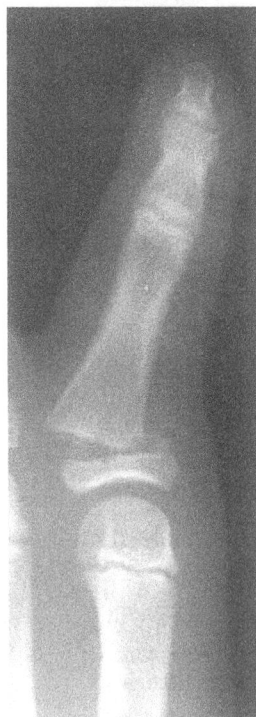

Figure 4.63
Salter-Harris Type II fracture separation of the epiphysis of the proximal phalanx.

Mallet finger

- sudden forced flexion of the distal interphalangeal joint may rupture the extensor tendon at the point of its insertion into the dorsal aspect of the base of the distal phalanx (fig 4.64a).

- flexion deformity of the distal interphalangeal joint. A bone fragment is present in a minority of cases of mallet finger (fig 4.64b).

- the anterior or palmar aspect of the joint capsule of the interphalangeal joint is a dense fibrous structure called the palmar plate.

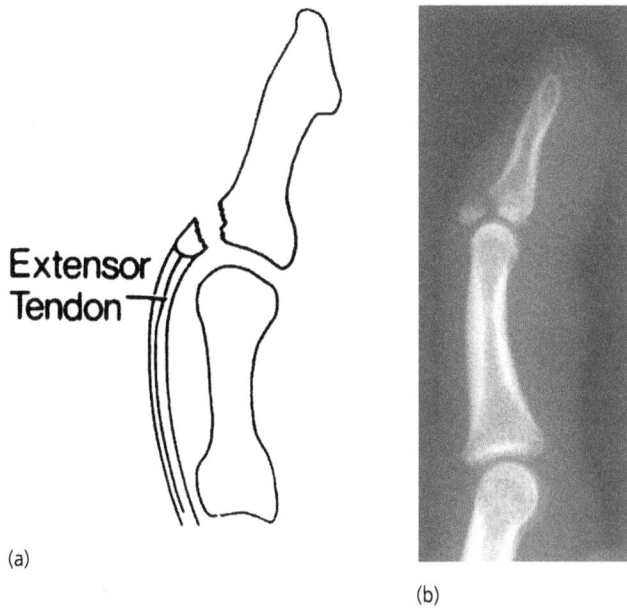

(a)

(b)

Figure 4.64
Mallet finger (a) line diagra; (b) lateral radiograph showing avulsion of the dorsal aspect of the base of the terminal phalanx with a mild flexion deformity.

Avulsion of the anterior (palmar) plate of the joint capsule

- the anterior or palmar aspect of the joint capsule of the interphalangeal joint is a dense fibrous structure called the palmar plate.

- a hyperextension injury can result in avulsion of the palmar plate with a small fragment of bone. The base of the middle phalanx is the commonest site for this injury (fig 4.65).

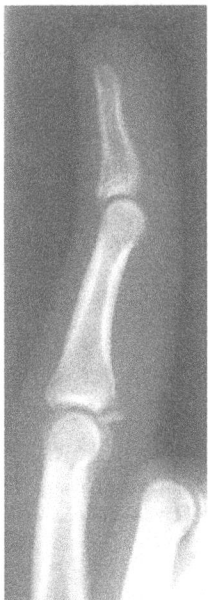

Figure 4.65
Palmar plate avulsion from the base of the middle phalanx.

Collateral ligament rupture

- valgus or varus injuries to the small joints of the fingers can cause avulsion of a medial or lateral collateral ligament.

- the usual site is on the ulnar side of the base of the proximal phalanx of the thumb (fig 4.66). It is due to avulsion of the ulnar collateral ligament. If the avulsion does not include a bony fragment then stress views will be required to demonstrate the ligamentous injury.

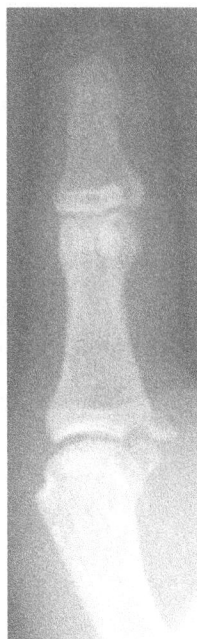

Figure 4.66
Avulsion of the ulnar collateral ligament from the base of the proximal phalanx of the thumb.

Dislocated interphalangeal joints

- most dislocations of the fingers are caused by forced hyperextension. The distal segment is usually displaced backwards (dorsally) from the proximal (fig 4.67).

- the dislocations are frequently associated with avulsion of the volar plate which may cause obstruction to reduction.

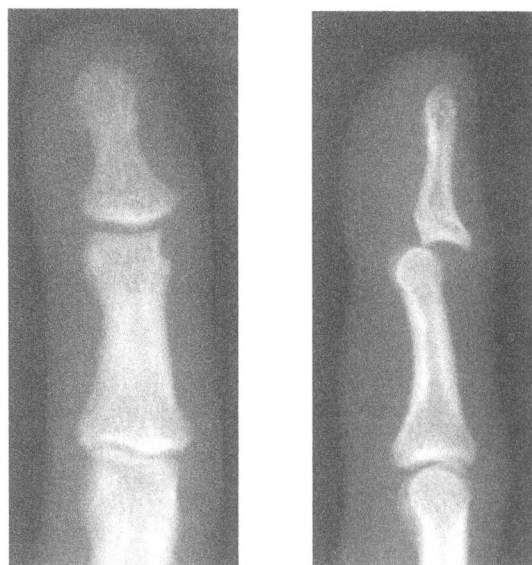

(a)

(b)

Figure 4.67
Dorsal dislocation of the distal interphalangeal joint not visible on the PA view (a) but easily identified on the lateral view (b).

Foreign bodies and complex injuries

- penetrating injuries to the hand frequently deposit foreign bodies in the soft tissues. If these are sufficiently dense (e.g. metallic) they can be identified on radiographs (fig 4.68). It is helpful to put a radiodense marker on the skin prior to obtaining the radiograph to identify the site of entry.

- complex injuries to the hand may result from major trauma from machinery or gunshots (fig 4.69). Radiographs will identify the extent of bony injury and presence or absence of foreign bodies but cannot assess the soft tissue injuries.

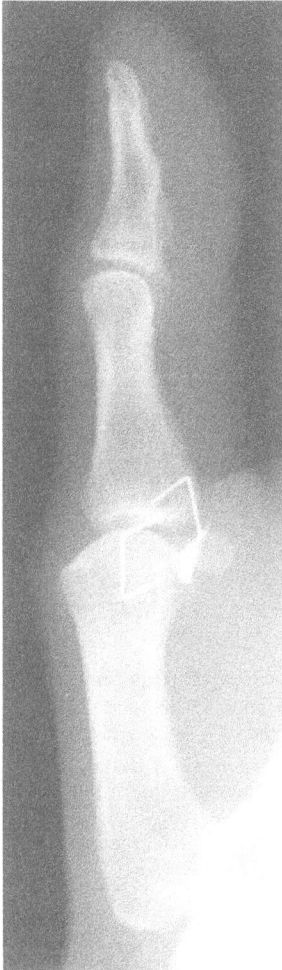

Figure 4.68
Metallic foreign body in the soft tissues. The two staples are on the skin surface identifying the site of the puncture wound.

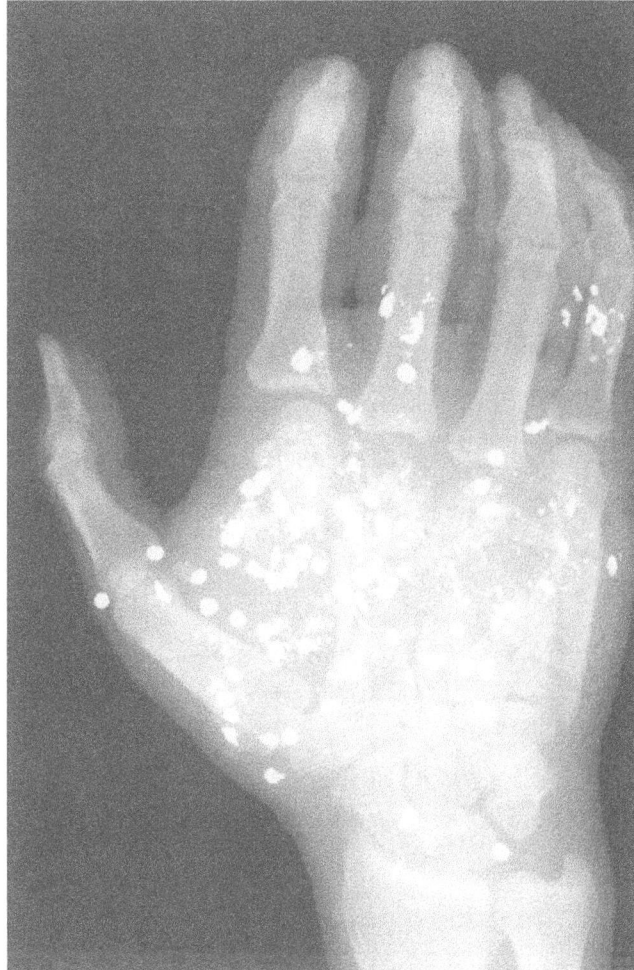

Figure 4.69
Severe injury due to a gunshot wound. Multiple metallic gunshot with underlying fractures of the second to fifth metacarpals. A lateral projection is needed to localize these fragments and further examine the bone injury.

4.5 **Spinal Trauma**

- there is a wide and complex spectrum of injuries to the spine. Radiographs are used to show the extent of bony injury and assess whether a fracture or fractures are "stable" or "unstable". It is important that, in a case of suspected spinal injury, the radiographs are obtained with the minimum amount of patient movement.

- a stable fracture is one that can be expected to retain its position without immobilisation. An unstable fracture is one that, without immobilisation, may deteriorate in position thereby causing progressive neurological compromise.

- the spine is considered to be made up of three functional columns (fig 4.70). If two or more of these columns are involved in trauma then the injury should be considered to be potentially unstable. Remember that trauma to the columns may cause a combination of bony (fractures) and soft tissue injuries (ligamentous/disc disruption), of which the latter is not seen on the radiograph.

- with major trauma it is not unusual to sustain more than one fracture. Therefore, it is prudent not to stop looking at the spine radiographs when the first fracture is identified. CT, if available, is an excellent method of demonstrating the presence and extent of spinal fractures.

COLUMNS

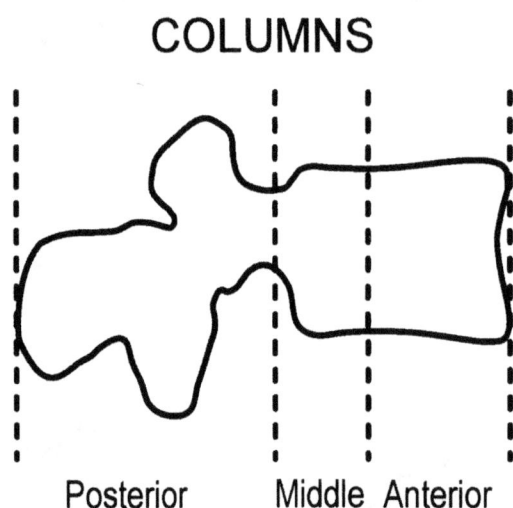

Posterior   Middle Anterior

Figure 4.70
Line diagram showing. The functional columns of the spine. Disruption of two or more columns results in an unstable fracture.

(modified from Lee Rogers *Radiology of Skeletal Trauma* 2nd Ed, Churchill Livingstone 1992)

4.5.1 **Cervical spine**

- the routine series of radiographs for cervical spine trauma are;

  — full length AP
  — lateral (to include T1, fig 4.71)
  — open mouth AP (odontoid view) to show the C1–C2 articulation (fig 4.72)

- it is important to exclude an occult cervical spine fracture with a lateral radiograph in any unconscious patient in whom trauma to the neck is suspected.

- the following features should be assessed when reviewing the films;

  — vertebral alignment
  — spinous processes alignment
  — vertebral body height
  — disc space height
  — prevertebral soft tissues

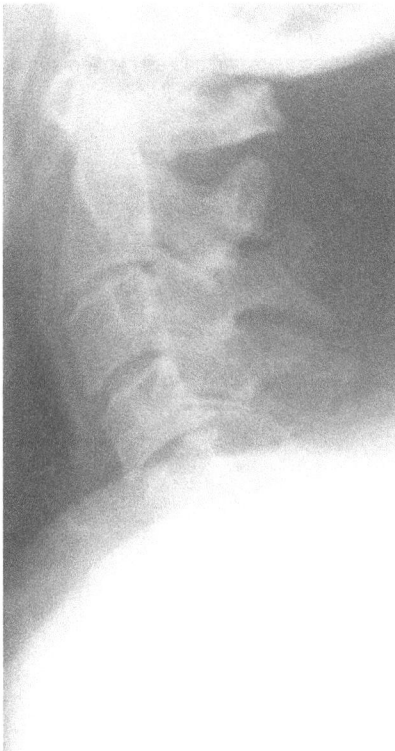 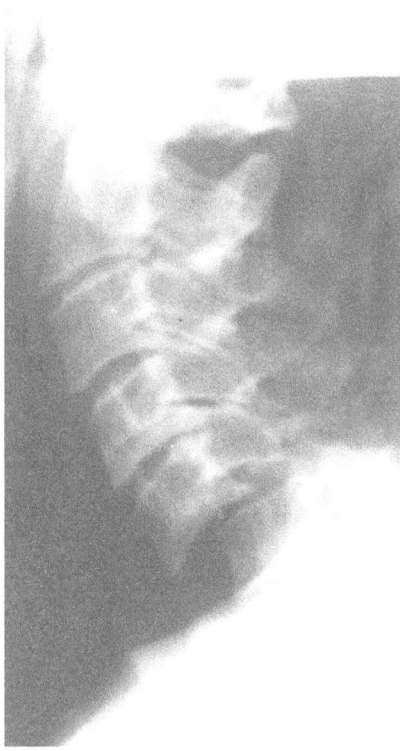

(a)   (b)

Figure 4.71
Lateral radiographs in an elderly patient with a history of trauma. (a) this film is inadequate as it only demonstrates down to C4; (b) the more penetrated film shows a dislocation at C5/6 with bilateral locked facets.

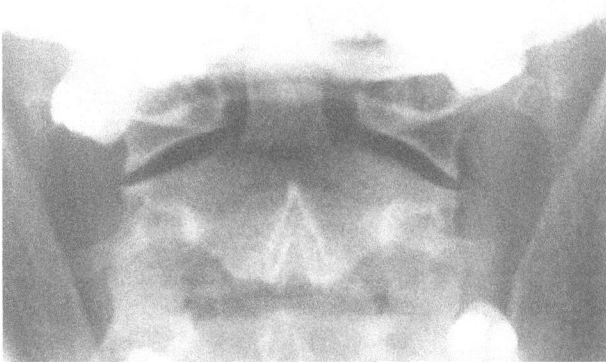

Figure 4.72
Open mouth (odontoid view) showing normal C1–C2 articulation. There is a fracture across the base of the odontoid process. Overlapping of the occiput or teeth can simulate an odontoid process fracture on this view.

Vertebral alignment

- 3 smooth unbroken lines (or arcs) should be present in the normal spine, which are (fig 4.73);

    — along the anterior margins of the vertebral bodies
    — along the posterior margins of the vertebral bodies
    — along the bases of the spinous processes (spinolaminar line)

- disruption of any or all of these lines should suggest significant trauma (fig 4.71).

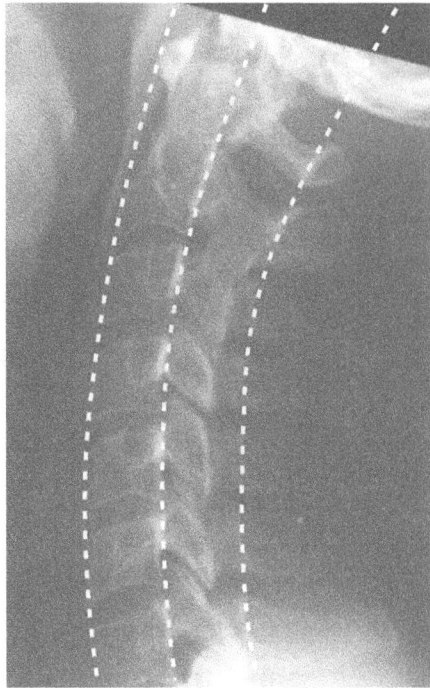

Figure 4.73
Lateral view of cervical spine with the three lines (arcs) that should be reviewed when assessing a lateral radiograph of the cervical spine in trauma.

Alignment of spinous processes

- the spinous processes should lie in a straight line on the AP view and be equidistant on the lateral view.

- splaying of the interspinous space on the lateral view will indicate ligamentous disruption and a degree of subluxation. Loss of alignment on the AP view suggests unilateral problems with abnormal rotation at the injured level e.g. unilateral facet dislocation.

Vertebral body and disc space height

- the vertebral bodies should have a relatively uniform square/rectangular shape and the disc spaces be of uniform height.

- loss of height of a vertebral body indicates a compression fracture.

- widening of a disc space indicates severe injury with disruption of the disc.

- narrowing of the disc space may be due to chronic disc damage, and is common in old age. However, subluxation of the vertebrae must be excluded when there has been an acute injury.

Prevertebral soft tissues

- on the lateral view the normal prevertebral soft tissues should be no more than 30% of the vertebral body width from C1 to C4 and no more than 100% of the vertebral body width at C5 to C7 (fig 4.74a).

- abnormal prevertebral soft tissue swelling is seen in approximately 50% of patients with bony injury. It is important to remember that absence of soft tissue swelling does not exclude a significant injury (4.74b).

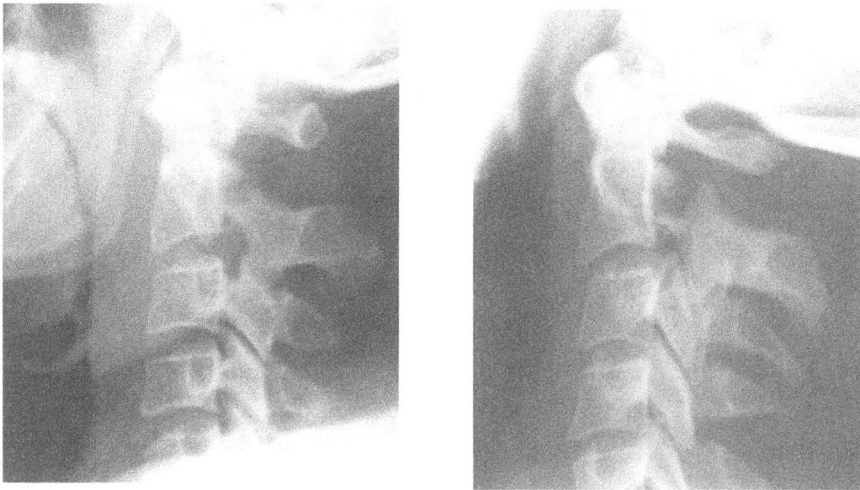

(a) (b)

Figure 4.74
Fractures of the pedicles of C2 (Hangman's fracture). (a) Undisplaced fractures with moderate prevertebral soft tissue swelling; (b) Displaced fracture but absence of prevertebral soft tissue swelling. Note that the lines along the anterior and posterior margins of the vertebral bodies are disrupted at C2/3.

Fractures of C1 (atlas)

- C1 (atlas) may be fractured by a vertical force acting through the skull. This results in a burst fracture splaying the lateral masses of C1 (Jefferson fracture).

- the fractures may only be visible on the open mouth/odontoid view (fig 4.75).

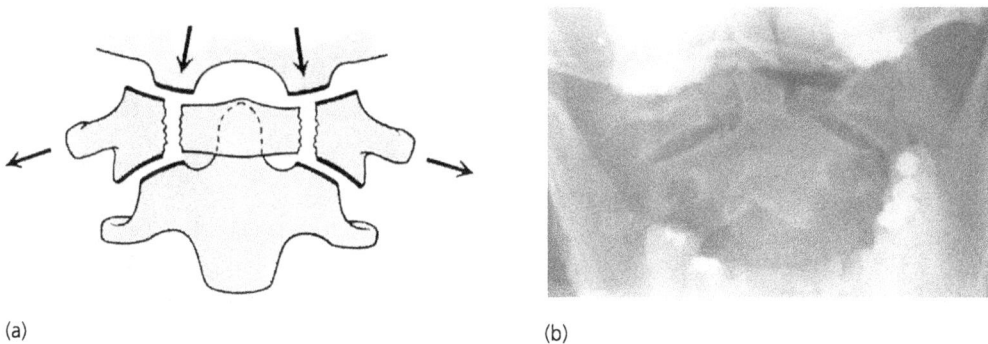

(a) (b)

Figure 4.75
Fractures of C1 (Jefferson fracture). Line diagram (a) an open mouth view (b) showing vertical compression force and lateral displacement of the lateral masses of C1 relative to C2.

(from Adams & Hamblen, *Outline of Fractures* 10th ed, Churchill Livingstone 1992, with permission)

Fractures of C2 (axis)

- fractures of C2 (axis) may involve the odontoid process (55%, figs 4.72 and 4.76) or the pedicles (Hangman's fracture, 25%, fig 4.74).

- subluxation of C1 on C2 (atlantoaxial subluxation) may be seen with a displaced fracture (fig 4.76a) but is more commonly associated with inflammatory conditions such as rheumatoid arthritis (see Chapter 6.2.4).

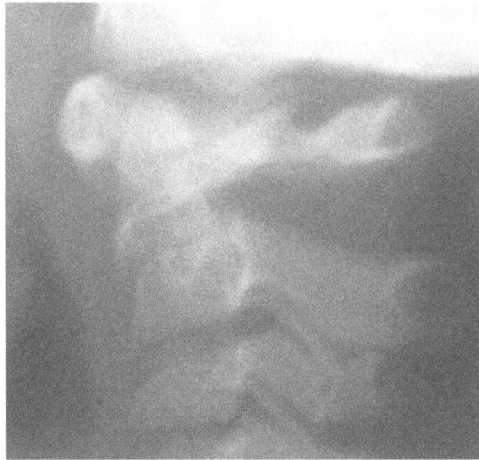
(a)

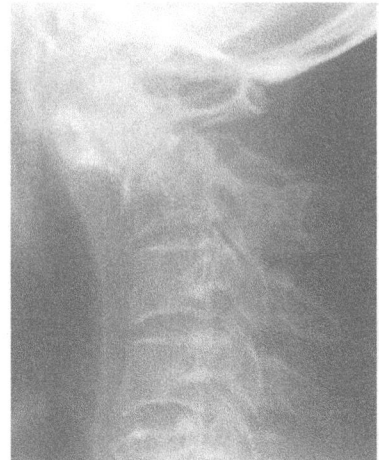
(b)

Figure 4.76
Fractures of the base of the odontoid process in (a) a child and (b) an adult. In the adult the odontoid is angulated with atlantoaxial subluxation.

Unilateral and bilateral locked facets

- when a vertebral body is displaced anteriorly so that 50% or more overrides the vertebral body below this is usually due to bilateral locking (dislocation) of the facet joints (figs 4.71b, 4.77 and 4.78). Lesser degrees are due to unilateral locking of the facets. C5/6 and C6/7 are the commonest levels for unilateral facet dislocation.

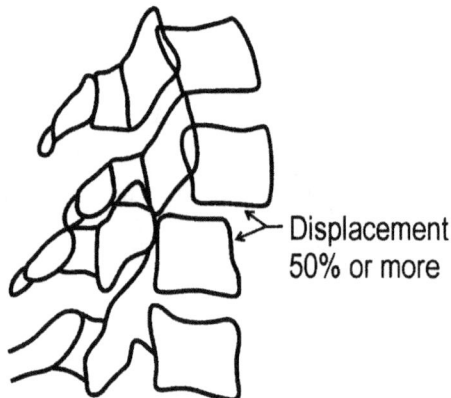

Bilateral Locked Facets

Figure 4.77
Line diagram of a lateral radiograph showing bilateral facet dislocation.

(modified from Lee Rogers *Radiology of Skeletal Trauma* 2nd Ed, Churchill Livingstone 1992)

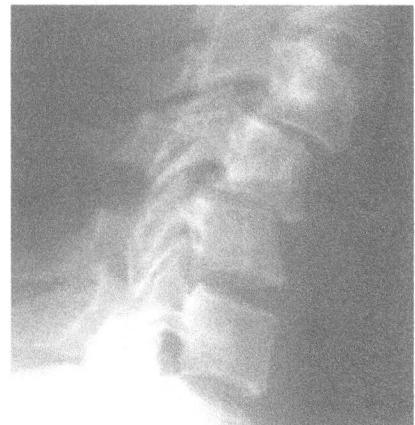

Figure 4.78
Unilateral facet dislocation.

Fracture of the spinous process

- isolated fracture of the spinous process of the lower cervical or upper thoracic spine is usually a rotational injury. It can be painful but is not of much clinical significance, and no specific treatment is needed (fig 4.79).

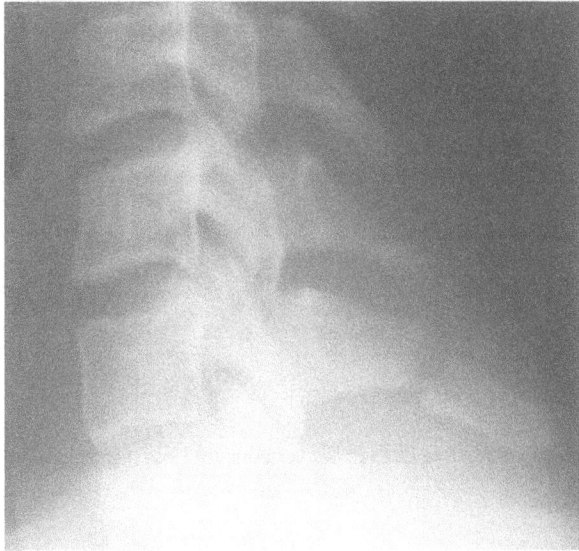

Figure 4.79
Fracture of the spinous process of C7.

4.5.2 **Thoracic spine**

- the thoracic spine is an unusual site for fractures unless the spine is osteoporotic.

- thoracic spine fractures are usually stable because of the support of the thoracic cage. Instability is more likely if there are multiple rib fractures.

- a clue to trauma on the AP film is widening of the interpedicular distance (burst fracture) and a paraspinal soft tissue mass due to a haematoma. On a chest film a haematoma may be mistaken for lymphadenopathy, a paraspinal abscess or an enlarged/ruptured major vessel.

4.5.3 **Lumbar spine**

- 60% of thoracolumbar fractures are at T12 to L2, and 90% from T11 to L4.

- 75% are compression fractures (anterior wedging or depression of the superior vertebral endplate) with intact posterior elements. Care needs to be taken to assess the posterior elements on both the AP and lateral films (fig 4.80).

- 20% are fracture dislocations (involvement of the posterior elements as well as the vertebral body, fig 4.81).

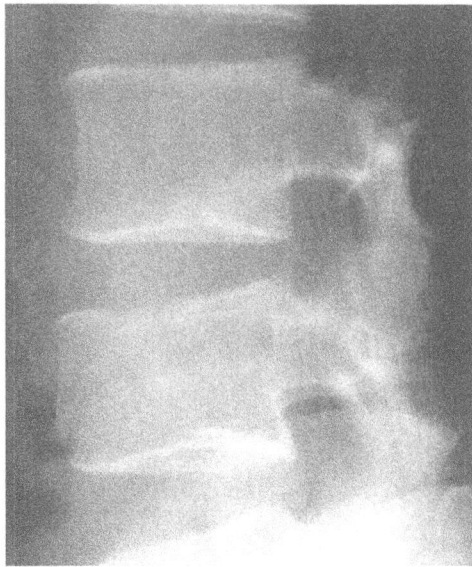

(a)

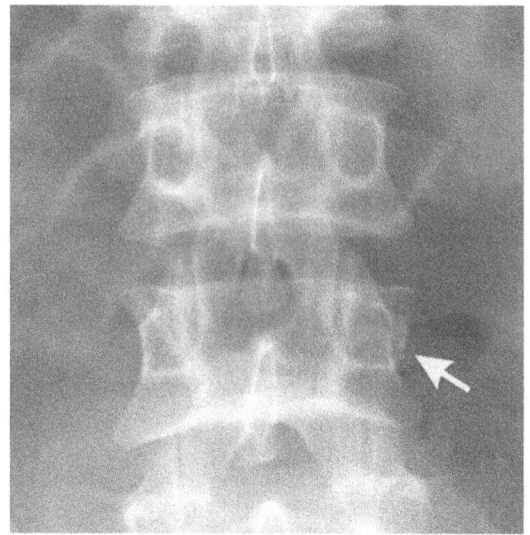

(b)

Figure 4.80
(a) Lateral view which appears to show a simple wedge fracture of a lumbar vertebra; (b) close inspection of the AP shows that there is also a fracture of the left pedicle (arrow).

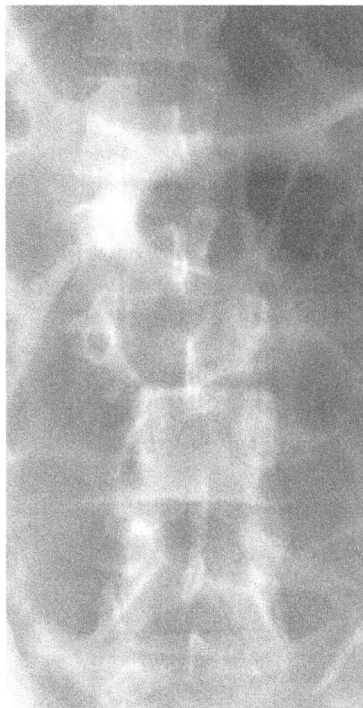

(a)

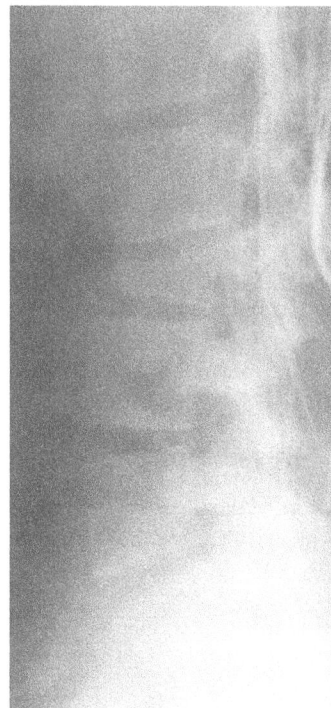

(b)

Figure 4.81
Complex fracture-dislocation of L3, (a) AP and (b) lateral. The posterior elements are obscured on the lateral by bedding as the radiograph was obtained with minimal movement of the patient, who was lying in bed.

Burst fracture

- a burst fracture includes anterior wedging of the vertebral body with a posteriorly displaced fragment (the burst fragment) from the posterosuperior lip of the vertebral body (fig 4.82). This is important because the burst fracture is displaced into the spinal canal and may injure the spinal cord and nerves.

- look very carefully at every simple wedge compression fracture to make sure it is not a burst fracture.

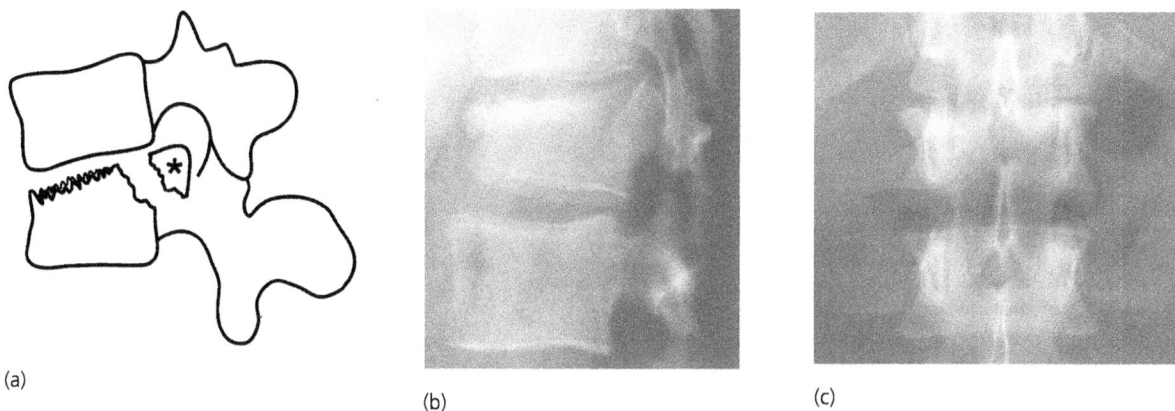

(a)   (b)   (c)

Figure 4.82
Burst fracture. (a) line diagram showing the wedge compression of the superior part of the vertebral body and the posteriorly displaced fragment; (b) lateral and (c) AP view showing a typical burst fracture

(modified from Lee Rogers *Radiology of Skeletal Trauma* 2nd Ed, Churchill Livingstone 1992)

Fracture of the posterior elements

- this fracture is a transverse fracture through the posterior elements (spinous process, pedicles, facets and transverse processes, fig 4.83). The vertebral body or disc may or may not be involved.

- it is a hyperflexion injury often associated with lap-type seatbelts.

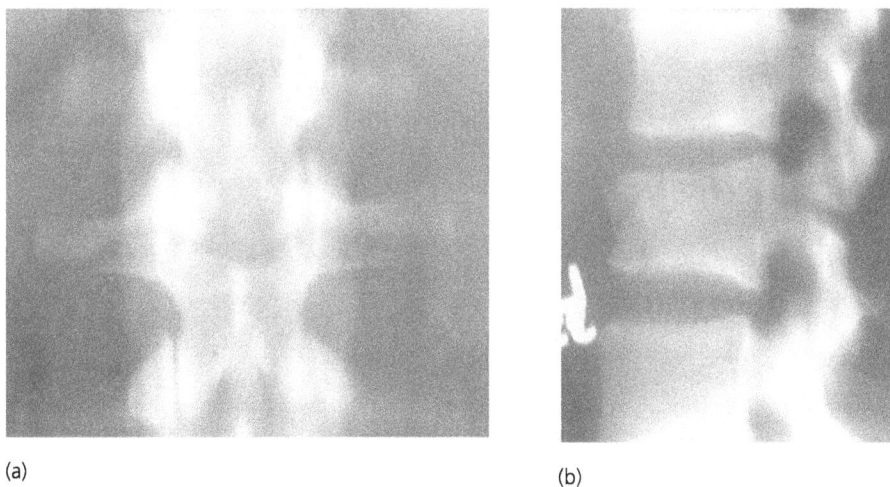

(a)   (b)

Figure 4.83
(a) AP and (b) lateral tomograms showing a transverse fracture through the body and posterior elements of L1.

Transverse process fractures

- fractures of one or more transverse processes are quite common (fig 4.84). They result from avulsion due to the action of the paraspinous muscles or direct trauma. They are often very painful, but easy to recognize. The psoas muscle may show a bulge because of haematoma.

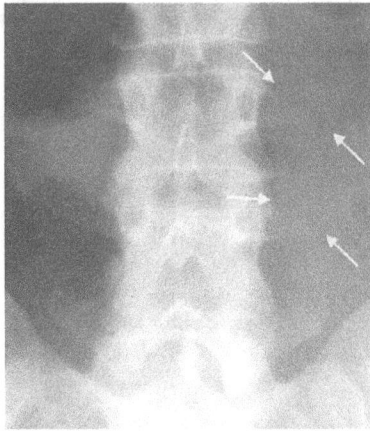

Figure 4.84
AP showing fractures of the left transverse processes of L3 and L4 (arrows).

Spondylolysis

- spondylolysis is the term for a fracture or separation of the pars interarticularis, which is the neck of the posterior elements between the pedicle and the lamina. It is best visualised on oblique views of the lumbar spine.

- spondylolysis most often occurs at L5, usually bilateral. It is considered as a stress fracture rather than due to an acute episode of trauma. The reason may be a congenital defect or weakness of the pars interarticularis (see Chapter 4.8.1).

- may be associated with anterior slipping of the affected body (i.e. L5 slipping forward on S1). This condition is called spondylolisthesis (see Chapter 4.8.1).

4.6 **Pelvic Trauma**

- the pelvis is a ring of bones made up of a strong posterior arch (iliac bones, sacroiliac joints and sacrum) and a weaker anterior arch (ischial and pubic bones). Fractures are commoner in the weaker anterior arch. Because it is like a ring the pelvis often fractures in 2 or more places (similar to the mandible).

4.6.1 **Sacral fractures**

- isolated traumatic fractures of the sacrum are usually transverse due to a direct blow.

- they can be difficult to identify on radiographs. Look for disruption of the superior margins of the anterior sacral foramina on the AP and evidence of deformity on the lateral (fig 4.85a).

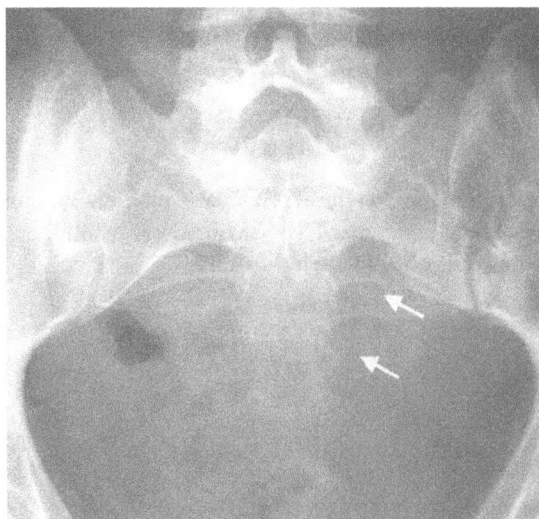

Figure 4.85
Fractures of both the posterior and anterior arches of the pelvis in the same patient. (a) vertical fracture of the left side of sacrum indicated by the disruption of the anterior sacral foramina.

- the sacrum is also a common site for insufficiency type stress fractures in postmenopausal women.

4.6.2 **Pubic fractures**

- pubic fractures are the commonest pelvic fracture. They involve the superior or inferior pubic ramus or both (fig 4.85b). If isolated they are of little clinical significance. It is however prudent to review the posterior arch of the pelvis on the radiographs to ensure there is no further fracture or disruption of one of the sacroiliac joints (fig 4.85a).

- the pubic rami are also a site for insufficiency stress fractures and decalcified zones often seen in osteomalacia.

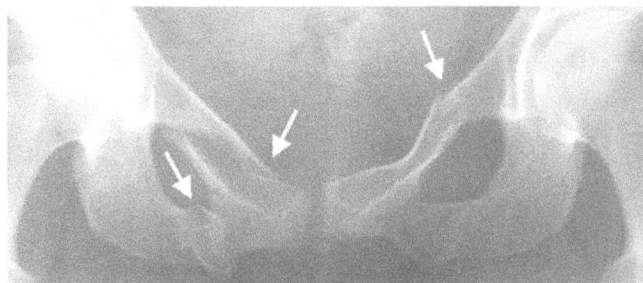

Figure 4.85
(b) right superior and inferior and left superior pubic rami fractures.

4.6.3 **Apophyseal avulsion injuries**

- an apophysis is the ossification centre of a bony outgrowth, such as the tibial tuberosity or the iliac crest

- pelvic apophyseal avulsions can occur in children and adolescents at one of 4 sites (fig 4.86):
    — iliac crest
    — anterior superior iliac spine
    — anterior inferior iliac spine
    — ischial tuberosity

- the amorphous new bone formation that develops at the site of an avulsion may be mistaken for a malignant bone tumour.

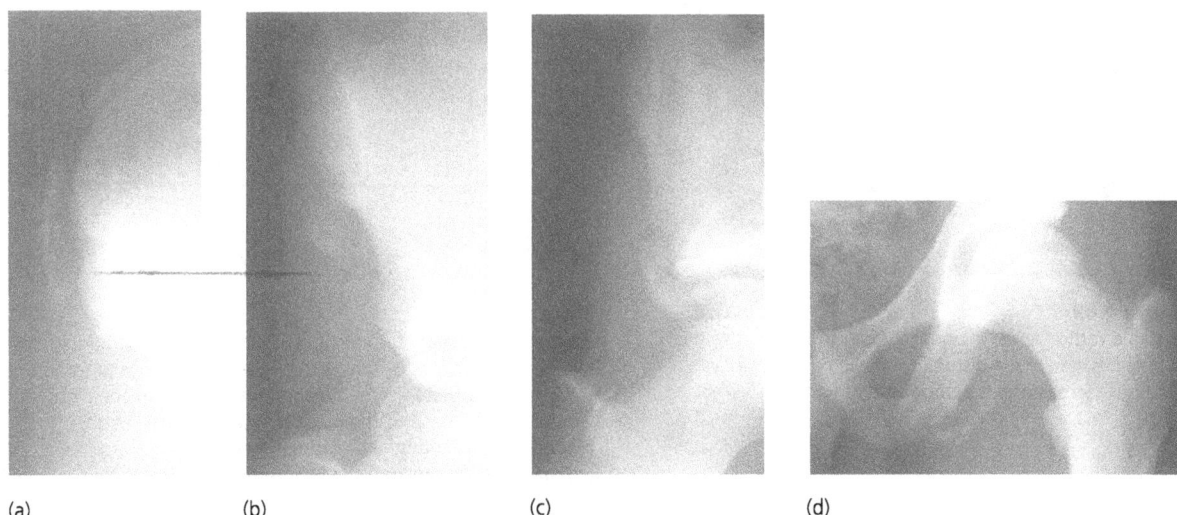

(a)   (b)   (c)   (d)

Figure 4.86
Pelvic apophy-seal avulsion fractures in children (a) iliac crest; (b) anterior superior iliac spine; (c) anterior inferior iliac spine; (d) ischium.

4.6.4 **Unstable pelvic fractures**

* unstable pelvic fractures occur when there is disruption of the pelvic ring in two or more places (fig 4.85).

* the most common fracture pattern is a vertical shear. This is usually a sacral fracture plus superior and inferior pubic rami fractures on the same side (fig 4.87). Numerous variations exist including iliac wing fractures and soft tissue trauma with disruption (widening) of the sacroiliac joints and pubic symphysis (4.88 and 4.89).

* another form of unstable fracture is the "straddle fracture" which results from falling astride an object. This injury causes bilateral superior and inferior pubic rami fractures (fig 4.90).

* unstable fractures are associated with a significant risk of visceral injury and haemorrhage (fig 4.90). Anterior pelvic arch fractures can damage the urethra and bladder.

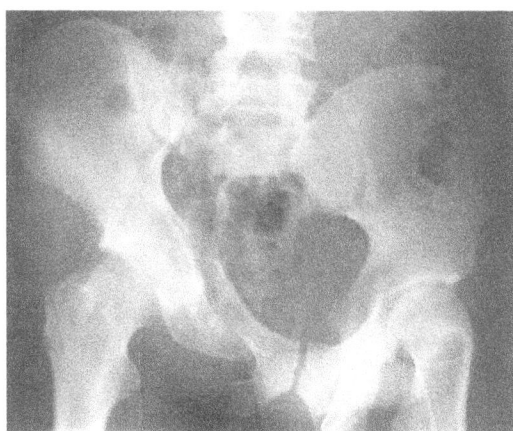

Figure 4.87
Displaced unstable vertical shear fractures of the pelvis. There are fractures of the right superior and inferior pubic rami as well as the sacral ala on the same side.

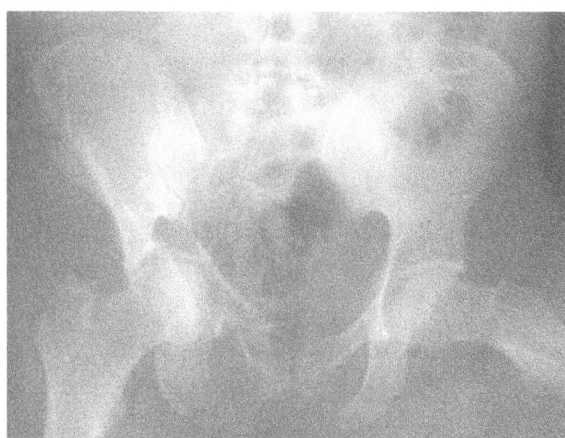

Figure 4.88
Unstable vertical shear fractures of the pelvis. Unlike figure 4.87 the fracture of the posterior arch extends across the iliac blade and does not involve the sacrum.

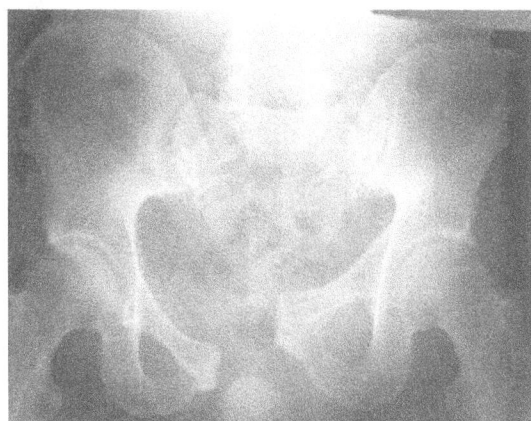

Figure 4.89
Unstable vertical shear injury of the pelvis. In this case the trauma has resulted in disruption of the pubic symphysis and right sacroiliac joint without fractures.

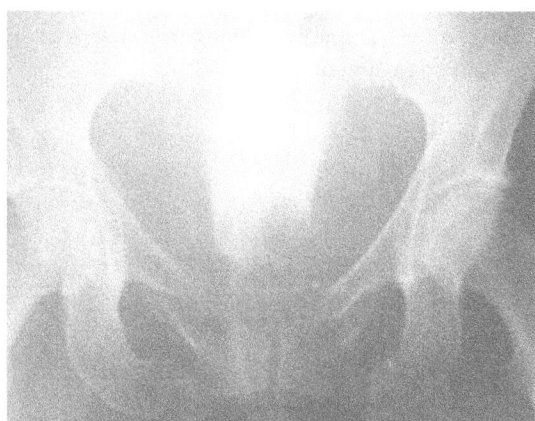

Figure 4.90
Bilateral superior and inferior pubic rami fractures (straddle injury). This film was obtained during an intravenous urogram (IVU) with a catheter in the bladder. The balloon of the catheter is overlying the base of the bladder. The remainder of the bladder is opacified by the contrast medium. The abnormal elongated appearance to the bladder is due to extrinsic compression from intrapelvic haemorrhage.

4.7 **Lower Limb Trauma**

4.7.1 **Hip trauma**

Dislocations and Fracture-dislocations of the Hip

- 3 types

> — posterior dislocation or fracture-dislocation
> — central fracture-dislocation
> — anterior dislocation (very rare)

- it is important to recognize hip dislocation as delayed treatment significantly increases the risk of avascular necrosis.

- posterior dislocation is the commonest form of hip dislocation. It is frequently associated with a fracture of the posterior rim of the acetabulum (fig 4.91).

- in central fracture-dislocation the femoral head is driven through the medial wall of the acetabulum (fig 4.92). Central fracture-dislocation may also occur when there is destruction of the acetabulum from a malignant tumour, most commonly a metastasis or infection, e.g. tuberculosis.

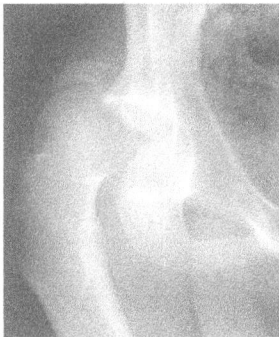

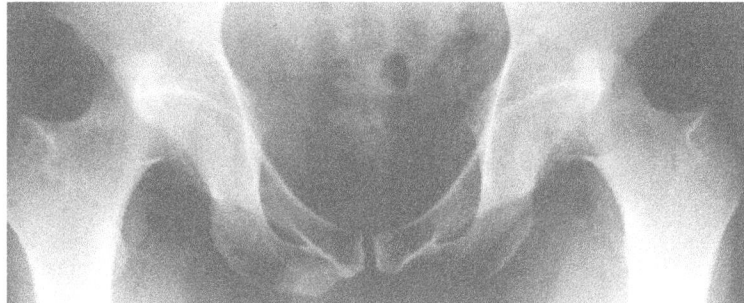

(b)

(a)

Figure 4.91
Posterior dislocation of the hip (a) unilateral with a fracture of the posterior lip of the acetabulum;
(b) bilateral.

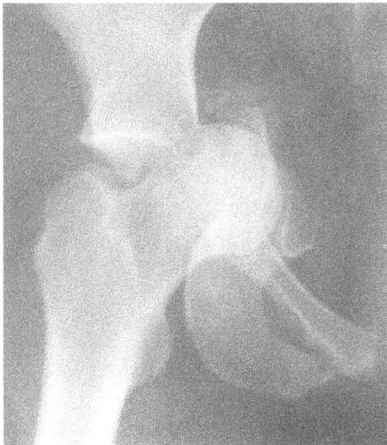

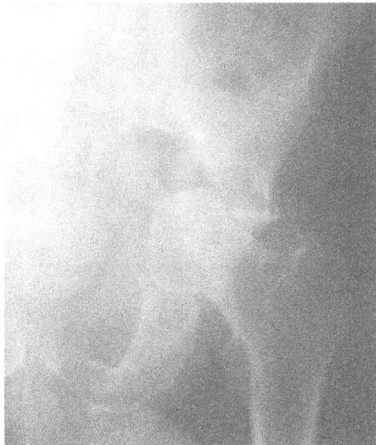

(a)   (b)

Figure 4.92
Central fracture-dislocation of the hip. (a) traumatic; (b) due to underlying metastasis from breast carcinoma.

Hip fractures

- hip (proximal femoral) fractures are rare in young and middle aged patients. They are common in the elderly due to underlying osteoporosis (fig 4.93).

- subcapital (across the neck beneath the head of the femur) fractures are twice as common as intertrochanteric (between the trochanters).

- impacted fractures may be difficult to see on the radiographs.

- femoral neck is also a site for stress fractures and decalcified zones in osteomalacia.

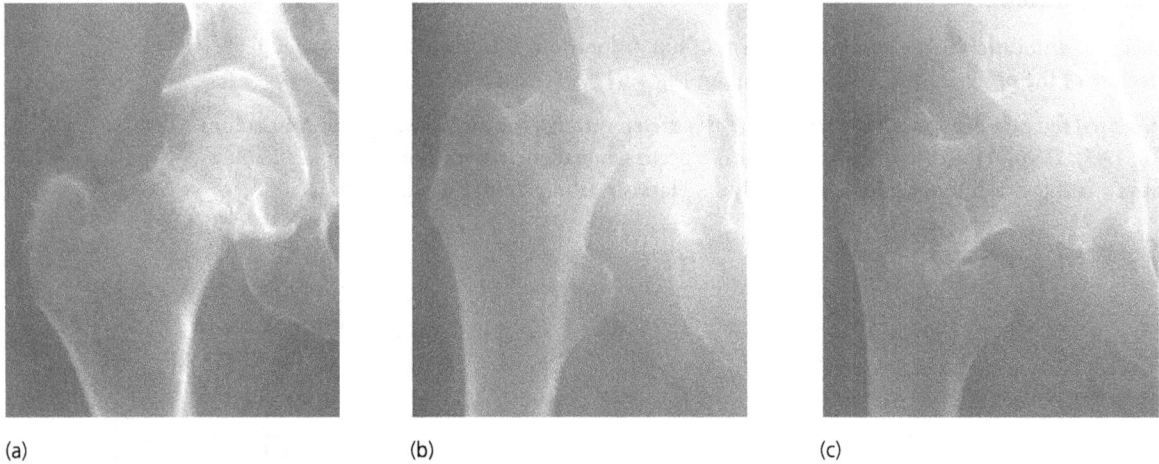

(a) (b) (c)

Figure 4.93
Fractures of the proximal femur. (a) impacted subcapital fracture several days after injury. Sclerosis due to callus (healing bone) is developing at the fracture site; (b) displaced subcapital fracture; (c) intertrochanteric fracture.

Avulsion fractures

- avulsion injuries from the proximal femur may impact the greater and lesser trochanters (fig 4.94). Isolated avulsion of the lesser trochanter in an adult is usually due to an underlying tumour, most commonly a metastasis (fig 4.94b).

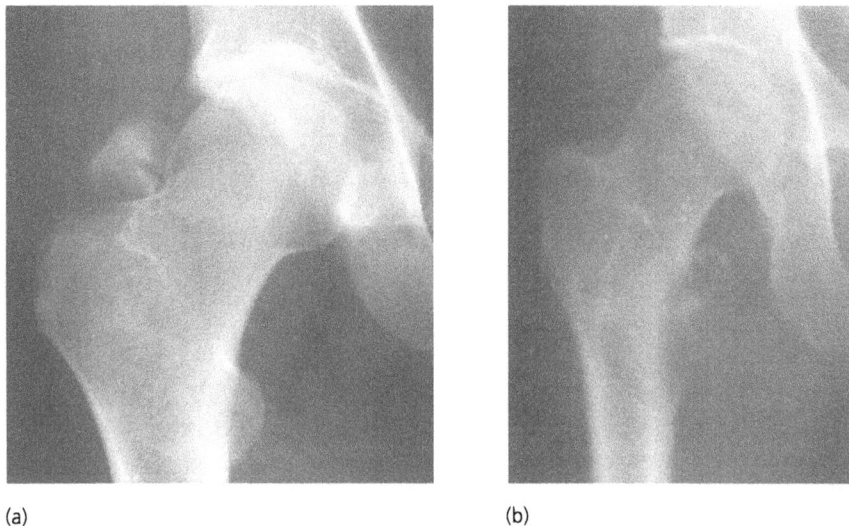

(a) (b)

Figure 4.94
(a) Traumatic avulsion of the greater trochanter; (b) avulsion of the lesser trochanter because of weakening of the bone from an underlying metastasis from breast carcinoma.

Slipped upper femoral epiphysis

- slipped upper femoral epiphysis (also known as slipped capital femoral epiphysis) occurs in adolescence. The femoral head gradually slips posteriorly, medially and inferiorly with respect to the neck (fig 4.95).

- it is generally thought that the slip occurs in adolescence due to shear stresses when the growth plate is relatively weak.

- it affects boys more commonly then girls and is bilateral in approximately 30% of the cases. It is more common in some parts of the world than in others.

- the radiographic appearances on the AP may be subtle and include;
    — decreased height of the femoral epiphysis
    — blurring of the growth plate
    — medial migration results in loss of intersection of the lateral epiphysis when a line is drawn along the outer lateral cortex of the femoral neck

- the slip is readily apparent on the "frog-lateral" projection.

- treatment requires pinning of the growth plate to prevent deterioration of the slip.

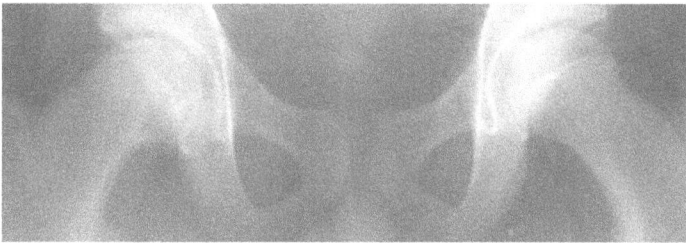

(a)

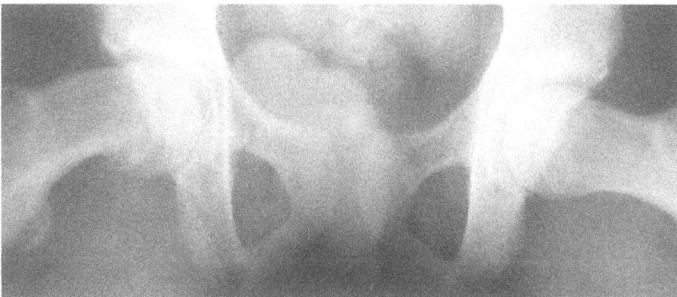

(b)

Figure 4.95
Slipped upper femoral epiphysis (a) AP showing flattening of the right femoral epiphysis and loss of definition of the growth plate; (b) the frog-lateral view confirms the slip.

Neurogenic ossification

- occasionally paraplegic patients or those unconscious for a prolonged period of time may develop para-articular ossification. This condition, known as neurogenic ossification, is most commonly seen affecting the soft tissues around the hip joints and can result in fixed deformities (fig 4.96).

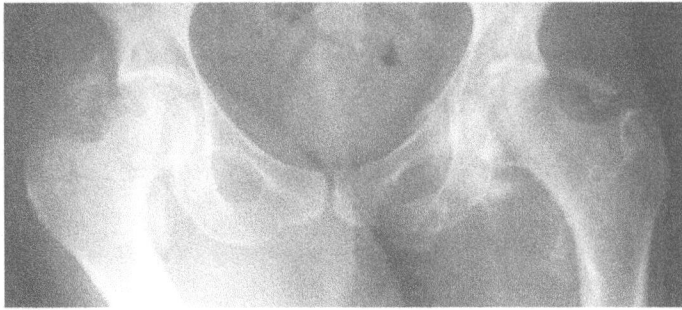

Figure 4.96
Neurogenic ossification developing in the soft tissues around the hip joints. Healing fractures of the left pubic rami. This patient had been unconscious for several weeks following a road traffic accident 3 months before this radiograph was obtained.

4.7.2 **Fractures of the femoral shaft**

- fractures of the femoral shaft occur at any age, usually from severe trauma. They can occur at any site with equal incidence in the upper, mid and lower thirds (fig 4.97).

- the pattern of fracture is variable, including transverse, oblique, spiral and comminuted.

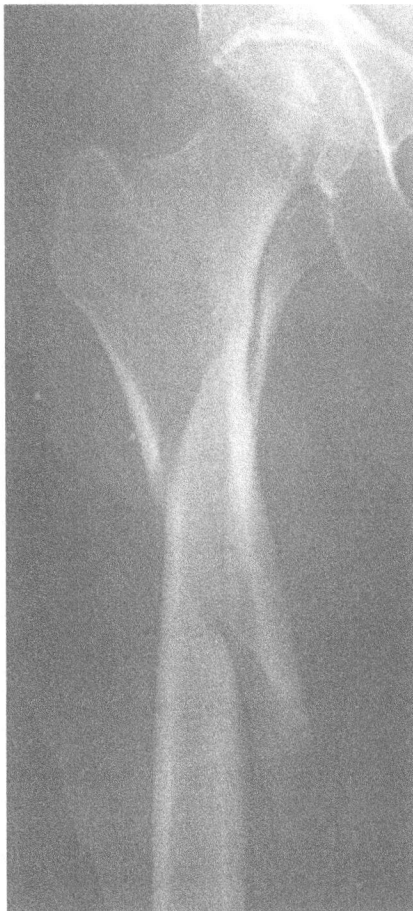

Figure 4.97
Spiral fracture of the proximal third shaft of femur.

4.7.3 **Injuries of the knee**

Fractures and dislocations of the patella

- fractures of the patella may be caused by two types of injury;

    — violent contraction of the quadriceps muscle (single fracture with displacement, fig 4.98). If the tendon ruptures, instead of a fracture, the patella will be displaced inferiorly into the knee joint (fig 4.99).
    — direct blow over patella (comminuted fracture, fig 4.100).

- observe that the patella may have one or two separate ossification centres that do not unite, and then may be mistaken for fragments after trauma. To exclude this, take a radiograph of the uninjured knee, because bipartite patella is often bilateral.

- dislocation of the patella may be acute or recurrent. The direction of the dislocation is usually lateral. In acute dislocation a fragment of the medial facet of the patella may be sheared off as it is driven into the lateral femoral condyle (fig 4.101). Recurrent dislocation is particularly common in young women.

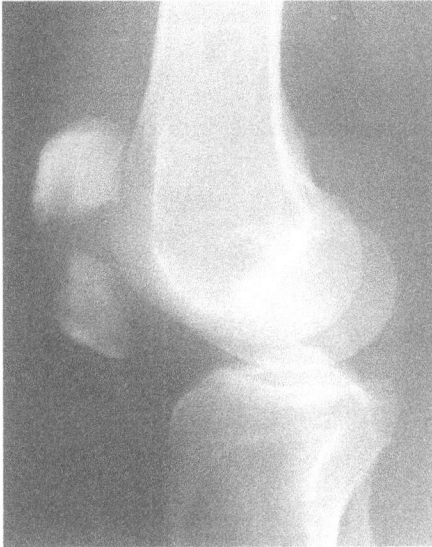

Figure 4.98
Transverse fracture of the patella due to forced contraction of the quadriceps muscle.

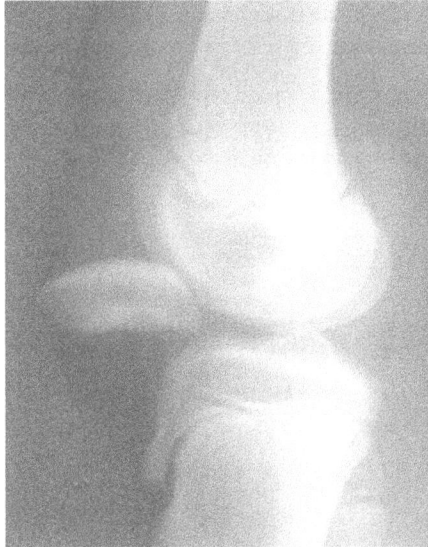

Figure 4.99
Rupture of the quadriceps attachment to the upper pole of the patella. As a result the patella is displaced inferiorly.

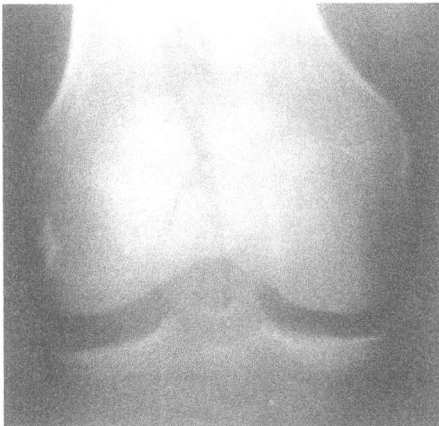

Figure 4.100
Comminuted fracture of the patella (stellate pattern) due to direct blow.

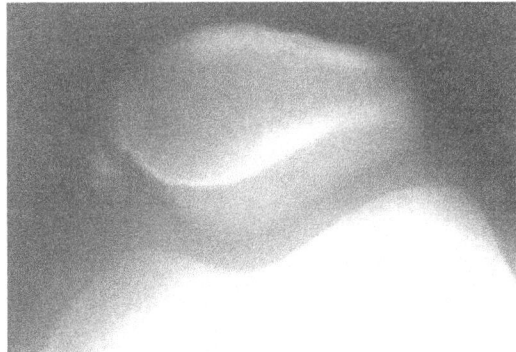

Figure 4.101
Recurrent lateral dislocation resulting in calcification adjacent to the medial pole of the patella on this skyline view.

Soft tissue injuries of the knee

- the knee joint is particularly susceptible to soft tissue injuries which may involve the menisci (cartilages), tendons (quadriceps and patella) and ligaments (cruciate, medial and lateral collateral). Intra-articular injuries, sometimes generally referred to as "internal derangement of the knee", may show little abnormality on radiographs apart from a joint effusion. Full assessment of the intra-articular structures requires either diagnostic arthroscopy or MRI. However, occasionally, subtle signs on the radiographs may give a clue to the nature of the underlying injury. These include;

- the two cruciate ligaments (anterior and posterior) fasten the distal femur to the proximal tibia. Most cruciate ruptures are not visible on radiographs. If the insertions of the ligaments are avulsed with a fragment of bone the diagnosis can be made (fig 4.102).

- avulsion of the lateral capsular ligament produces a characteristic linear fragment avulsed from the lateral margin of the tibial plateau (fig 4.103a). This is usually associated with a rupture of the anterior cruciate ligament (fig 4.103b).

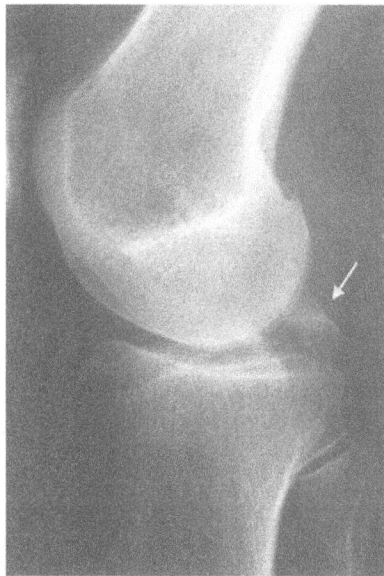

Figure 4.102
Avulsion of the posterior cruciate ligament insertion into the posterior tibia (arrow).

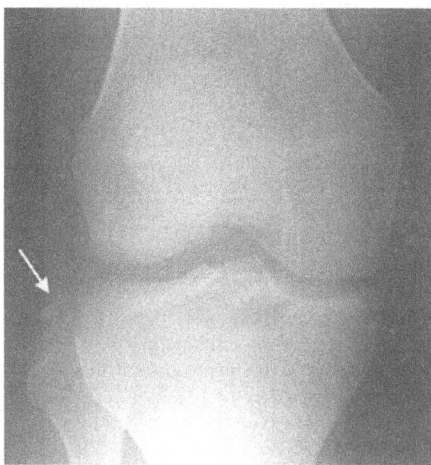

(a)

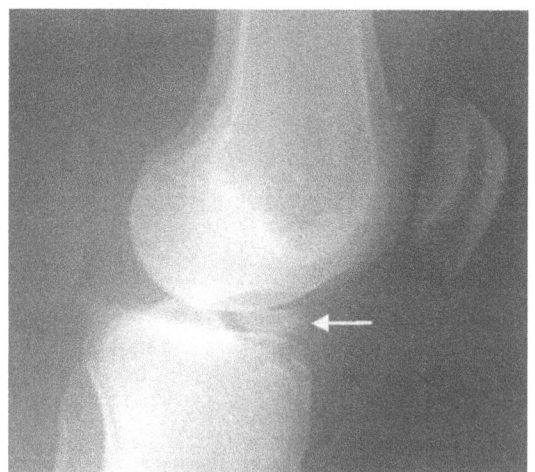

(b)

Figure 4.103
(a) avulsion of lateral capsular ligament from the lateral margin of the tibial plateau (arrow); (b) avulsion insertion of anterior cruciate ligament (arrow).

- chronic ligamentous injuries may result in some irregular ossification at the site of injury (fig 4.104 and 4.105). Stress views may be required to show the extent of instability (fig 4.105).

    — do not mistake the fabella (fig 3.41 and 3.42) for a fragment of bone.

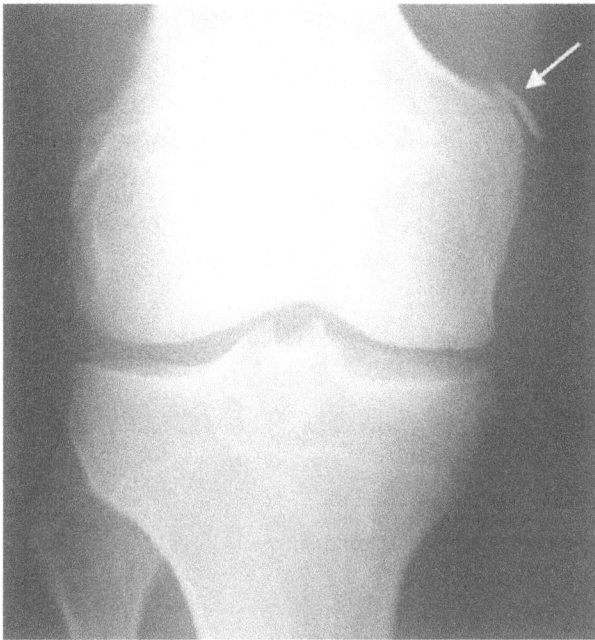

Figure 4.104
Chronic avulsion of the origin of the medial collateral ligament from the medial femoral condyle (arrow).

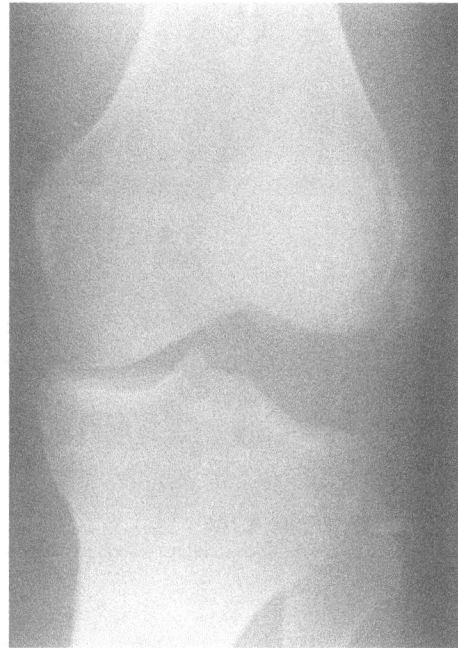

Figure 4.105
Stress view of knee showing widening of the lateral joint space due to chronic rupture of the lateral collateral ligament.

Fractures of the proximal tibia

- fractures of the proximal tibial condyles (tibial plateau) are included under the category of knee injuries as the they extend into the joint and present with pain and swelling of the knee.

- most fractures involve only the lateral condyle (fig 4.106). Less common are fractures of the medial condyle (fig 4.107) and occasionally both condyles are fractured together.

- the fractures are most frequently seen in elderly women. It is a typical injury when a pedestrian is struck from the side by a car or other vehicle.

- injury results in variable depression (inferior migration) of one or more bone fragments.

- if the degree of displacement is minimal and the bones osteoporotic (reduced bone density) the fractures may be subtle on radiographs. A clue to the diagnosis is the identification of fat and blood in the joint. When a fracture extends into a joint, marrow fat can be released into the joint cavity. If a horizontal-beam lateral radiograph is obtained the low density fat will layer out superior to the higher density intra-articular blood (haemarthrosis). This can be seen as a fluid level in the suprapatellar pouch and is called a lipohaemarthrosis (fig 4.107, b, c).

- a lipohaemarthrosis in the knee is most commonly seen with fractures of the proximal tibia but can also be seen with any intra-articular fracture e.g. femoral condyle fractures. It can only be seen if the radiograph is obtained with a horizontal beam.

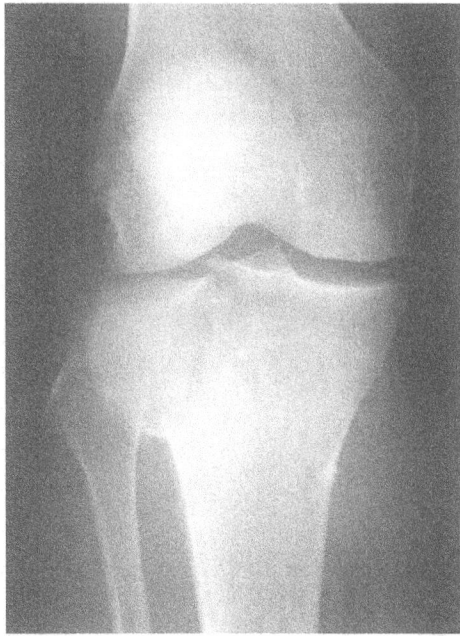
(a)

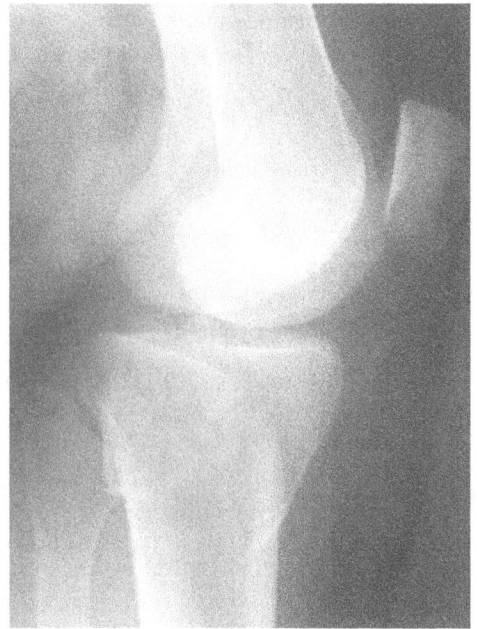
(b)

Figure 4.106
(a) AP and (b) lateral views of a depressed fracture of the lateral tibial condyle.

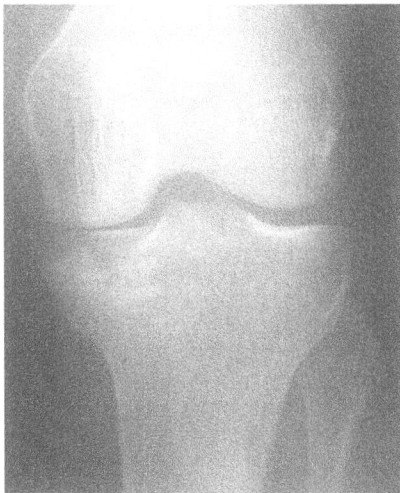
(a)

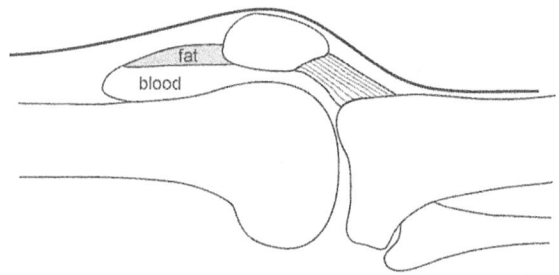
(c)

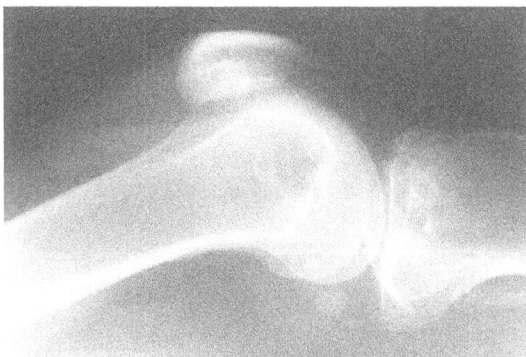
(b)

Figure 4.107
(a) AP and (b) horizontal-beam lateral views of depressed fracture of the medial femoral condyle. Note the lipohaemarthrosis in the suprapatellar pouch on the lateral projection. (c) schematic diagram showing a lipohaemarthrosis (i.e. blood and fat in the distended bursa)

(modified from Lee Rogers *Radiology of Skeletal Trauma* 2nd Ed, Churchill Livingstone 1992)

4.7.4 **Fractures of the shafts of the tibia and fibula**

- most fractures of the shafts of the tibia and fibula affect both bones together (fig 4.108). Isolated fractures are less common.

- there is a spectrum of fractures from the undisplaced (fig 4.109) to the displaced and comminuted (fig 4.110).

- as the tibia is relatively superficial it is the commonest site for an open fracture. Road accidents, especially with motor-cycles are one of the commonest causes of major fractures of the tibia and fibula.

- in children acute injury may result in buckle and greenstick fractures of both the tibia and fibula (fig 4.111). A subtle undisplaced spiral fracture may be seen in toddler's (young children at the age of starting to walk). The child is reluctant to bear weight on the injured leg. This is known as the toddler's fracture.

- the proximal tibial shaft is a common site for fatigue type stress fractures in children and adolescents (see Chapter 4.8).

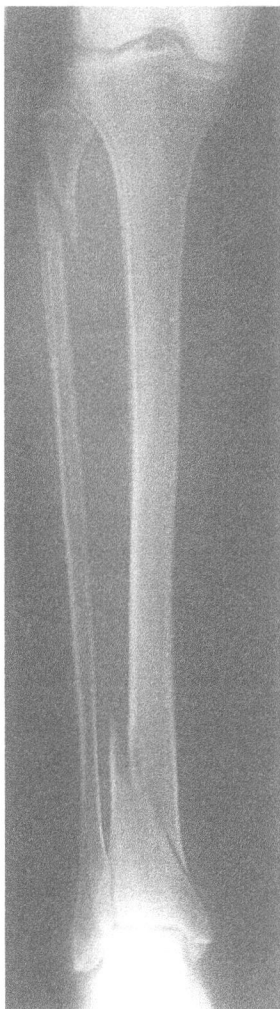 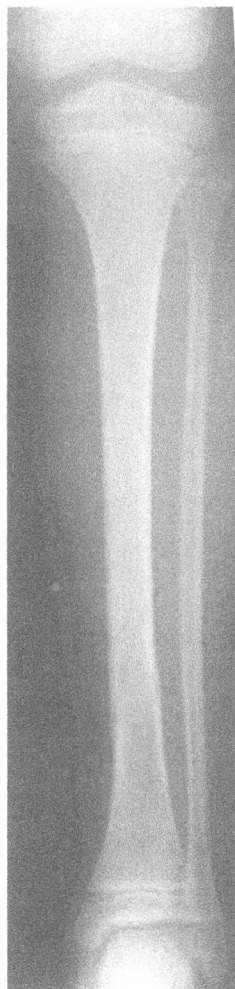 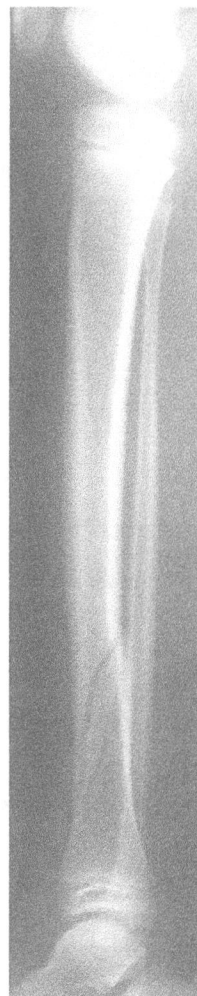

(a)   (b)

Figure 4.108
Spiral fractures of the distal
tibia and proximal fibula.

Figure 4.109
(a) AP and (b) lateral views of a child with an
undisplaced spiral fracture of the tibial shaft.

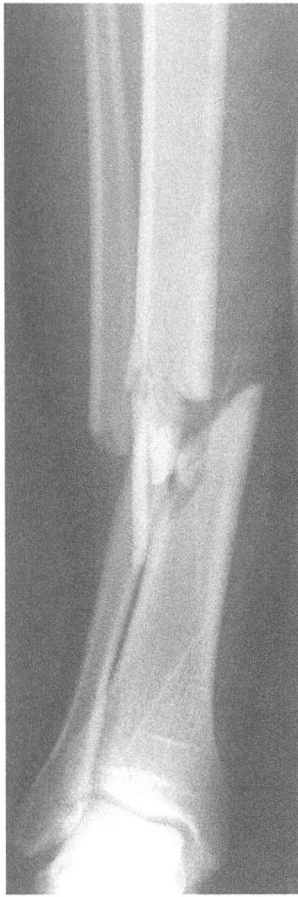
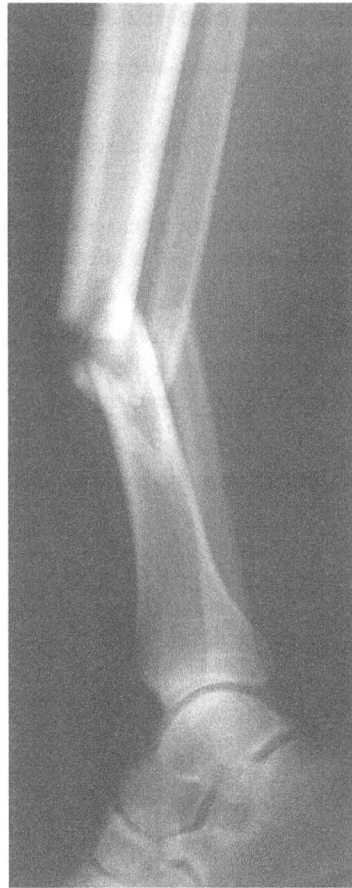

(a)   (b)

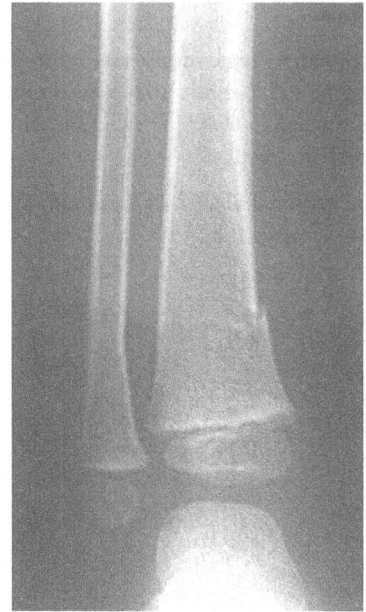

Figure 4.110
(a) AP and (b) lateral views of displaced comminuted fractures of the tibia and fibula.

Figure 4.111
Child with a greenstick fracture of the distal tibia.

4.7.5 **Fractures of the ankle**

- there are numerous different fractures and fracture-dislocations of the ankle. They are usually classified according to the mechanism of injury and the pattern of the fracture. These fractures are loosely grouped together under the general title "Pott's fracture".

- often a fracture of the ankle is visible on only one view. This applies particularly to spiral fractures of the distal fibula and fractures of the posterior lip of the distal tibia, which are normally best seen on the lateral view.

- the following should be assessed when reviewing radiographs for ankle trauma;

  — is there soft tissue swelling which may indicate the site of injury?
  — is there a fracture, and if so, more than one?
  — is there any diastasis of the distal tibiofibular joint?
  — is there any displacement of the talus with respect to the tibia and fibula?

- diastasis of the distal tibiofibular joint and displacement of the talus indicates the presence of subluxation/dislocation in addition to fractures.

- figures 4.111 to 4.115 show some of the most common ankle fractures.

- in children and adolescents fracture separations of the distal tibial growth plate are common (fig 4.116).

- significant ligamentous injuries may occur in the absence of fractures. Stress views (usually AP) may be required to demonstrate the extent of ligamentous laxity (fig 4.117).

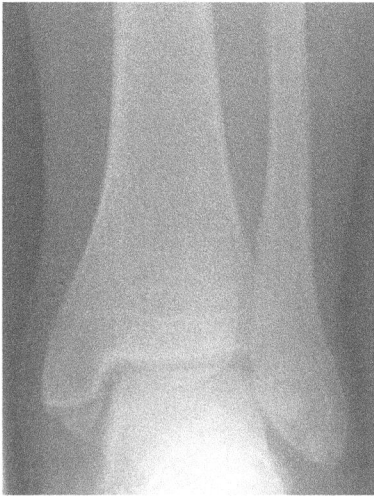

Figure 4.112
Isolated avulsion of the medial malleolus.

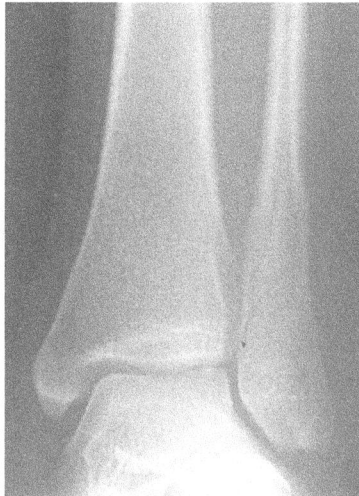

(a)

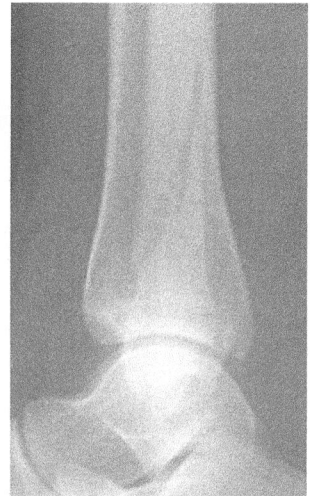

(b)

Figure 4.113
(a) AP and (b) lateral views of an undisplaced spiral fracture of the distal fibula. These fractures may be invisible on the AP.

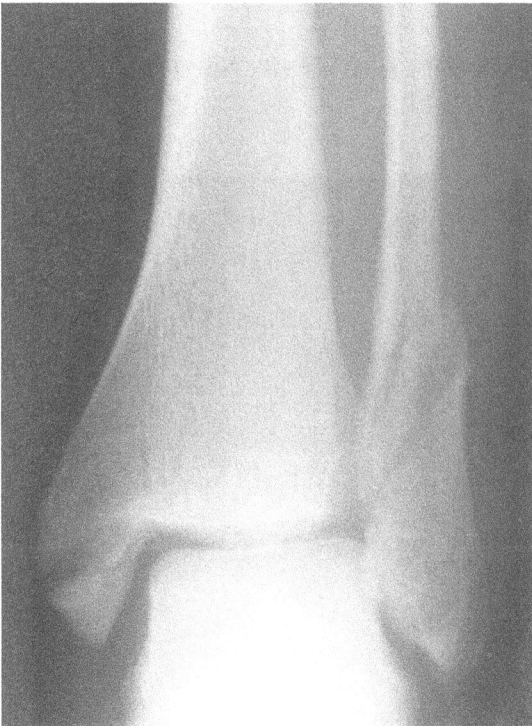

(a)

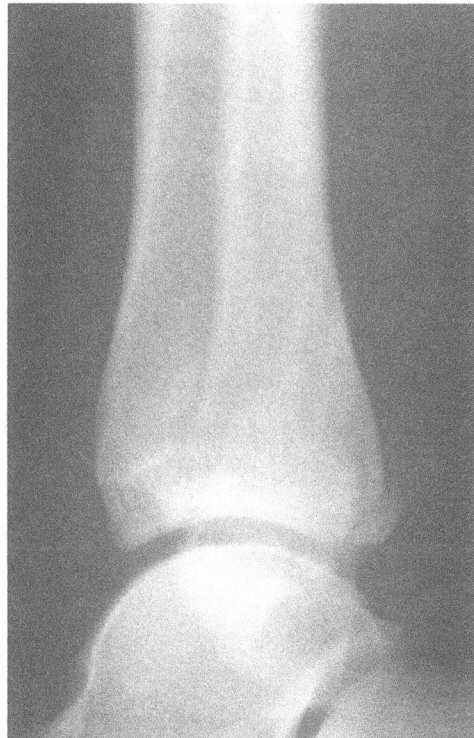

(b)

Figure 4.114
(a) AP and (b) lateral views of fractures of the medial malleolus, distal fibula and posterior lip of the tibia.

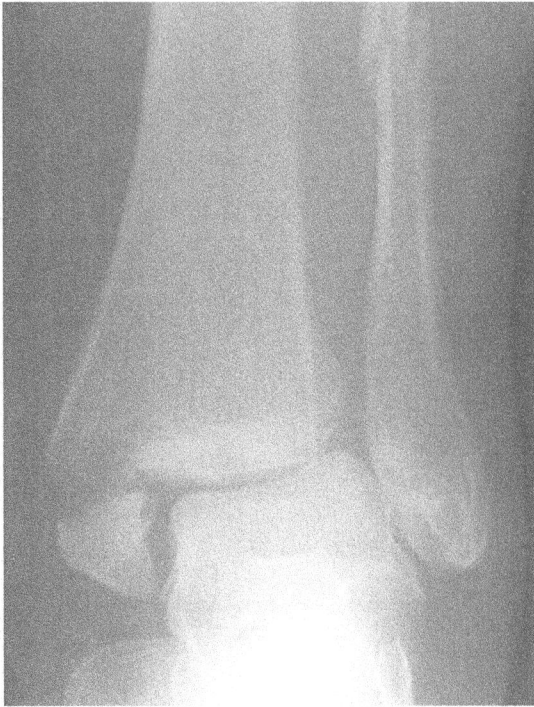
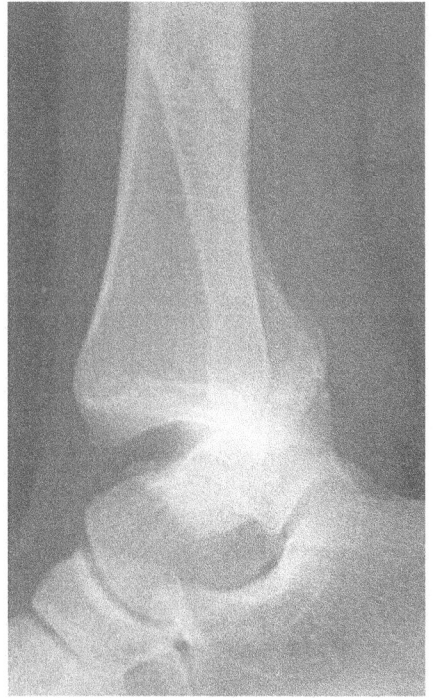

(a)   (b)

Figure 4.115
(a) and (b) lateral views of a fracture-dislocation with fractures of the medial malleouls, shaft of fibula and anteromedial displacement of the tibia on the talus.

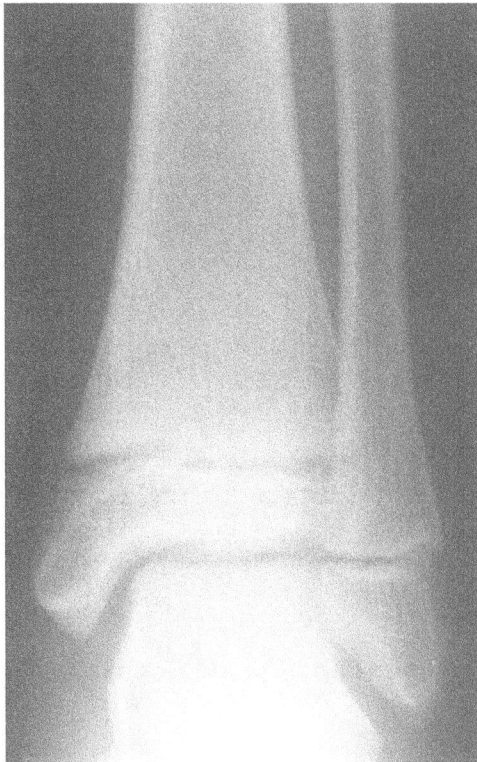
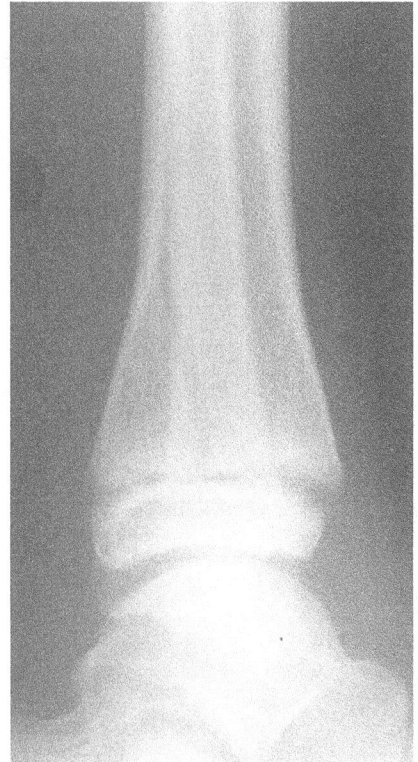

(a)   (b)

Figure 4.116
Fracture separation of the distal tibial growth plate. The AP view (a) is normal. On the lateral (b) there is an oblique fracture across the posterior aspect of the tibia with minor separation of the growth plate anteriorly.

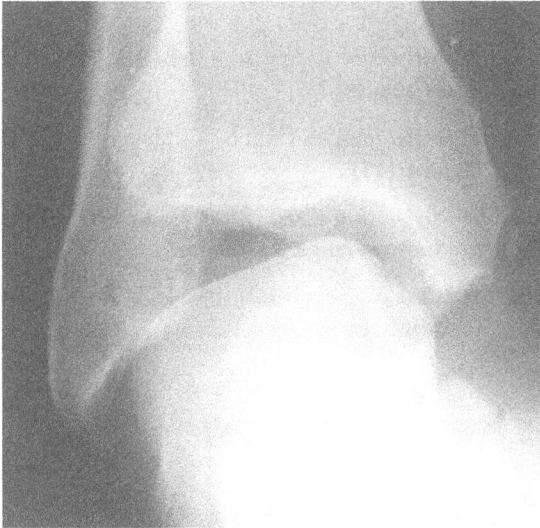

Figure 4.117
Stress view showing widening of the lateral ankle joint indicating rupture of the lateral ligaments.

4.7.6 **Fractures of the foot**

Talus

- fractures of the talus are less common than of the calcaneus.

- falls from a height may result in vertical fractures through the body or neck (anterior) of the talus, and are best seen on the lateral view (fig 4.118).

- avascular necrosis of the proximal fragment is a well recognized complication of a fracture through the neck of the talus.

- osteochondral fractures of the dome (articular surface) are also possible. If the fragment is inverted or displaced union will not occur (fig 4.119).

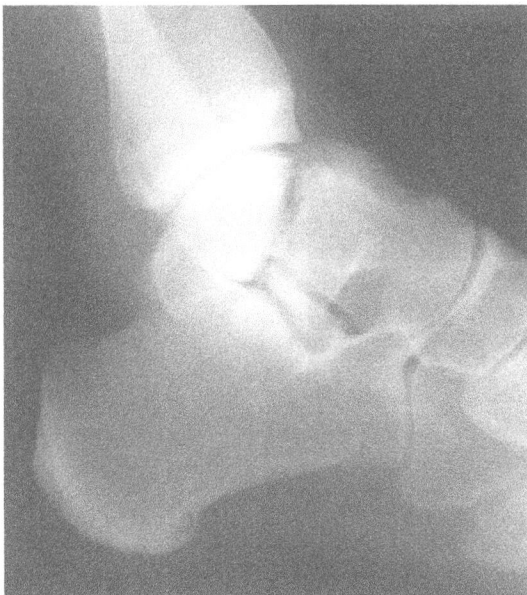

Figure 4.118
Vertical fracture through the body of the talus.

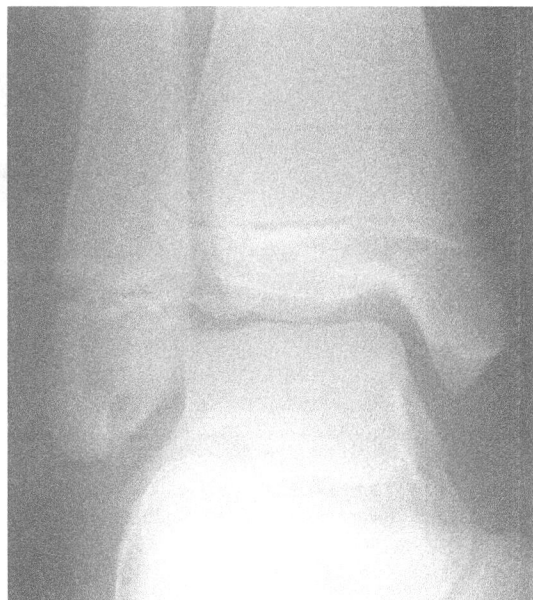

Figure 4.119
Avulsion fracture of the tip of the lateral malleolus and osteochondral fracture of the lateral dome of the talus. The fragment has become inverted so that union will not occur.

Calcaneus

- the majority of fractures of the calcaneus result from a fall or a jump from a height. Some are bilateral and some are associated with thoracolumbar fractures.

- most calcaneal fractures extend into the posterior subtalar joint and will be visible on the lateral view with varying degrees of depression (fig 4.120 and 4.121).

- subtle depressed fractures may only be identified by noting a reduction in Boehler's angle (fig 4.120), which should not be less than 25 degree (normal range: 25–40 degree).

- extra-articular fractures of the calcaneus include fractures of the tuberosity, avulsion fractures of the insertion of the achilles tendon (fig 4.122) and stress fractures (fig 4.123).

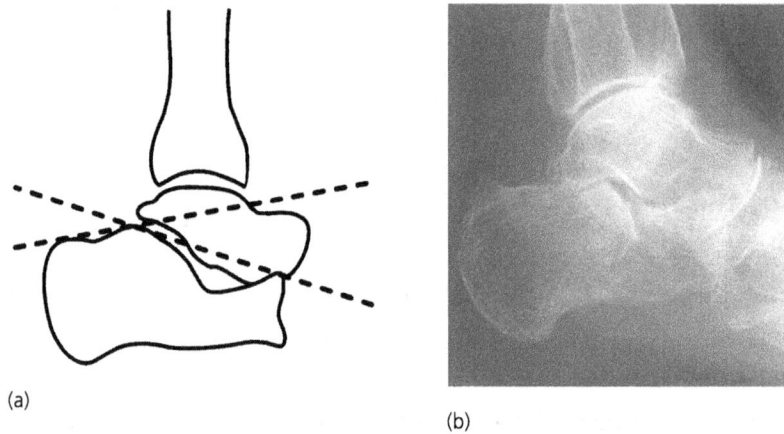

(a)

(b)

Figure 4.120
(a) schematic diagram showing Boehler's angle; (b) lateral view showing flattening of Boehler's angle indicating a depressed fracture of the calcaneus. (modified from Lee Rogers *Radiology of Skeletal Trauma* 2nd Ed, Churchill Livingstone 1992)

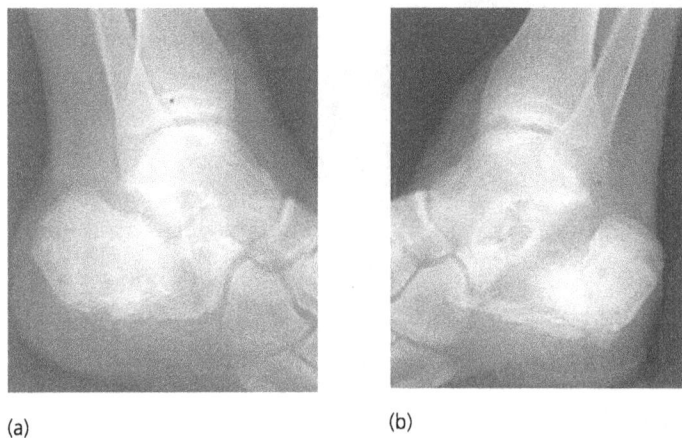

(a)

(b)

Figure 4.121
Bilateral, severely comminuted depressed fractures of the calcanei (a), (b).

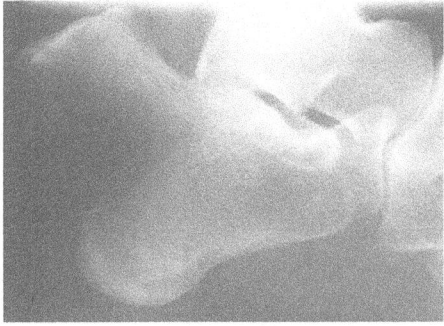

Figure 4.122
Avulsion of the posterosuperior aspect of
calcaneus pulled off by the achilles tendon.

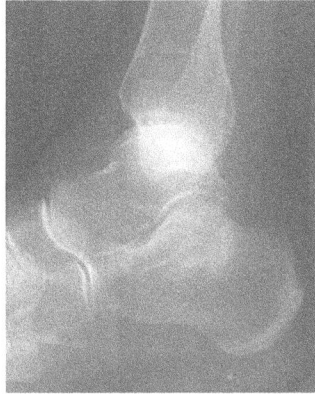

Figure 4.123
Fatigue type stress fracture of the
calcaneus indicated by the vertically
oriented band of sclerosis
superiorly.

Navicular

- fractures of the navicular bone are rare. The most commonly seen is a flake fracture from the dorsal surface followed in frequency by a fracture of the medial tuberosity.

- more severe trauma can result in vertical or horizontal fractures of the body of the navicular (fig 4.124) or talonavicular joint dislocation (fig 4.125).

- the navicular is also a typical site for a fatigue type stress fracture in runners. It can be extremely difficult to identify on radiographic examination. The healing fracture will produce a line of trabecular sclerosis.

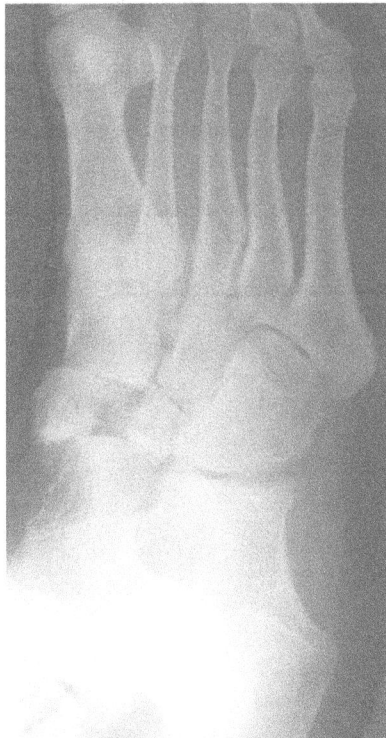

Figure 4.124
Displaced vertical fracture of the navicular.

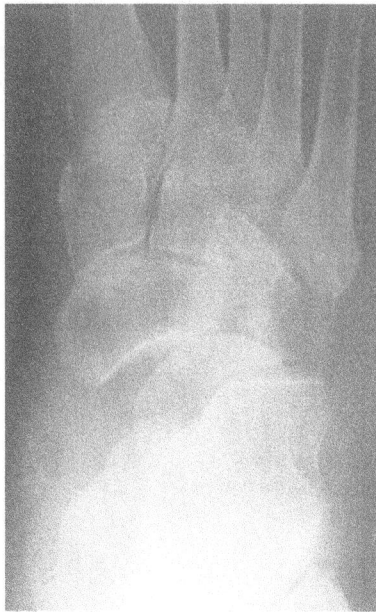
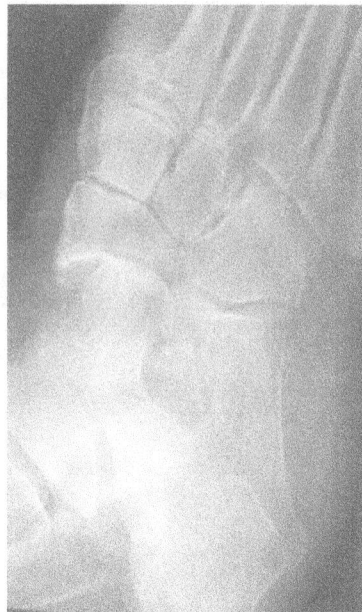

(a)   (b)

Figure 4.125
(a) PA and (b) oblique views of a talonavicular joint dislocation.

Tarsometatarsal

- severe trauma to the midfoot can result in tarsal fractures and dislocations.

- tarsometatarsal dislocations are easily overlooked on radiographs. It is important to be aware of the normal alignment at these joints. Some basic rules are;

  — on the *AP view* the medial margin of the base of the second metatarsal should be in line with the medial margin of the middle cuneiform.
  — on the *oblique view* the medial margin of the third metatarsal should be in line with the medial margin of the lateral cuneiform.
  — if a fracture of the base of one of the medial four metatarsals is seen, suspect also a fracture-dislocation (fig 4.126).

- the tarsometatarsal dislocation with lateral dislocation of the 2nd to 5th metatarsals is usually associated with several avulsion/chip fractures (fig 4.126).

- a chronic dislocation is a common manifestation of a diabetic neuropathy (fig 4.127).

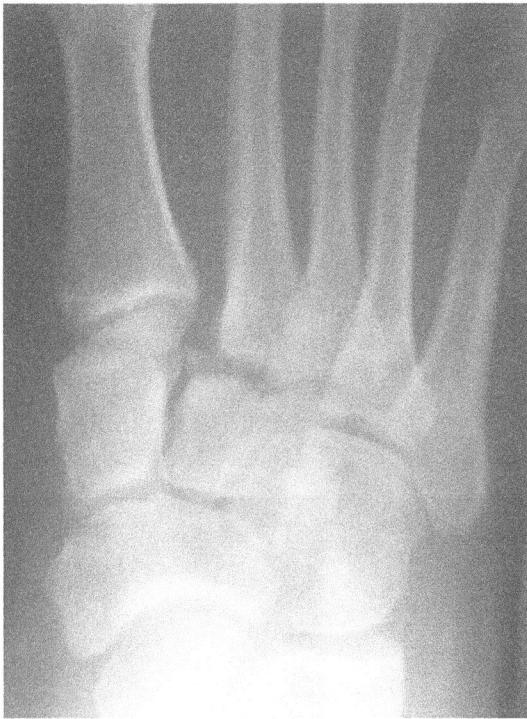

Figure 4.126
Tarsometatarsal fracture-dislocation. There is widening between the bases of the first and second metatarsals and a fracture with lateral displacement of the base of the second metatarsal on the intermediate cuneiform.

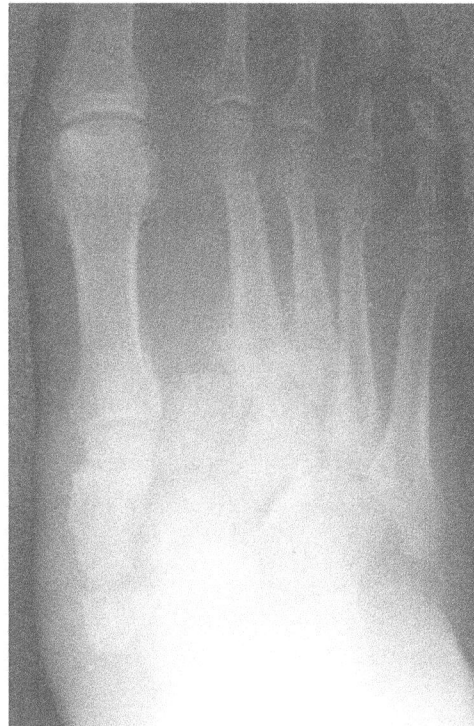

Figure 4.127
Chronic tarsometatarsal fracture-dislocation secondary to a diabetic neuropathy.

Forefoot

- most metatarsal and phalangeal fractures are caused by direct trauma from an object falling on the forefoot. A twisting injury is a less common cause of metatarsal injury with the exception of the base of the 5th metatarsal. This common fracture is the result of avulsion by the tendon of the peroneus brevis muscle (fig 4.128). In the child the normal longitudinally oriented epiphysis at the base of the 5th metatarsal should not be mistaken for a fracture. The fracture is typically transverse.

- figures 4.129 and 4.130 show the spectrum of metatarsal fractures.

- the neck of 2nd and less commonly the 3rd metatarsal is a common site for a fatigue type stress fracture ("march" fracture).

- chronic stress, particularly in young women, is thought to be the cause of sclerosis and fragmentation of the second metatarsal head followed by irregular healing and premature degenerative change (fig 4.131).

- examples of trauma to the toes are shown in figure 4.132.

- the forefoot is a common site for penetrating injury and the introduction of foreign bodies (fig 4.133).

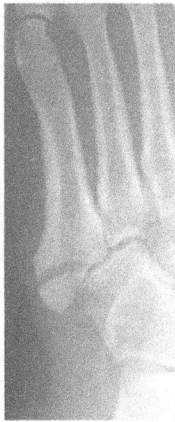

Figure 4.128
Fracture of the base of fifth metatarsal.

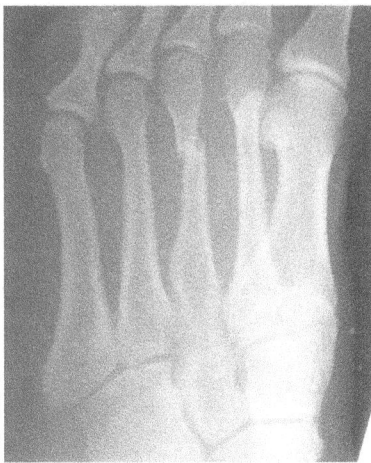

(a)

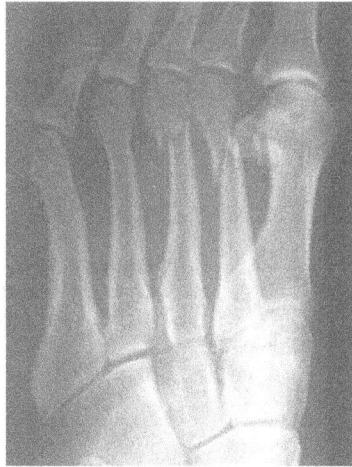

(b)

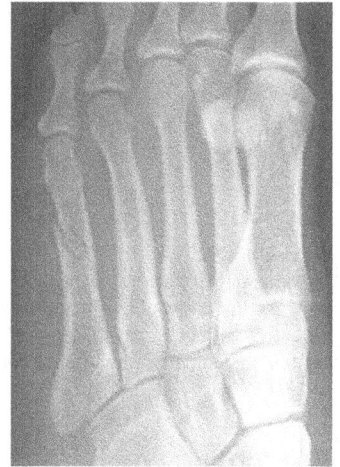

(c)

Figure 4.129
(a) transverse fracture of the third metatarsal; (b) oblique fractures of the second and third metatarsals; (c) incomplete spiral fracture of the fifth metatarsal.

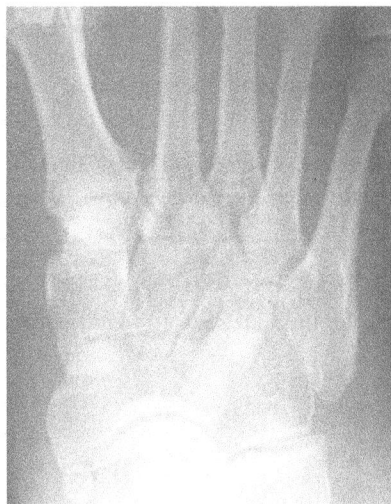

(a)

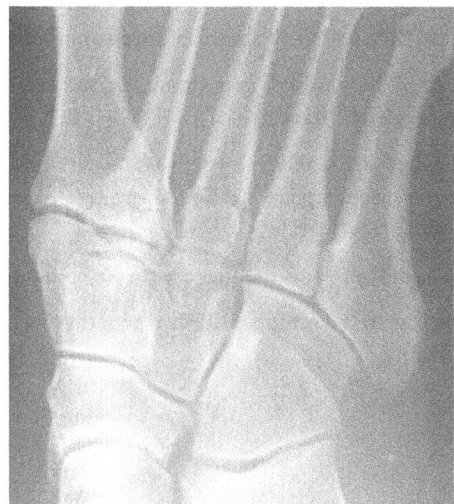

(b)

Figure 4.130
(a) PA and (b) oblique views of undisplaced fractures of the bases of the second and third metatarsals.

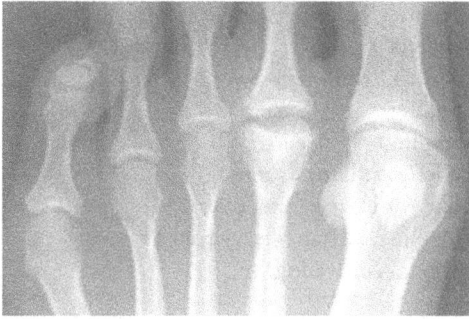

Figure 4.131
Osteochondritis Dissecans. Fragmentation of the head of the second metatarsal.

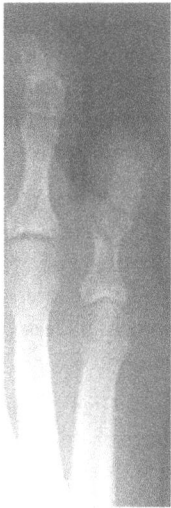

(a)

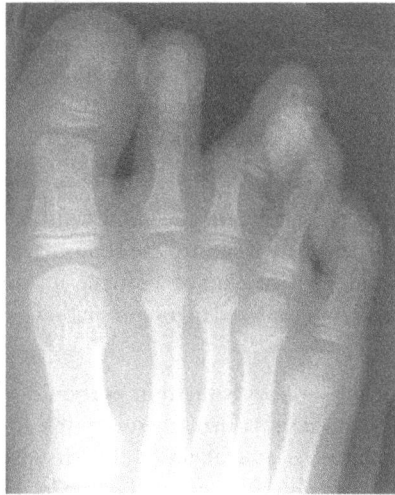

(b)

Figure 4.132
(a) oblique fracture of the proximal phalanx; (b) dislocated fracture proximal to the interphalangeal joint.

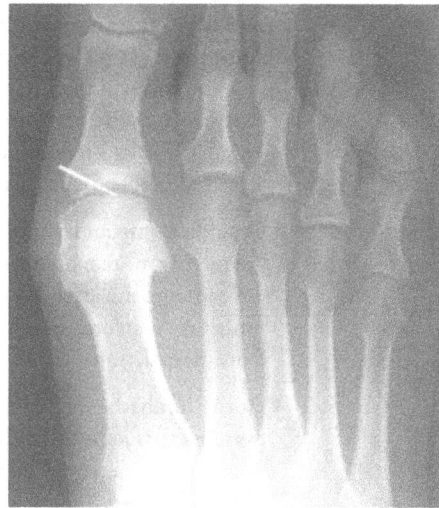

Figure 4.133
Foreign body. Fragment of a needle embedded in the foot A second (lateral) radiograph is needed to localize the needle.

4.8 **Stress Fractures**

- bones may eventually fracture if subject to repeated injury even if each traumatic episode is insufficient in itself to cause a fracture. The cumulative effect of repeated trauma is weakening of the microscopic structure of bone thereby causing a *stress fracture*.

- there are two types of stress fractures known as *fatigue fractures* and *insufficiency fractures.*

- patients with a stress fracture will frequently have normal radiographs at the time of onset of symptoms. It may take from one to three weeks before radiographic changes develop. The older the patient the longer the period before abnormality becomes visible. Therefore, normal radiographs early after the onset of symptoms do **not** exclude a stress fracture. The patient should be re-examined after some 10 days if symptoms persist.

4.8.1 **Fatigue fractures**

- a *fatigue fracture* is defined as a stress fracture that occurs due to the repeated application of abnormal loads on normal bone i.e. excess stress on a normal skeleton.

- fatigue fractures may affect almost every bone. The important factor is the nature of the activity which produces the symptoms. Athletes in training and recruits undergoing military training are particularly susceptible to develop fatigue fractures.

- Typical sites of fatigue fractures and causation include (fig 4.134 to 4.137);

— metatarsal shaft	(marching/ballet)
— calcaneus	(toddlers*)
— tibia	(toddlers*/running)
— distal fibula	(running)
— proximal fibula	(jumping)
— femur (neck and shaft)	(ballet/gymnastics/running)
— pars interarticularis of the vertebra	(ballet/lifting/cleaning floors)
— ribs	(coughing/carrying heavy packs)
— lower cervical/upper thoracic spinous processes	(digging, cultivating)

toddler = infant just learning to walk

- the radiographic appearances of a fatigue fracture depend on the location and time between injury and the X-ray examination. Initial radiographs may be normal. If affecting predominantly cortical bone the first sign will be a single lamella of periosteal new bone formation (fig 4.135 and 4.136). In time this will mature to produce localized cortical thickening (hyperostosis). The underlying fracture may or may not be evident as a thin dark line traversing the cortical thickening (fig 4.137). In predominantly cancellous bone the fracture is seen as a band of focal sclerosis oriented perpendicularly to the long axis of the bone (4.138).

- in adolescents and young adults the early radiographic abnormalities of a fatigue fracture are frequently mistaken for a sarcoma, particularly if a history of abnormal activity is lacking. Follow-up radiographs after 10–14 days will show healing of a fatigue fracture provided the cause is stopped. A sarcoma or other tumour can be expected to progress rapidly with evidence of increased bone destruction.

- in the lumbar spine, pars interarticularis which is the thin portion of the posterior arch of the vertebra that joins the pedicle to the lamina, is particularly susceptible to fatigue fracture. In some individuals, there may be a congenital defect or weakness of the pars interarticularis predisposing for the fracture. This is known as *spondylolysis*. Almost all occur in the lower two levels in the lumbar spine. It is best demonstrated on oblique views of the lumbar spine (fig 4.139). If associated with forward slipping of the proximal vertebra the condition is known as *spondylolisthesis* (fig 4.140). It is often a chance finding and may not be related to trauma. Treatment is often not necessary.

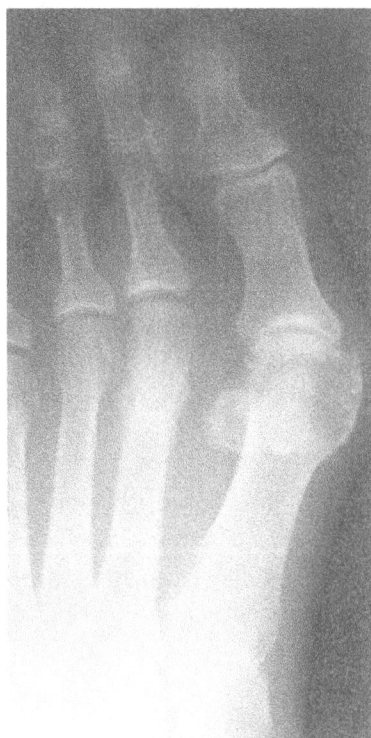

Figure 4.134
Fatigue fracture of the neck of second metatarsal ("march" fracture).

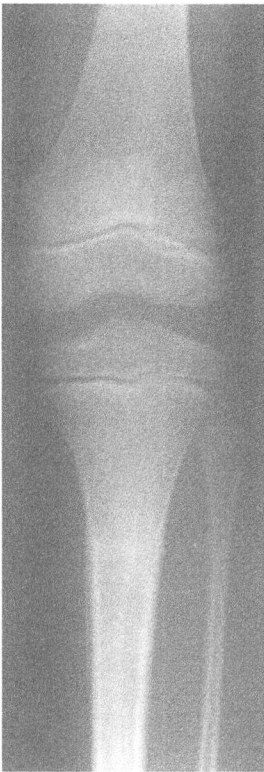
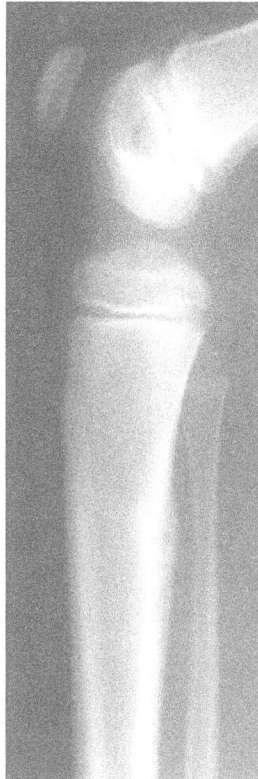

(a)   (b)

Figure 4.135
(a) AP and (b) lateral views of a fatigue fracture of the proximal
tibial diaphysis in a child.

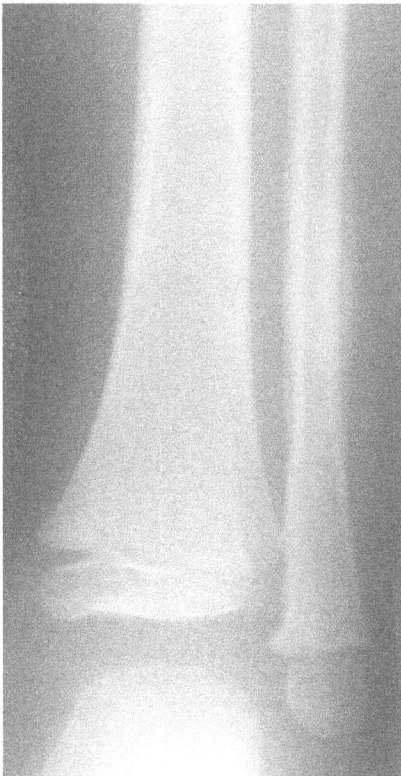

Figure 4.136
Fatigue fracture of the distal fibula in a child.

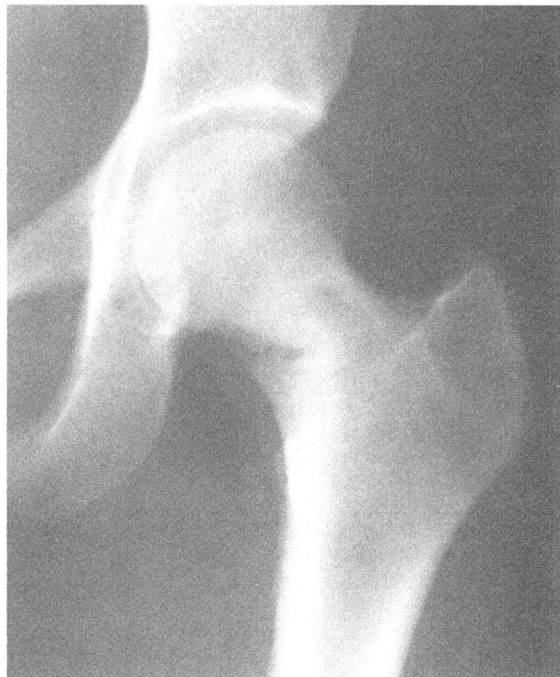

Figure 4.137
Fatigue fracture of the neck of femur.

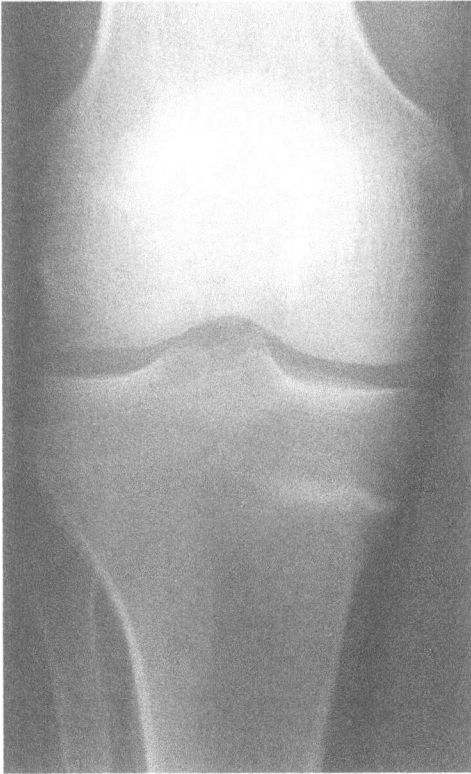

Figure 4.138
Stress fracture indicated by the horizontal focus of sclerosis in the medial aspect of the proximal tibia.

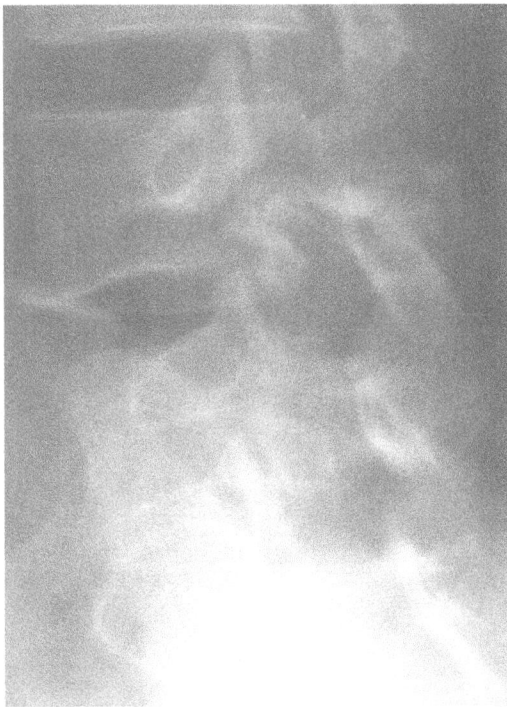

Figure 4.139
Oblique view of the lower lumbar spine showing a fracture through the pars interarticularis (spondylolysis) of L4.

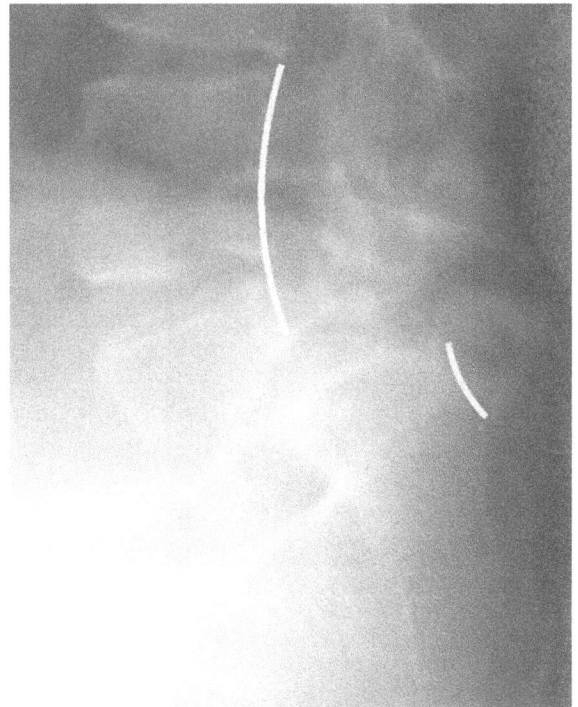

Figure 4.140
Severe anterior slipping (spondylolisthesis) of L5 on S1 due to bilateral pars interarticularis fractures of L5. The lines drawn along the posterior borders of the vertebral bodies show the pronounced anterior slip of L5 relative to S1.

4.8.2 **Insufficiency fractures**

- an *insufficiency fracture* is defined as a stress fracture that occurs with normal physiological loading on bones with abnormal elastic resistance i.e. normal stress on bones weakened by a pre-existing condition.

- conditions predisposing to insufficiency fractures include;

    — osteoporosis (from any cause)
    — rheumatoid arthritis
    — rickets/osteomalacia
    — hyperparathyroidism
    — scurvy
    — Paget's disease (osteitis deformans)
    — congenital bone disorders (e.g. fibrous dysplasia, osteogenesis imperfecta)
    — changes induced by radiation (radiotherapy)

- the most common insufficiency fractures occur in osteoporotic bone. A common example is the wedge collapse of one or more thoracic vertebrae in post-menopausal women (4.141). Other frequent sites, particularly in patients with rheumatoid arthritis or those on steroid therapy, are the pelvic ring (fig 4.142), tibia, fibula and calcaneus (fig 4.143).

- pelvic insufficiency fractures occur usually in the body of the pubis (near the symphysis), pubic rami, medial wall of acetabulum and the sacrum (fig 4.142).

- the first radiographic sign is a band of medullary sclerosis extending to involve the cortex with a minimally displaced fracture (fig 4.143). Delayed healing is common and the combination of lysis (decalcification) at the fracture site and surrounding callus formation may be mistaken for malignancy, usually a metastasis.

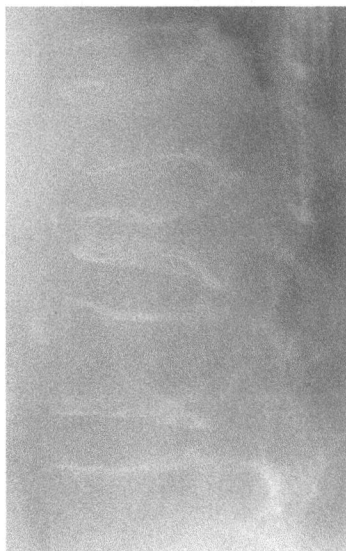

Figure 4.141
Insufficiency fractures of the lumbar vertebrae due to osteoporosis.

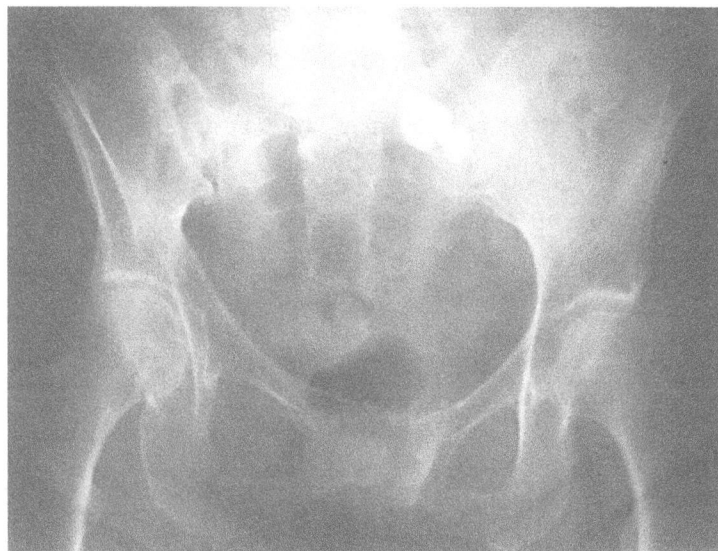

Figure 4.142
Insufficiency fractures of the left pubis and right side of the sacrum in an osteoporotic postmenopausal woman.

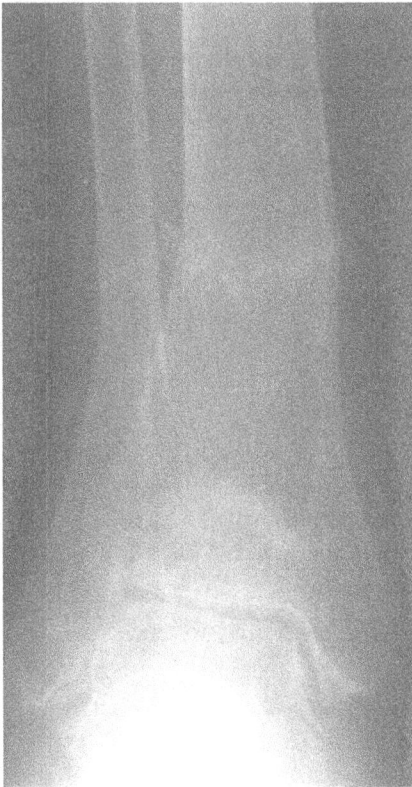

(a)

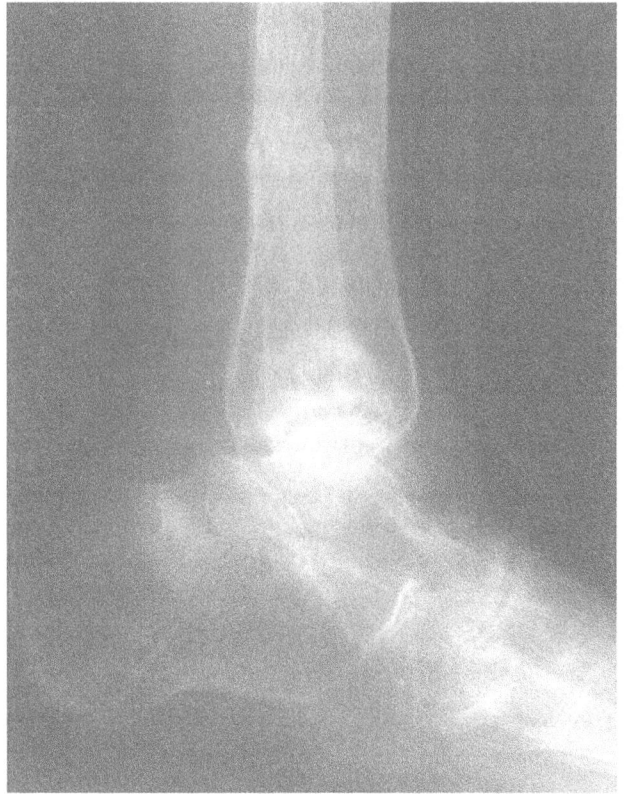

(b)

Figure 4.143
(a) AP and (b) lateral views of the ankle in a woman on long term steroid therapy for rheumatoid arthritis. There are insufficiency fractures of the distal tibial and fibular shafts, distal tibial metaphysis and calcaneus.

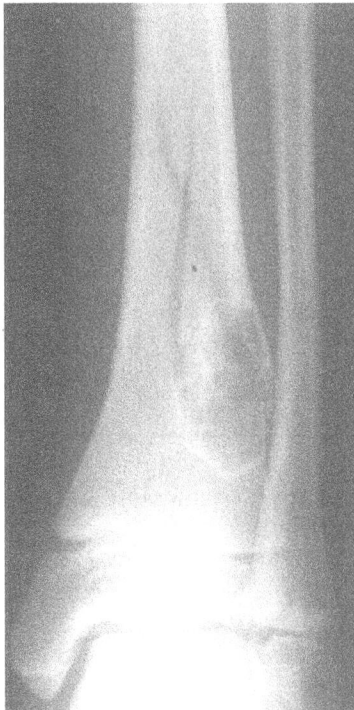

Figure 4.144
Child with an undisplaced pathological fracture through a benign bone tumour (non-ossifying fibroma).

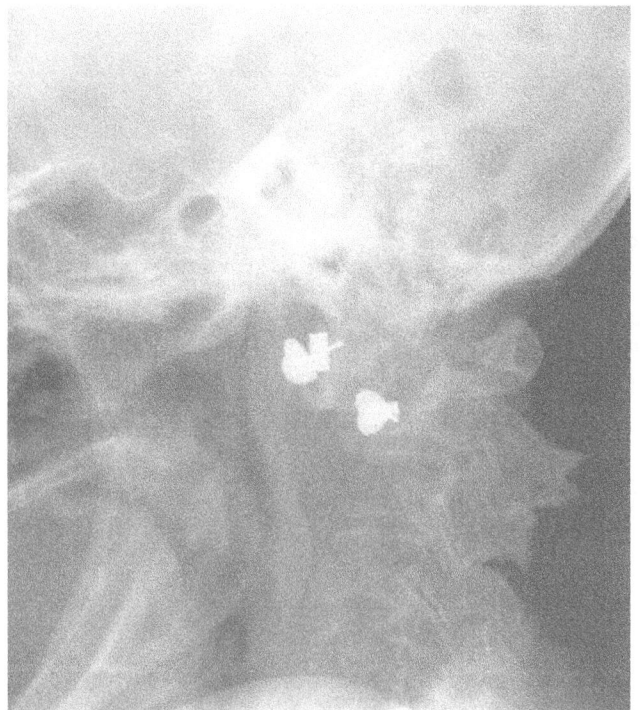

Figure 4.145
Atlantoaxial subluxation due to a pathological fracture of C2 due to infiltration from a breast metastasis. There are also metastases in the skull vault and mandible. The metallic "foreign bodies" are ear ornaments.

4.9 **Pathological fractures**

- the term ***pathological fracture*** can be applied to any fracture through a localised abnormality of bone. However, it is frequently used for fractures through neoplastic lesions i.e. tumours of bone, both benign (fig 4.144) and malignant (fig 4.145).

- in elderly people, the most common cause of a pathological fracture is a metastasis (fig 4.145). Pathological fractures will also occur through primary bone tumours but these are rarer than metastases.

- pathological fractures tend to affect weight bearing bones. A bone will be at significant risk of a pathological fracture if greater than half of the diameter is destroyed by the pathological process. Prophylactic stabilization such as internal fixation should then be considered.

- pathological fractures may also occur at sites of severe bone infections due to delayed or inadequate treatment.

Infection

Definitions

- infection is the result of pathogenic organisms invading and multiplying in the body, and it is important to know which organisms are common locally, as this will significantly influence the differential diagnosis of a musculoskeletal infection. In addition, climate and general living conditions need to be taken into account.

- pre-existing conditions may increase the risk to the patient of developing musculoskeletal infection. These include;

   — sickle cell disease
   — intravenous drug abuse
   — immunosuppression (e.g. HIV)
   — diabetes
   — malnourishment, protein deficiency

- infections of the musculoskeletal system can be subdivided by site;

   — bone infection (osteomyelitis)
   — joint infection (septic arthritis)
   — soft tissue infection (cellulitis and/or soft tissue abscess)
   — mixed (two or more of the above)

5.1 **Introduction of Infectious Agents into the Bone**

- bone may be infected by:

— haematogenous spread (via the bloodstream from infection elsewhere)
— contiguous infection (infection spread from adjacent soft tissues)
— direct implantation (either due to trauma or surgery).

- haematogenous spread is common in children and usually starts in the metaphysis. Because of the pattern of blood supply to bone, epiphyseal involvement is usually seen in infants only, whereas in older children, evidence of infectious spread from the metaphysis through the growth plate helps to differentiate infection from tumour.

5.2 **Pyogenic Osteomyelitis**

- the commonest causative organism in children and adults is *Staphylococcus aureus*. In neonates most such infections are caused by *Streptococcus Type B*.

- osteomyelitis in patients with sickle cell disease an increased incidence of salmonella infection is seen, whereas in drug abusers, *Staphylococcus* is most common although an increased incidence of *Pseudomonas* and *Seratia* infections are also seen.

5.2.1 **Acute osteomyelitis**

- if bone infection is suspected, immediate ultrasonography will show localised periosteal oedema at the site of most pain long before radiographic changes appear. Needle aspiration relieves the pressure and pain and allows for identification of the organism and antibiotic sensitivity. This early procedure frequently prevents further development of infection and spread.

- radiographs appear normal in the first 1 to 2 weeks of the infection (fig 5.1a).

- the first abnormal radiographic sign is soft tissue swelling and obliteration of the normal intermuscular fat planes due to the oedema. These changes should also be clinically apparent, i.e. the patient is presenting with a hot and swollen limb.

- after some 2 weeks a periosteal reaction and underlying bone destruction (lysis) involving the medulla and cortex start to develop, and there will be loss of density in the surrounding bone due to the hyperaemia (fig 5.1b).

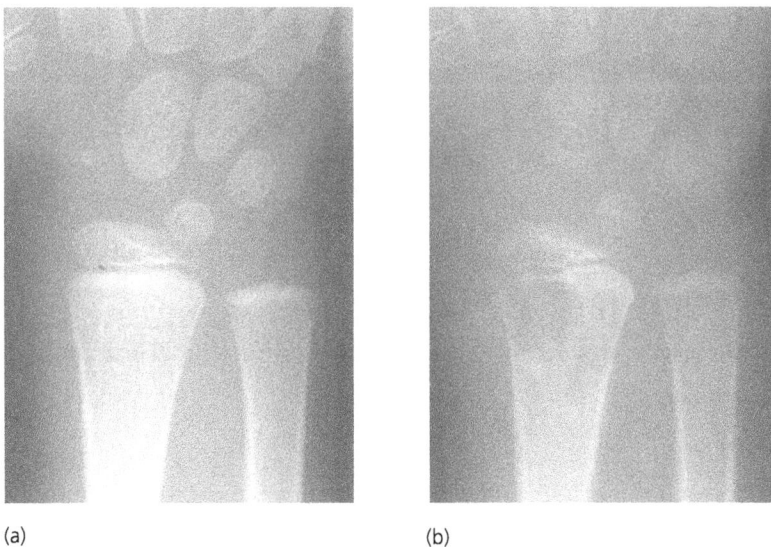

(a)   (b)

Figure 5.1
Child with acute osteomyelitis of the distal radial metaphysis (a) normal radiograph at first examination; (b) 9 days later there is a destructive lesion in the metaphysis. The rate of progression suggests infection as it is too rapid for even the most malignant of tumours.

- at this stage the lesion can resemble a malignant bone tumour (fig 5.2). However, infection tends to progress more rapidly than tumour, i.e. increasing destruction in infection is evident over days rather than weeks (fig 5.1). A serpiginous (serpent-like) pattern of bone destruction is typical of osteomyelitis.

- if the osteomyelitis is treated promptly healing will be indicated by the reduction in soft tissue swelling, increased sclerosis within the bone (i.e. healing of the lysis) and thickening of the periosteal reaction.

- eventually, a sequestrum and involucrum may develop. A sequestrum is a fragment of necrotic bone, usually linear, isolated from the surrounding living bone by granulation tissue (fig 5.3). It may harbour bacteria, leading to chronic osteomyelitis. An involucrum is the new bone that develops around the sequestrum (fig 5.4).

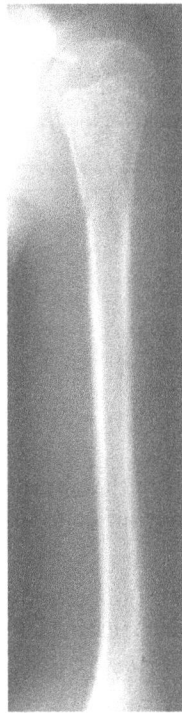

Figure 5.2
Child with acute osteomyelitis of the proximal humerus. The appearances in this case are indistinguishable from a sarcoma.

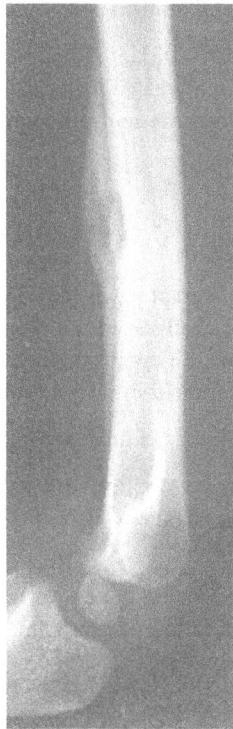

Figure 5.3
Child with a cortically based abscess containing a sequestrum.

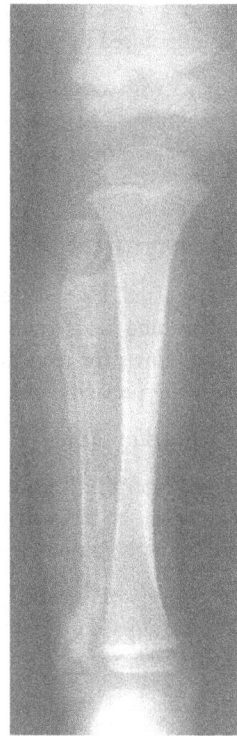

Figure 5.4
Child with extensive osteomyelitis of the fibula. The new bone formation around the old shaft of the fibula represents the involucrum.

5.2.2 **Subacute osteomyelitis**

- due to the gradual development of an abscess within a bone (also known as Brodie's abscess).

- commonest age group – children.

- commonest site – metaphysis.

- commonest bone affected – tibia.

- the clinical features can be misleading: local pain but little evidence of soft tissue swelling and localised soft tissue inflammation.

- the radiographic changes vary from small abscess cavity close to the growth plate (fig 5.5) to a more extensive metaphyseal cavity with a sclerotic margin (due to reaction in the surrounding bone, fig 5.6).

- the differential diagnosis includes benign bone tumours e.g. eosinophilic granuloma (Langerhans cell histiocytosis), or chronic infection from tuberculosis or fungus.

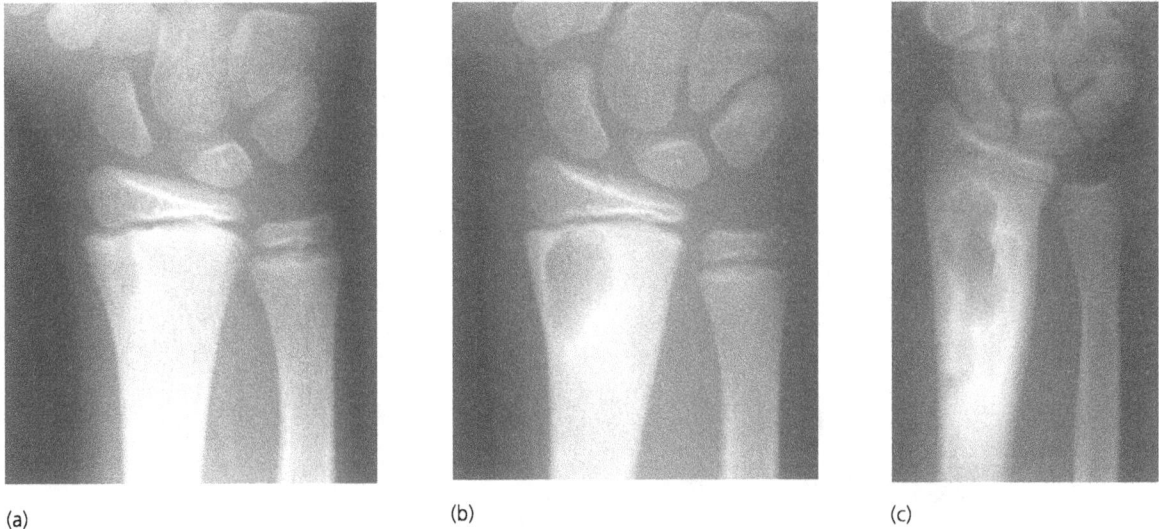

(a) (b) (c)

Figure 5.5
Progress of untreated subacute osteomyelitis (Brodie's abscess) in a child (a) when first examined; (b) 5 months later; and (c) 5 years later.

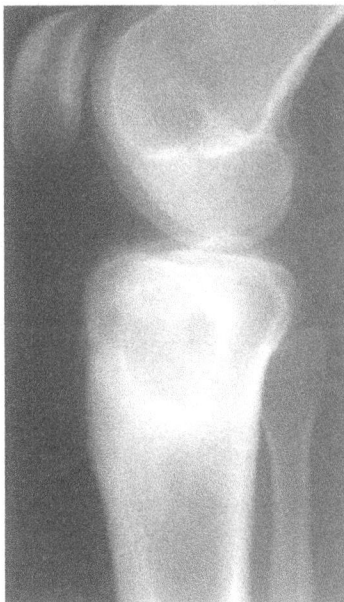

Figure 5.6
Typical subacute osteomyelitis (Brodie's abscess) in the proximal tibia. The only slightly unusual feature is that the patient is an adult. Tuberculosis must be excluded.

5.2.3 **Chronic osteomyelitis**

- if the infection persists for months or years the degree of host bone reaction exceeds the destruction from the infection and chronic osteomyelitis develops. The radiographic features include increasing sclerosis with lytic foci, sequestra and involucrum formation (fig 5.7).

  — in the form known as sclerosing osteomyelitis of Garré, there is marked sclerosis with cortical thickening and little or no lysis (fig 5.8).

- chronic osteomyelitis may periodically become more active. It can be difficult to identify reactivation of infection on radiographs. Features suggestive of active infection include;

    — change in appearance since previous radiographs (i.e. increasing lysis)
    — immature periosteal reaction (i.e. thin and linear)
    — presence of sequestra
    — presence of draining sinuses (also found in mycotic and tuberculous infection)

- complications of chronic osteomyelitis include,

    — reactivation of infection
    — deformity (due to premature fusion of growth plate or pathological fracture)
    — joint involvement with degenerative joint disease and ankylosis (fusion) (fig 5.9)
    — rare development of malignancy in chronic draining sinus tract (or in tropical ulcer, see Chapter 5.2.4).

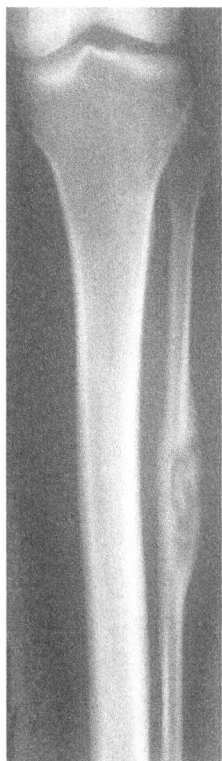

Figure 5.7
Adult with osteo-myelitis of the fibular shaft. The abscess cavity contains a sequestrum.

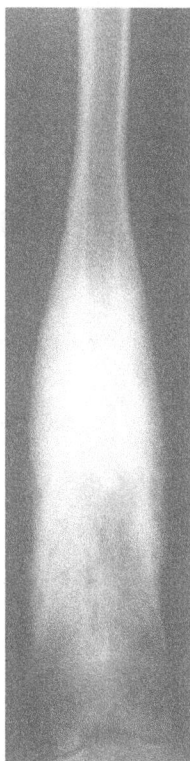

Figure 5.8
Sclerosing form of chronic osteomyelitis (of Garré).

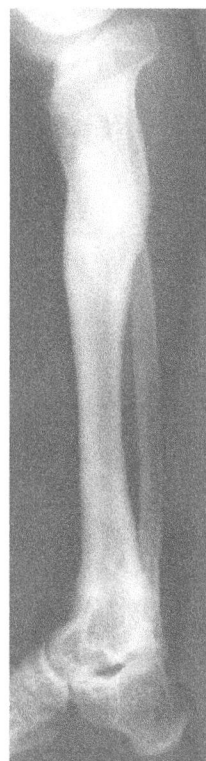

Figure 5.9
Adult showing complications of chronic osteomyelitis. There is deformity of the proximal tibia and ankylosis (fusion) of the ankle joint.

5.2.4 **Tropical ulcer**

- an acute localized necrosis of the skin and subcutaneous tissues which is endemic in, but not confined to, tropical regions. Almost all such ulcers develop below the knee.

- superimposed infection may lead to destruction of the deeper soft tissues and involvement of bone. Destructive changes within the bone indicate chronic osteomyelitis (fig 5.10).

- healing or reactive change within the bone can result in a bowing deformity and focal cortical thickening resembling a cortically based osteoid osteoma or healed stress fracture (fig 5.11).

- in some cases malignancy may develop within the ulcer, and in several tropical countries this is a common form of skin cancer.

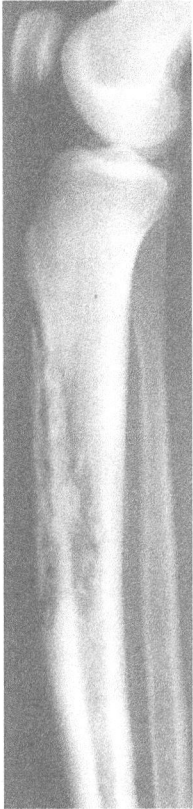

Figure 5.10
Adult with chronic osteomyelitis of the anterior tibia below a tropical ulcer.

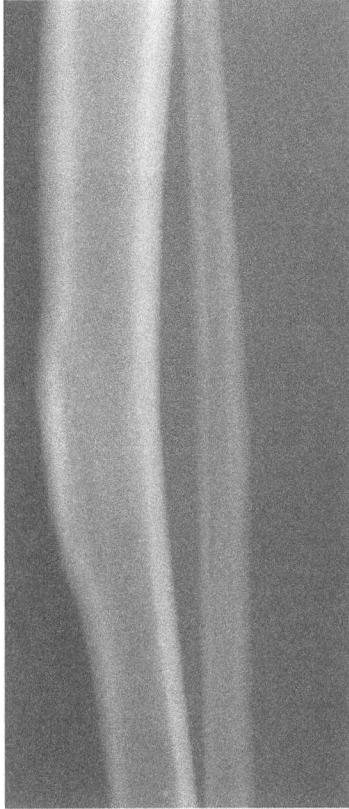

Figure 5.11
Bony prominence of the anterior aspect of the mid-tibial shaft resulting from a healed tropical ulcer.

5.3 **Septic Arthritis**

- an infection within a joint (septic arthritis) may arise from haematogenous spread or from an adjacent focus of osteomyelitis. The latter is most commonly seen in infants under 12 months of age where the purulent effusion can cause joint subluxation/dislocation (fig 5.12).

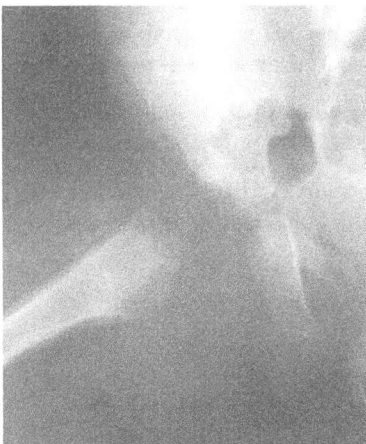

Figure 5.12
Infant with acute osteomyelitis of the proximal femur. Note that there is also involvement of the hip joint with dislocation. A line drawn along the shaft of the femur passes through the ilium and NOT the acetabulum, as would be normal.

- the radiographic features of a septic arthritis include (fig 5.13);

    — soft tissue swelling around the joint and effusion into the joint
    — localised osteoporosis (due to increased blood flow)
    — joint space loss
    — articular erosions
    — ankylosis, eventually, when healed
    — a late feature

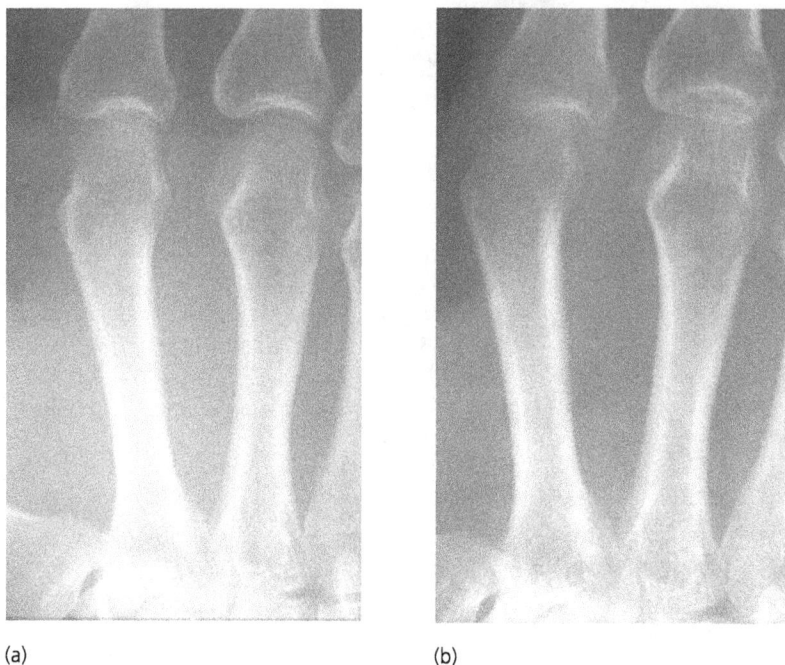

(a)   (b)

Figure 5.13
Adult with rapid progression of septic arthritis of the 2nd metacarpopha-langeal joint due to a human "bite". (a) at presentation there is some localized loss of bone density and early narrowing of the joint; (b) 11 days later there has been marked progression of the joint destruction.

5.4 **Mycobacterial Infections**

5.4.1 **Tuberculosis (TB)**

- the incidence of skeletal TB is varies considerably from place to place and over time, and factors such as antibiotic resistance and increased infections in immunocompromised individuals, especially HIV-positive, are influencing the occurrence of disease.

- it is assumed that skeletal TB develops by haematogenic spread. Chest radiography shows active disease in less than 50% of the cases, as the organism may lay dormant and become active later.

- lesions may be single or multifocal. Multifocal lesions are most common in the spine (see Chapter 5.8).

- irrespective of the site, tuberculosis may have a slower clinical course and a less rapid host reaction than other infections. Thus, the diagnostic procedures are often delayed, and when performed, the radiographic changes are mostly extensively developed.

- many may, however, behave like any acute infections mimicking pyogenic osteomyelitis.

Tuberculous osteomyelitis

- tends to arise in the metaphysis and occasionally the epiphysis.

- predominantly lytic, honey-combed appearance with limited response from host bone (fig 5.14). Periosteal reaction and surrounding sclerosis are **not** prominent features. Sequestra are uncommon.

- when one or more of the tubular bones of the hand are involved together with florid soft tissue swelling it is known as tuberculous dactylitis (fig 5.15). This is most commonly seen in children and, and is known as "spina ventosa"when associated with bony expansion (fig 5.16). It is important to recognize that other conditions may present with a dactylitis (see Table 5.1).

- multifocal TB in a middle aged or elderly patient can easily be mistaken for metastatic disease.

Table 5.1 **Causes of Dactylitis (inflamed finger/toe).**

Pyogenic osteomyelitis (especially salmonella)
Sickle cell anaemia
Tuberculosis (spina ventosa)
Fungal infections (e.g. mycetoma, sporotrichosis)
Leprosy
Tumour (osteoid osteoma, metastasis, Ewing's sarcoma)
Syphilis, yaws
Sarcoidosis

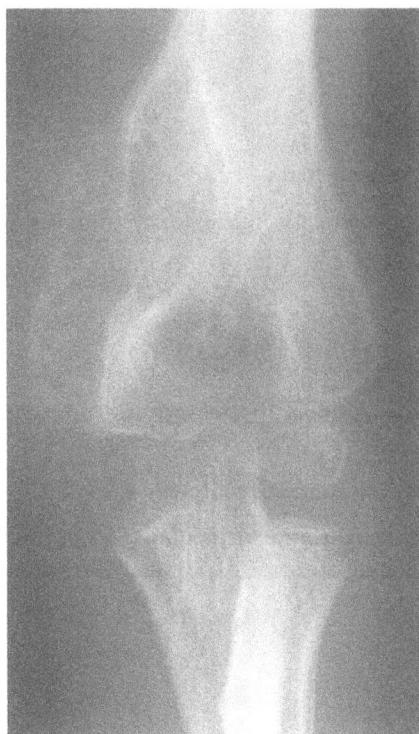

Figure 5.14
Child with TB osteomyelitis of the distal humerus.

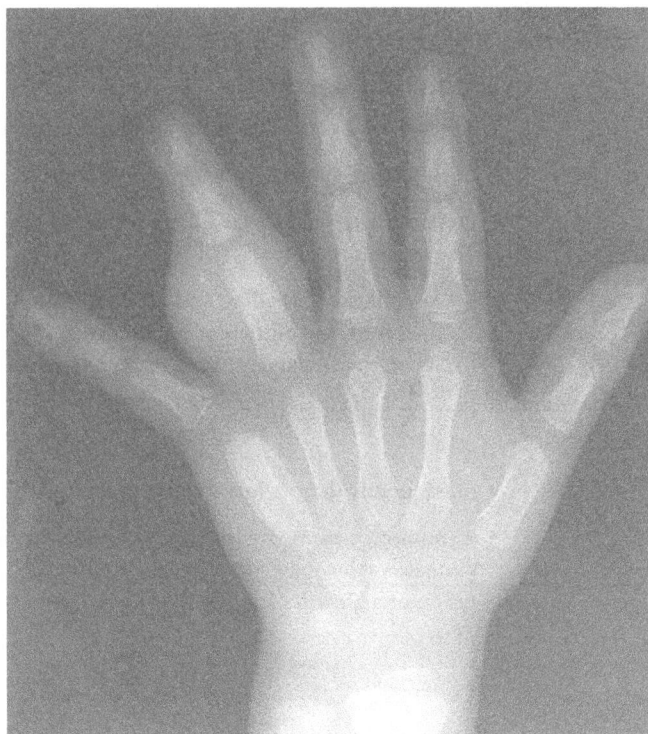

Figure 5.15
Child with multifocal TB. There is involvement of the 5th meta-carpal and proximal phalanx of the 4th finger. There is a dactylitis of the 4th finger.

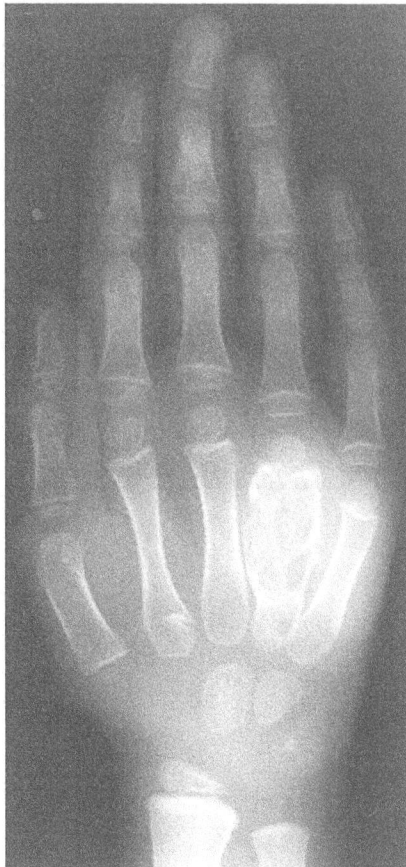

Figure 5.16
Child with TB of the 4th metacarpal S(spina ventosa). Other bone infection foci are likely.

Tuberculous arthritis

• TB arthritis usually affects major joints, especially hip and knee.

• the infection may be synovial or develop from an adjacent bony focus.

• the early signs of synovial TB are similar to those of any monarticular inflammatory arthropathy. The features include (fig 5.17);

    — soft tissue swelling and joint effusion
    — severe juxta-articular osteoporosis
    — relative enlargement of the epiphyses due to hyperaemia

• the next radiographic change to develop is loss of the white line indicating the articular cortex (fig 5.18).

• subsequently there is loss of joint space due to cartilage destruction and fine erosions (fig 5.19).

• if antibiotic treatment is delayed or ineffective, abscess formation with calcification (fig 5.20) and ultimately joint ankylosis will occur. Another complication in children is deformity due to premature fusion of a growth plate (fig 5.21).

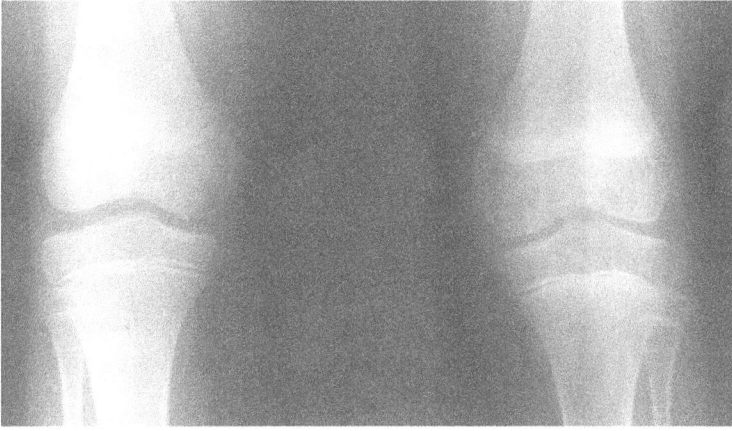

Figure 5.17
Synovial TB of the left knee. There is loss of bone density and enlargement of the epiphyses due to the hyperaemia. Compare with the normal knee.

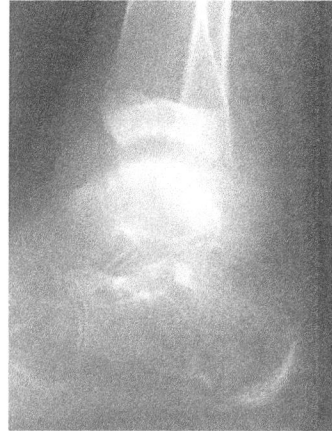

Figure 5.18
Child with TB arthritis of the ankle. There is severe loss of bone density, soft tissue swelling and loss of definition of the articular cortices of the ankle joint.

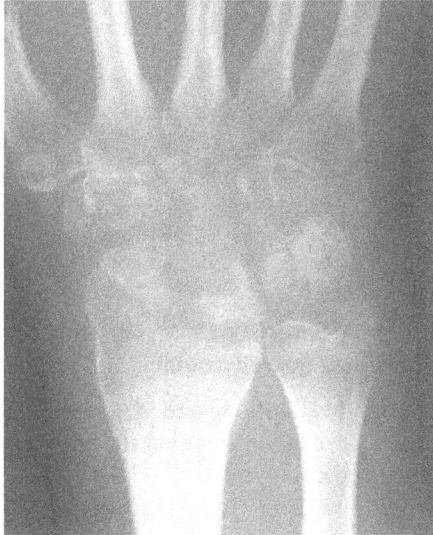

Figure 5.19
Advanced TB arthritis of the wrist with loss of bone density and erosions of the carpal bones.

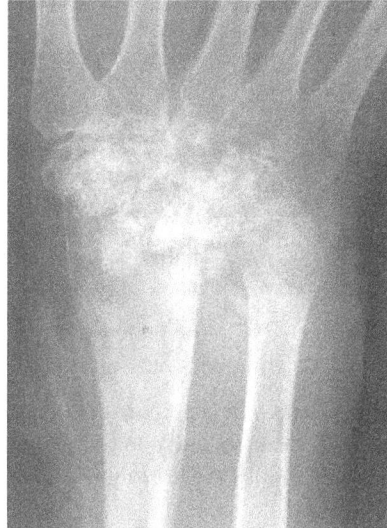

Figure 5.20
Late stage TB arthritis of the wrist with destruction of the carpal bones and calcification in the abscess.

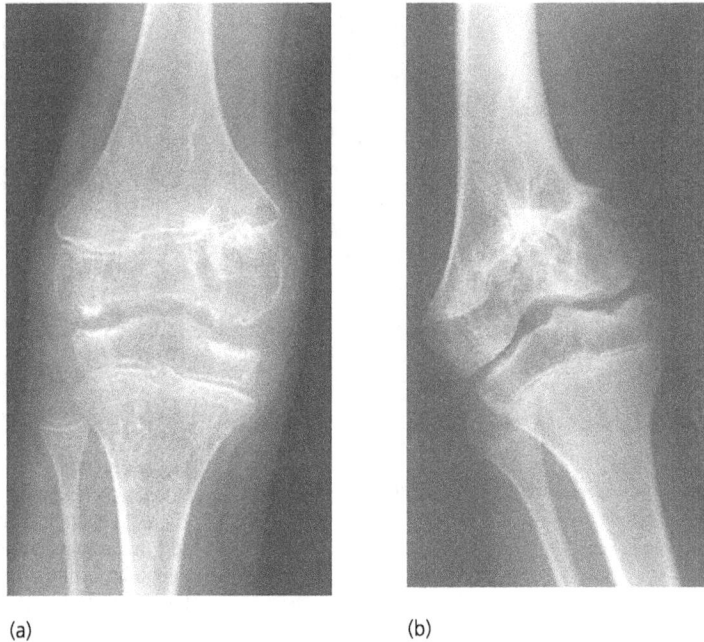

(a)   (b)

Figure 5.21
Child with TB arthritis of the knee (a) in the active phase there is severe loss of bone density, irregular enlargement of the epiphyses and erosions; (b) 7 years later there is a severe varus deformity due to premature fusion of the medial aspect of the distal femoral growth plate.

5.4.2 **Leprosy**

- leprosy (Hansen's disease) is a chronic infection caused by *Mycobacterium leprae*, mainly affecting peripheral nerves and skin.

- the radiographic changes can be classified as:

  Specific changes – due to the presence of granulomata in the bones, well defined cyst-like lesions in the phalanges, prominent nutrient foramina, osseous destruction, and deformity (fig 5.22a).

  Nonspecific (neurovascular) changes – terminal phalangeal resorption, secondary infection (osteomyelitis), fractures, and bony resorption (fig 5.22b). Due to loss of sensation and impaired/damaged blood supply, the deformities of feet and hands can become severe.

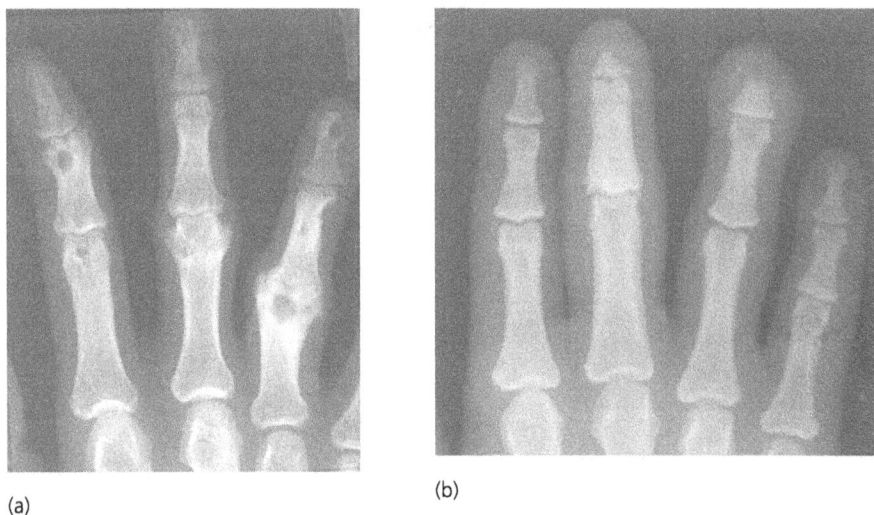

(a)   (b)

Figure 5.22
Leprosy (a) specific changes with cyst-like lesions, prominent nutrient foramina and destruction with deformity of the ends of the proximal phalanges; (b) non-specific changes with terminal phalangeal resorption due to a neuropathy.

5.5 Treponemal Infections

5.5.1 Syphilis

- infection with the spirochete, *Treponema pallidum*, occurs in 2 forms – congenital and acquired. Both progress through different stages. Bone infection is usually multiple, always following clinical findings.

Congenital syphilis

- results from transplacental infection of the foetus.

- in those that surviving and growing up, osseous lesions are typically seen in the long bones with metaphyseal defects and periosteal new bone formation (fig 5.23).

- involvement of the hands and feet is uncommon but can produce a nonspecific dactylitis (fig 5.24, see Table 5.1).

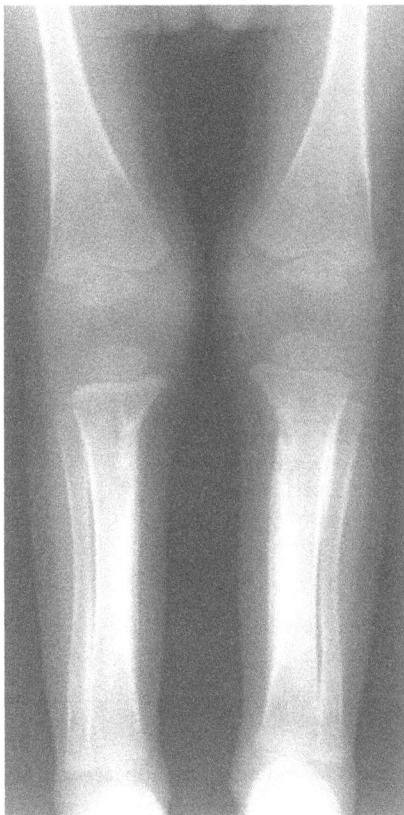

Figure 5.23
Child with congenital syphilis. There is periosteal new bone formation and metaphyseal defects of the medial aspect of the proximal tibiae.

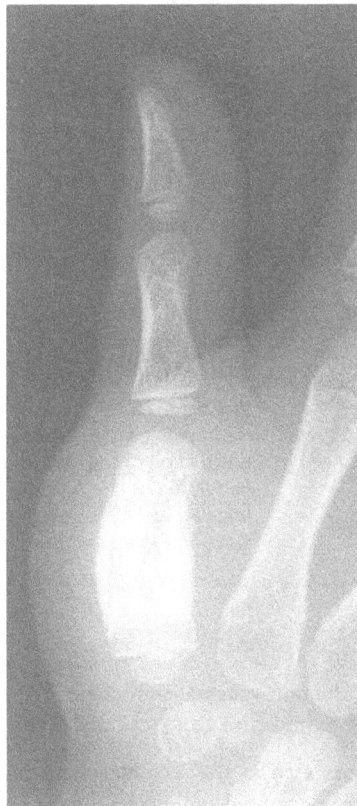

Figure 5.24
Child with dactylitis of the 1st metacarpal due to congenital syphilis. The features are non-specific.

Acquired syphilis

- any bone may be affected, including the skull bones. Usually a mixed pattern of sclerosis and lysis with periosteal new bone formation (gummatous osteitis, fig 5.25) is seen. Longstanding cases with periods of healing and reactivation of disease can be associated with bone deformity e.g. tibial bowing and anterior thickening (sabre tibia).

- chronic syphilis (tabes dorsalis) can be associated with neuropathic joints most commonly in the lower limbs (fig 5.26, see Chapter 6.6).

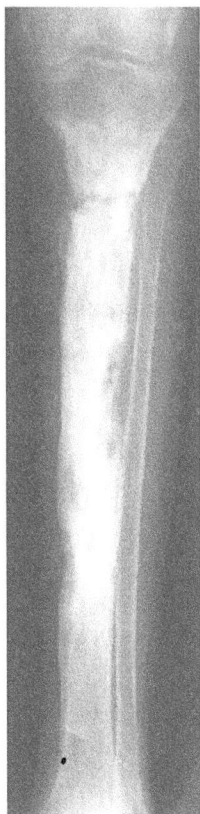

Figure 5.25
Adult with acquired syphilis of the tibia. There is a mixed pattern of lysis and sclerosis.

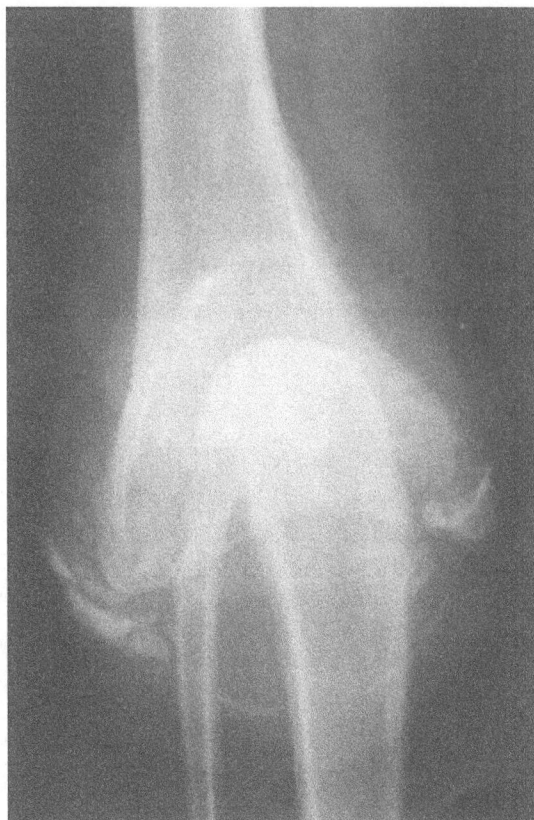

Figure 5.26
Neuropathic knee secondary to neurosyphilis, with total destruction of the joint and bone fragmentation.(From Pettersson, H and Allisson, D: The Encyclopaedia of Medical Imaging, Vol III, ISIS Medical Multi-Media/The Nicer Institute, Oslo, 1999, with permission)

5.5.2 Yaws

- it is caused by the non-venereal spirochete, *Treponema pertenue*, and is mainly seen in countries with warm and humid climate.

- bone changes are seen in the secondary and tertiary stages. The radiographic appearances are similar to those of acquired syphilis i.e. mixed pattern of lysis and sclerosis with florid periosteal new bone formation principally affecting the tubular bones (fig 5.27). Dactylitis may also develop (fig 5.28, Table 5.1 (pg. 111)).

- longstanding cases will show healing with marked thickening and bowing of the bone (fig 5.29 and 5.30). On radiographs it is often difficult to distinguish between yaws and syphilis.

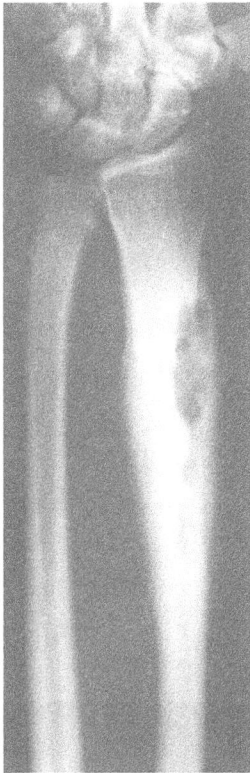

Figure 5.27
Yaws of the distal radius.
There is a mixed pattern of
lysis and sclerosis.

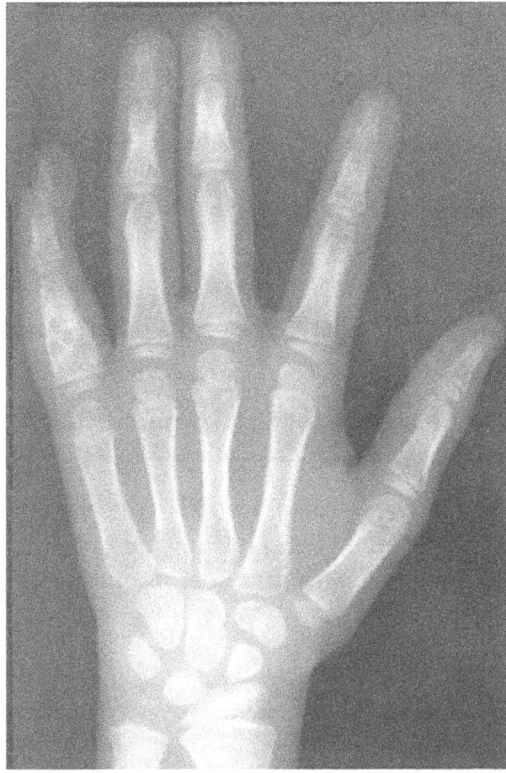

Figure 5.28
Child with a dactylitis of the little finger due to yaws.

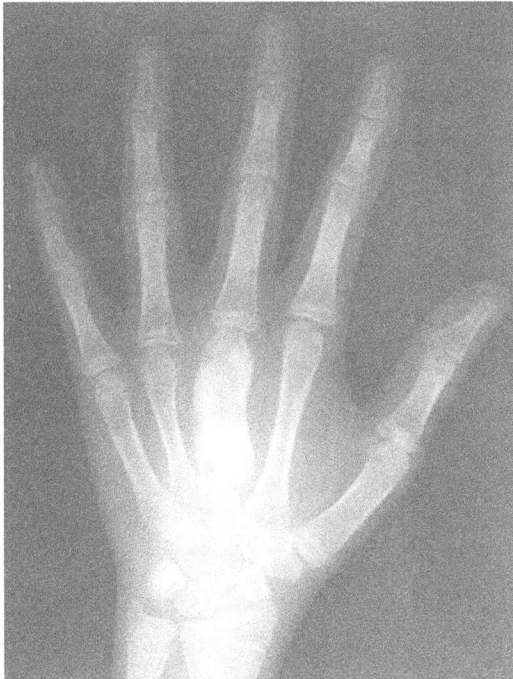

Figure 5.29
Child with a predominantly sclerotic lesion of the 3rd
metacarpal due to healed yaws.

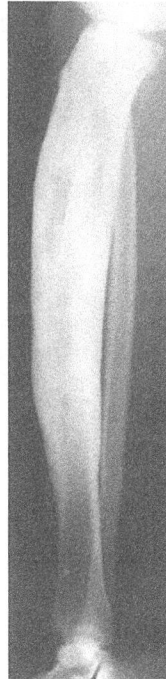

Figure 5.30
Sclerosis and
Anterior bowing of
the tibia in an adult
with healed yaws.

5.6 Fungal Infections

- fungal infections can involve bone and joints. Most important are;

  — blastomycosis
  — nocardiosis
  — coccidiomycosis
  — histoplasmosis
  — sporotrichosis
  — actinomycosis (a filamentous bacteria)

5.6.1 Mycetoma

- an indolent fungal infection, usually with secondary bacterial infection. Most are chronic. The infecting organism varies between different regions.

- there are multiple abscesses, fistulae and sinuses. It commonly affects the foot and ankle (Madura foot) and less commonly the arm and hand.

- there is gross soft tissue swelling, with bone destruction and periosteal new bone formation at a late stage (fig 5.31 and 5.32).

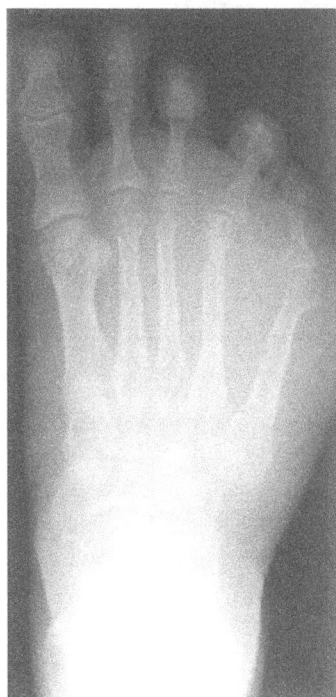

Figure 5.31
Madura foot. There is severe soft tissue swelling with early erosion of the 4th metatarsal.

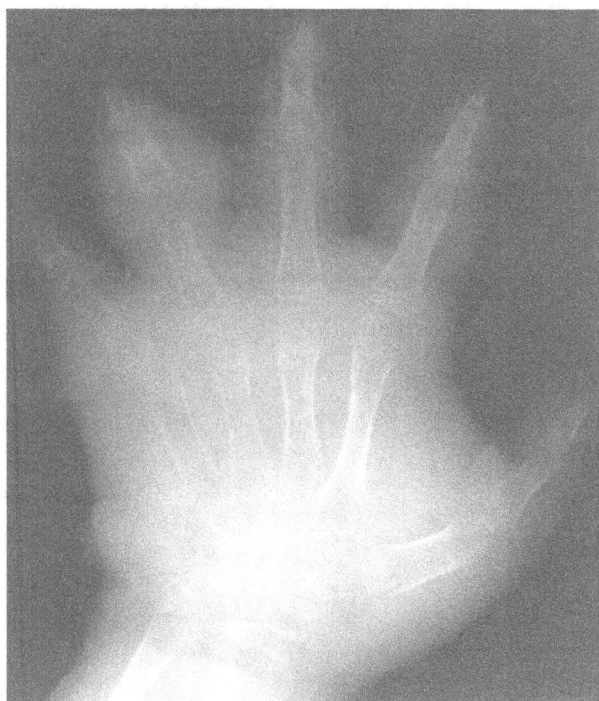

Figure 5.32
Child with mycetoma of the hand. There is severe soft tissue swelling, loss of bone density and a dactylitis of the 4th finger.

5.6.2 Coccidiaidomycosis

- it is a chronic granulomatous condition. Most commonly seen in the Southwestern parts of North America, but can also occur elsewhere in the world.

- bone lesions tend to be multiple with the predilection for the spine, pelvis, hands and feet. Bone lesions resemble pyogenic infections and joint lesions may resemble tuberculous arthritis.

5.7 **Parasitic Infections**

- parasitic infections are endemic in many parts of the world. Most of them affect soft tissues, but some also cause bone lesions. It is important to know which parasites are most common in a local environment.

5.7.1 **Hydatid disease (Echinococcosis)**

- a parasitic infection that it is commoner in temperate than in tropical zones. Often found in sheep, but also in several other species such as reindeers, dogs, wolves and foxes.

- there are two different forms of hydatid disease. The most common form is caused by *Echinococcus Granulosa* (cystic hydatid disease), whereas the type caused by *Echinococcus multilocularis* is much less widespread. Bone infection is uncommon in both varieties, but the latter can cause almost untreatable bone disease, especially affecting spine and pelvis (alveolar or multilocular hydatid disease).

- most common sites are spine, pelvis and long bones. Long bone lesions may mimic fibrous dysplasia.

- radiographic features are lytic, expansive, septated ("soap-bubble") medullary lesions without periosteal reaction or sclerosis (fig 5.33).

- complications include;

  — pathological fracture
  — secondary infection
  — spinal cord compromise from spinal involvement

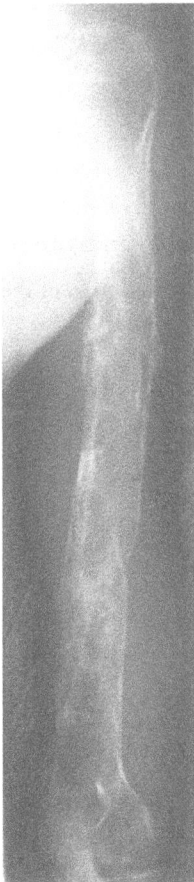

Figure 5.33
Hydatid disease. Extensive involvement of the humerus.

5.7.2 **Calcified helminthic infections**

- a variety of helminthic infections can produce soft tissue calcifications when the worm is dead. In endemic areas these are frequently an incidental finding on radiographs. Common examples follow below.

Cystercercus cellulosae (cysticercosis)

- due to ingestion of the ova of Taenia soleum.

- dead cysts within the muscles can calcify to produce oval, 10–15 mm long shadows oriented in the direction of the muscle fibres (fig 5.34).

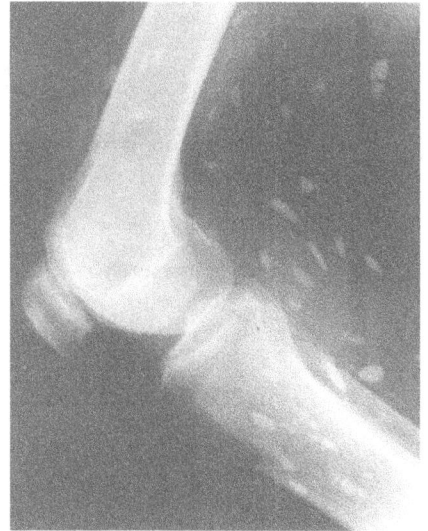

Figure 5.34
Typical calcification of cysticercosis

Dracunculus medinensis (guinea worm)

- as with cysticercosis, this parasite only becomes visible in soft tissues when the dead worm calcifies.

- fine linear or coiled calcification which, over time, may become fragmented by the action of the muscles (fig 5.35). Some may be very long.

- may cause abscess or joint infection when alive.

- similar linear spotty calcifications may also occur in the nerves of patients with leprosy. Although it resembles guinea worm, the patient will have other clinical and radiographic signs of leprosy.

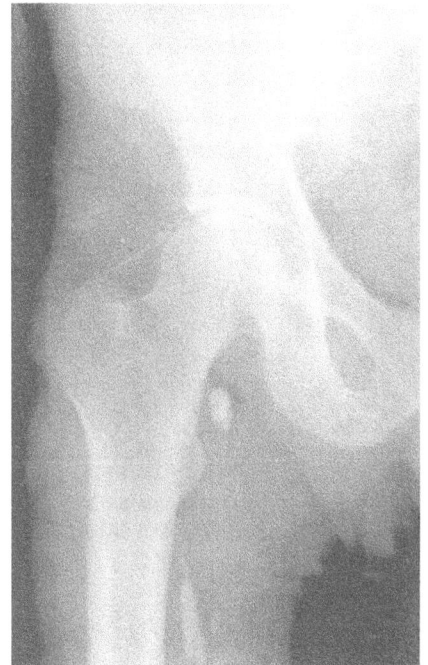

Figure 5.35
Typical calcification of guinea worm.

5.8 Infections of the Spine

- infections of the spine merit separate mention because of the special anatomy and the risk of serious damage to the spinal cord.

5.8.1 Pyogenic spinal infection

- there is a communication between the pelvic and thoracolumbar venous systems. Therefore, genitourinary infections may spread to the spine, and especially to the lower thoracic or lumbar spine.

- most infections of the spine are bacterial and caused specifically by staphylococci. Percutaneous aspiration or biopsy is, however, advised where possible to confirm the infective organism and to ensure that appropriate antibiotic treatment is given.

- although frequently referred to as a "discitis", spinal infection is a form of osteomyelitis which arises within the vertebral endplate (margin) and involves the disc secondarily. The term "discitis" is best reserved for the self-limiting condition arising in children (see Chapter 5.8.4).

- the radiographic appearances of a pyogenic spinal infection include (fig 5.36),

    — no changes for up to 6 weeks after onset of symptoms
    — first sign is reduced density and destruction of one vertebral endplate
    — disc space narrowing and destruction of the adjacent endplate follow
    — spreading of the infection causes increasing destruction of the vertebral bodies and development of a paravertebral soft tissue mass (e.g. psoas abscess)
    — healing is indicated by increasing sclerosis eventually with deformity if destruction was severe

- the differential diagnosis of discovertebral destruction also includes;

    — other infections e.g. tuberculous spondylitis (see Chapter 5.8.2) and brucellosis (see Chapter 5.8.3)
    — discovertebral pseudarthrosis in ankylosing spondylitis (see Chapter 6.3.1)
    — spinal trauma

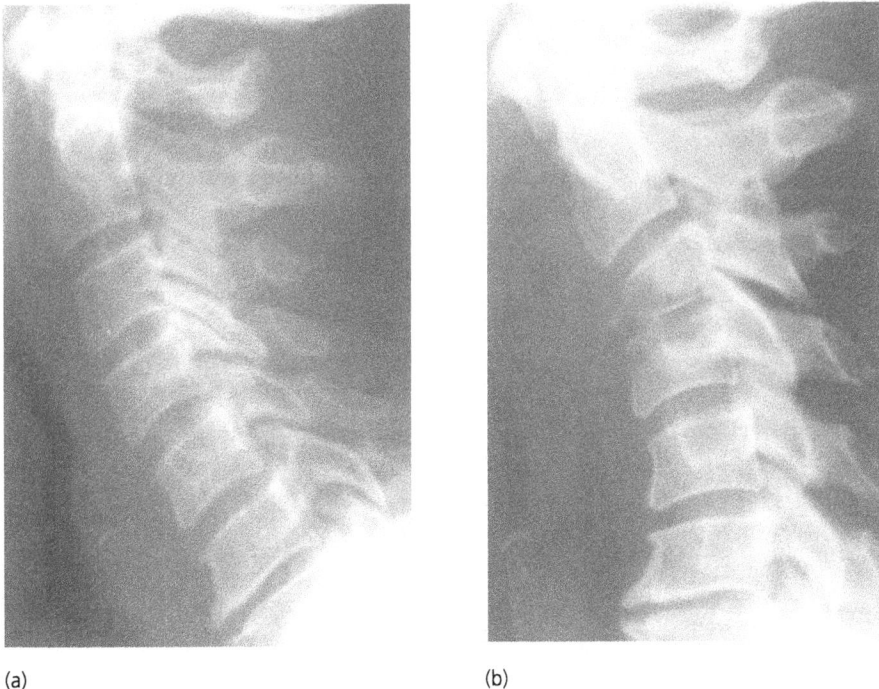

(a)   (b)

Figure 5.36
Pyogenic spinal infection at C3/4 (a) normal appearances at presentation; (b) destruction of the vertebral endplates and disc space narrowing 6 weeks later.

5.8.2 **Tuberculous spondylitis**

- the spine is one of the common sites for TB of the musculoskeletal system. It may progress more rapidly in immunosuppressed patients and may then resemble a pyogenic infection.

- 3 patterns of vertebral involvement of which the first (a) is the most common, can be seen;

  a. Discovertebral destruction – similar to pyogenic infection but the changes are often well established at presentation (fig 5.37). Disc involvement is a relatively late feature. Large paravertebral abscess with later calcification and multiple level involvement is often seen (5.38). Late cases often develop a severe angular spinal deformity (kyphotic gibbus), as the vertebrae collapse.

  b. Subligamentous – the infection begins anteriorly under the periosteum and spreads under the anterior longitudinal ligament. There are erosions of the anterior aspects of one or more vertebral bodies (fig 5.39). The disc space is preserved. Bony spurs may develop.

  c. Central – the infection develops within the vertebral body without involvement of the disc space (fig 5.40), until late in the course. The infected vertebra often collapses.

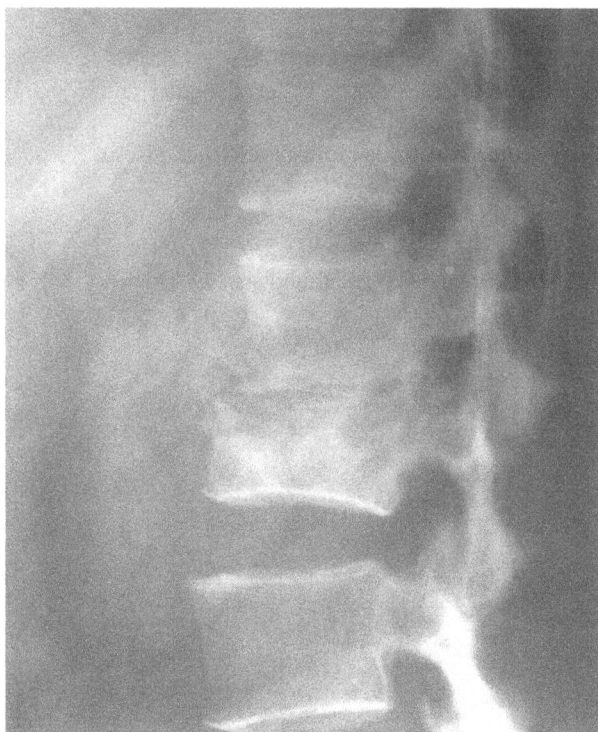

Figure 5.37
TB spondylitis with discovertebral destruction and the "ghost" of a paravertebral abscess extending anteriorly.

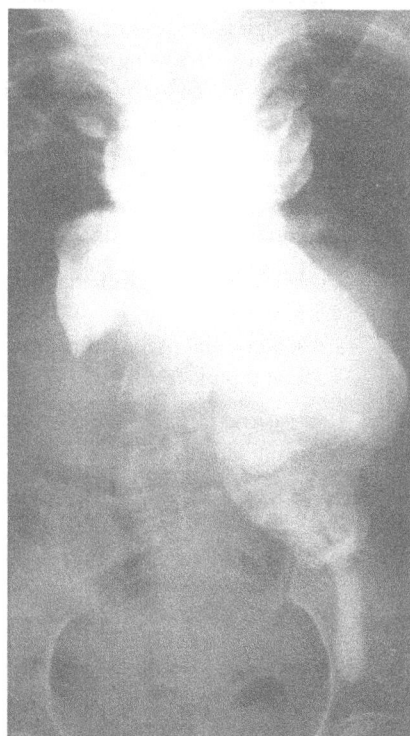

Figure 5.38
Chronic TB spondylitis of the thoracic spine. The spine is largely obscured by the massive bi-lateral calcified paravertebral/psoas abscesses. This does not always mean that the infection is now completely healed.

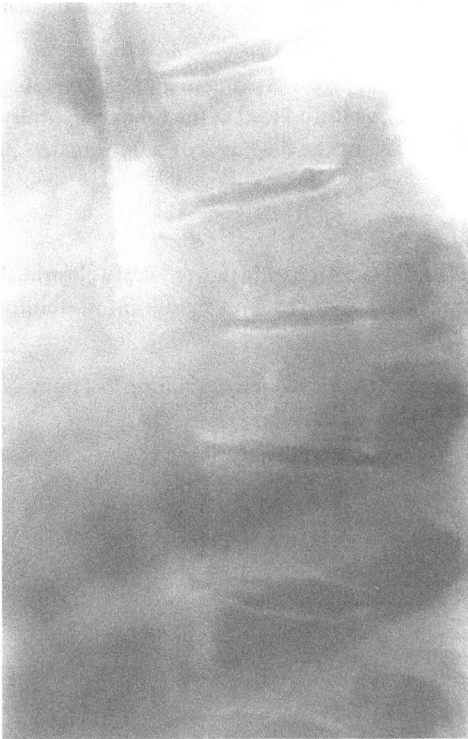

Figure 5.39
Anterior subligamentous TB spondylitis with erosion of the anterior aspects of two adjacent thoracic vertebrae.

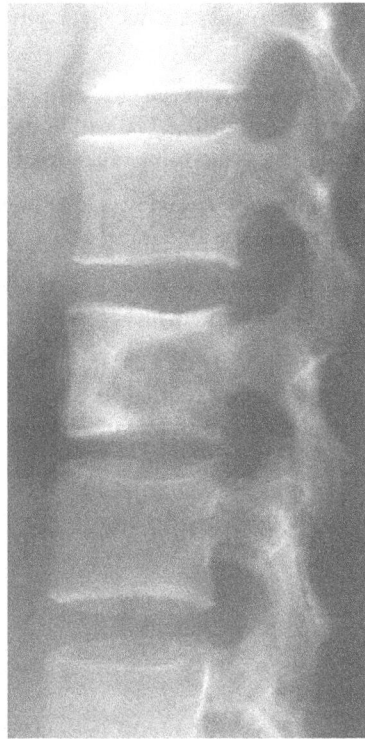

Figure 5.40
Central form of TB spondylitis confined to one of the lumbar vertebrae.

5.8.3 **Brucellosis**

• granulomatous condition also known as "undulant" or "Malta" fever. Transmission mostly from unpasteurised milk or direct contact with infected cattle.

• the bones are affected in 10% of the cases, most often the lumbar spine and pelvis.

• the radiographic appearances resemble pyogenic spinal infection although there tends to be a greater degree of bony sclerosis and large bridging osteophytes (marginal bony projections) when healing. Abscesses occur, but not as often as in tuberculosis.

5.8.4 **Discitis**

• a self-limiting inflammatory condition affecting intervertebral discs in children.

• probably a direct haematogenous infection of the disc (at this age the disc is vascularized).

• frequently no infective organism can be cultured.

• slow progression of radiographic changes with loss of disc height and vertebral endplate irregularity and sclerosis.

• clinical and radiographic follow up is necessary to exclude tuberculous infections.

5.9 **Soft Tissue Infections**

• infections of the soft tissues are mostly seen in;

— penetrating injuries
— intravenous drug abusers
— immunosuppression
— diabetes
— leprosy

- frequently the only radiographic sign is soft tissue swelling and obliteration of normal intermuscular fat planes.

- gas within the soft tissues can be identified as small dark (black) areas as compared to the greytones of surrounding soft tissues. Gas within the soft tissues may be introduced at the time of an injury or as a result of a gas forming organism. Features which favour the diagnosis of infection are:
  — gas appearing several days after injury
  — increase in the amount of gas

- wide spread gas formation tracking along muscle and fascial planes is highly suggestive of a clostridial infection (gas gangrene) which, if not treated promptly, is associated with significant morbidity and mortality.

- gas-forming infection is particularly liable to occur in uncontrolled diabetes, resulting in a number of small gas bubbles in an area of tissue necrosis (fig 5.41).

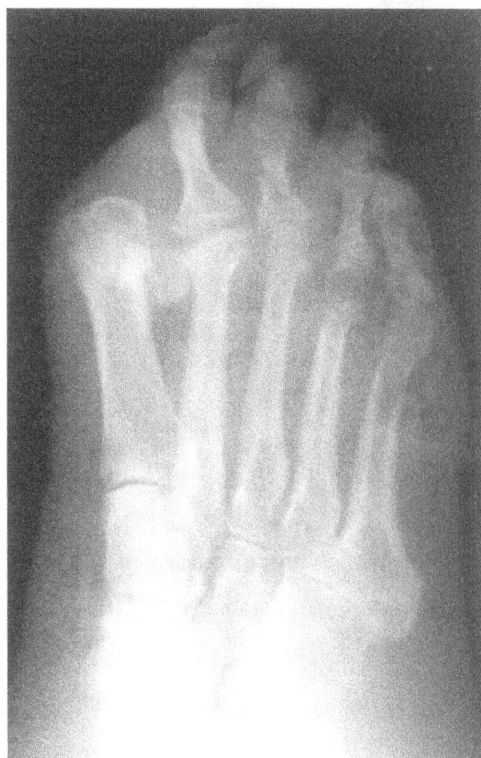

Figure 5.41
Diabetic with extensive gas forming infection of the soft tissues. Old amputation of the great toe. Recent fracture of the proximal phalanx of the 3rd toe.

5.10 Paget's Disease (Osteitis Deformans)

- a disease of unknown cause although infective origin is being considered (e.g. "slow" virus).

- it is a disease of the elderly and is common in the UK, parts of the USA, Australia and New Zealand but extremely rare in Africa and Asia.

- less than 20% of cases have single bone involvement. Overall, Paget's disease is found in the lumbar spine, followed by skull, pelvis and femur.

- 3 patterns of bone involvement are seen depending on the stage of the disease;

  a. Lytic phase – initial stage dominated by marked bone resorption. Lysis (loss of bone trabeculae) commences at a bone end and extends down the shaft. In a long bone the interface between the normal and abnormal tissue is sharply demarcated with a V-shaped configuration. In the skull large confluent area of lysis principally affecting the outer table (osteoporosis circumscripta) is seen.

b. Mixed phase – intermediate stage in which lytic areas start to be replaced by sclerosis (fig 5.42). There is also expansion of the affected bone with abnormally coarsened trabeculae.

c. Sclerotic phase – the bone becomes increasingly sclerotic (fig 5.43).

- pain may proceed any radiographic change.

- in the majority of people Paget's disease is asymptomatic and discovered as an incidental finding on a radiograph. Complications of Paget's disease include;
    — deformity (bowing of long bones as bone "soft", fig 5.43)
    — insufficiency fractures (usually transverse due to weakening of the bone)
    — degenerative joint disease adjacent to affected bones
    — malignant transformation (to an osteosarcoma, fig 5.44)

- despite recent advances in the treatment of bone sarcomas, malignant transformation in Paget's disease is rapidly fatal.

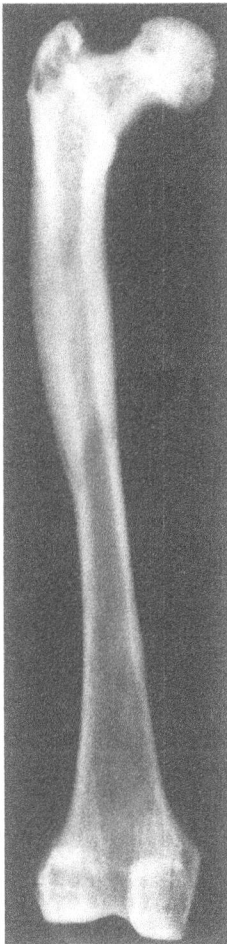

Figure 5.42
Specimen radiograph of the femur from the 1100 year old remains of an Anglo-saxon. There is sclerotic Paget's disease of the proximal femur. There is a small residual area of lytic Paget's distally with the typical V-shape.

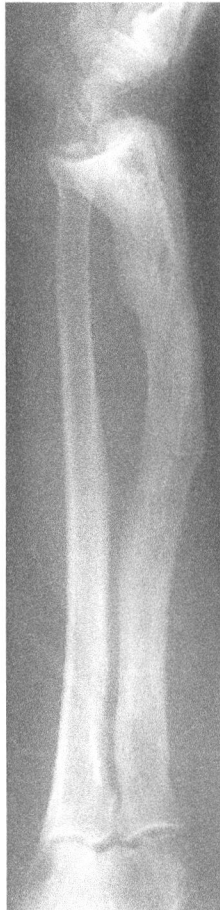

Figure 5.43
Sclerotic form of Paget's disease of the radius with bowing and a transverse fracture of the diaphysis.

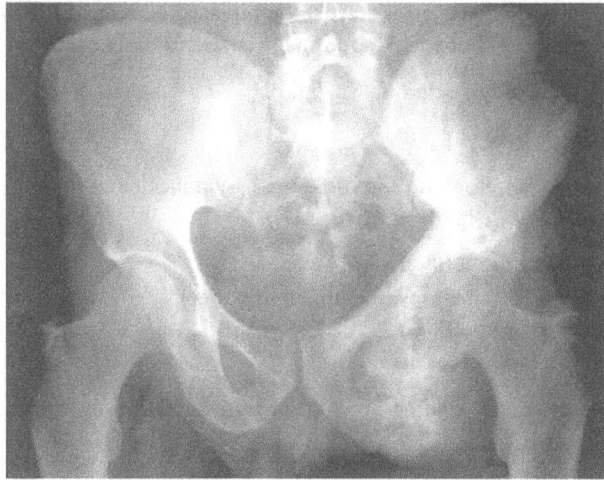

Figure 5.44
Extensive Paget's disease of the left hemipelvis. There is malignant transformation with an osteosarcoma arising from the left ischium.

5.11 **Sarcoidosis**

- a granulomatous disorder more common in young adults than in children or elderly.

- cause remains unknown but some evidence suggests infective aetiology.

- changes in the bones are found in less than 10% of the cases, and where present, focal bony destruction with a honeycomb or lattice-like appearance in the tubular bones of the hands and feet (fig 5.45) is seen.

- sclerotic bone involvement is very rare.

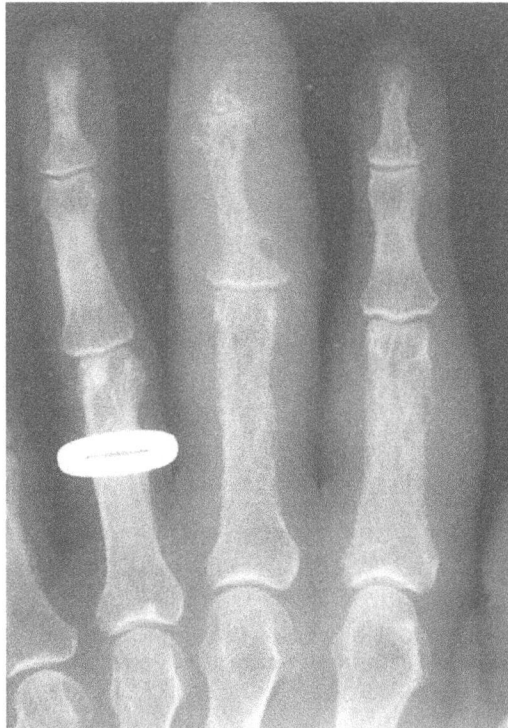

Figure 5.45
Sarcoidosis of the 2nd and 3rd fingers.

5.12 **Kaposi's Sarcoma**

- Kaposi's sarcoma is a multicentric vascular tumour with a viral aetiology.

- there is an increased incidence in immunosuppressed patients. Therefore, it is commonly found in AIDS patients.

- there are three clinical categories of Kaposi's sarcoma;

  a. Relatively slow progression is seen in older patients without immunosuppression living in temperate climates. If they then become immunosuppressed, the disease will progress rapidly, as in (b).

  b. Rapidly progressive/multifocal disease leading to death within 6 months to 3 years. This form is most common in younger people living in tropic countries, and often not associated with AIDS.

  c. Chronic disease associated with the development of other malignancies, especially lymphoma.

- radiographic features include;

  — multiple cutaneous nodules which may ulcerate
  — generalized oedema of the extremity
  — bone changes in advanced disease
  — osteoporosis
  — well defined cortical erosions
  — progression to bone destruction (fig 5.46)

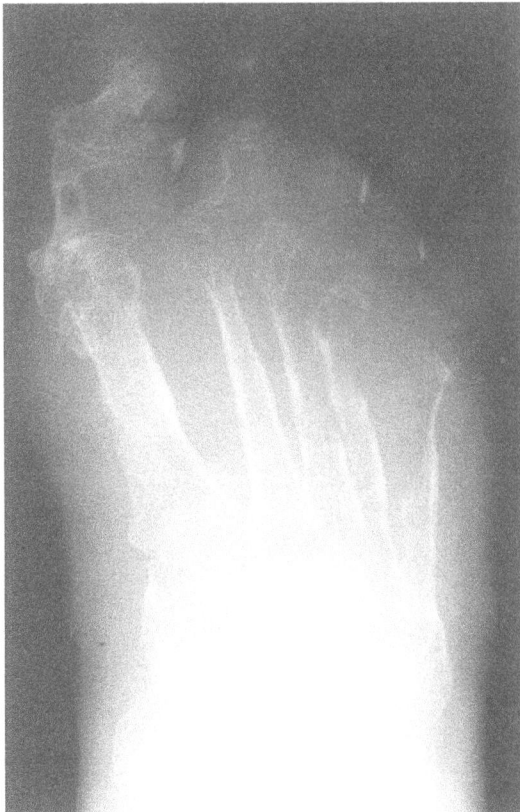

Figure 5.46
Kaposi's sarcoma of the foot. Advanced disease with extensive destruction of the forefoot. Much of the appearances are nonspecific but the cortical erosions along the 1st metatarsal are typical. This must be differentiated from Madura foot (Chapter 5.6.1)

Arthritis

Definitions

- the term *arthritis* refers to diffuse inflammatory and degenerative lesions of joints.

- there are 7 common types of arthritis;

  1. Degenerative joint disease (osteoarthritis)
  2. Rheumatoid arthritis
  3. Seronegative spondyloarthropathies
  4. Juvenile chronic arthritis
  5. Crystal-induced arthritis
  6. Neuropathic arthropathy
  7. Infective arthritis (pyogenic, tuberculous and fungal)

- the incidence of the different types of arthritis varies greatly between countries and continents.

- the first clinical sign of arthritis is a painful swollen joint. If there is a rapid onset of symptoms (within days or weeks) there is a strong possibility of infection (see Chapter 5).

- the interpretation of the radiographic examination of an arthritic joint should be approached in a systematic fashion looking for;

  — soft tissue changes
  — bone density changes
  — articular (joint) surface changes
  — bone alignment

- *soft tissue changes* usually means swelling but tissue loss is also important. In the fingers, fusiform (shaped like a spindle; pointed at both ends) periarticular (around the joint) swelling is typical of rheumatoid arthritis. Eccentric soft tissue swelling is typical of gout.

- *bone density* refers to how opaque (white) the bones appear on the radiograph. Is it increased or decreased? Increased bone density may be seen around joints in degenerative joint disease. If decreased, is it localised or generalized? If localised, is it periarticular? Periarticular reduced bone density often represents inflammatory disease, both infective and non-infective causes. Generalized reduced bone density may be due to a number of conditions including metabolic bone disease (see Chapter 7).

- *articular surface changes* refers to damage to the joint itself. Look for alterations to the joint space and the presence/absence of erosions. The *joint space* (the distance between two opposing bones) represents the two layers of radiolucent articular cartilage. Narrowing of the joint space indicates cartilage destruction. Inflammatory destruction often causes uniform narrowing across the entire joint, whereas nonuniform or asymmetric narrowing is typical of degenerative joint disease. *Erosions* (wearing away of bone) are foci of subchondral bone destruction. These are typically ill-defined and marginal in rheumatoid arthritis, whereas in gout they tend to be well-defined and periarticular.

- the *alignment* of bones across a joint may be altered in arthritis resulting in deformity or subluxation (incomplete dislocation). Ulnar subluxation of the metacarpophalangeal joints is typical of advanced rheumatoid arthritis. In the knee joint, medial joint compartment cartilage loss will result in outward bowing of the knee (varus deformity), whereas lateral compartment cartilage loss will result in inward bowing (valgus deformity).

6.1 Degenerative Joint Disease (Osteoarthritis, OA)

- *osteoarthritis* is defined as a non-inflammatory, localized degeneration of the hyaline cartilage in synovial joints. It is also known as *degenerative joint disease* which is the general phrase used to describe degenerative changes in any type of articulation (i.e. synovial, cartilaginous, or fibrous).

- numerous factors predispose to OA. Systemic factors include advancing age, genetic predisposition, physical activity including sport and occupation. Factors affecting a specific joint include trauma, pre-existing joint disease or deformity.

- the radiographic signs of OA are;
    - eccentric joint space narrowing leading to deformity
    - subchondral sclerosis (demineralization is **not** a feature of OA)
    - osteophyte formation
    - slow development over many years to decades

- an *osteophyte* is an outgrowth or excrescence of bone. Although they can occur in many conditions, they are typical of OA. The marginal osteophyte develops at the non-pressure segments of the joint to produce a bony lip or projection.

- *subchondral cysts* may be seen in OA and should not be mistaken for a neoplastic or infective process

- intra-articular *loose bodies* may be seen in longstanding OA as rounded fragments of bone within the joint. These should be distinguished from the more numerous osteocartilaginous loose bodies seen in synovial osteochondromatosis.

6.1.1 OA of the hip

- common site for OA, frequently bilateral, often asymmetric.

- 75% of the cases show superior joint space loss (figure 6.1).

- less common is medial joint space loss.

- thickening of the medial neck of femur is common (fig 6.1).

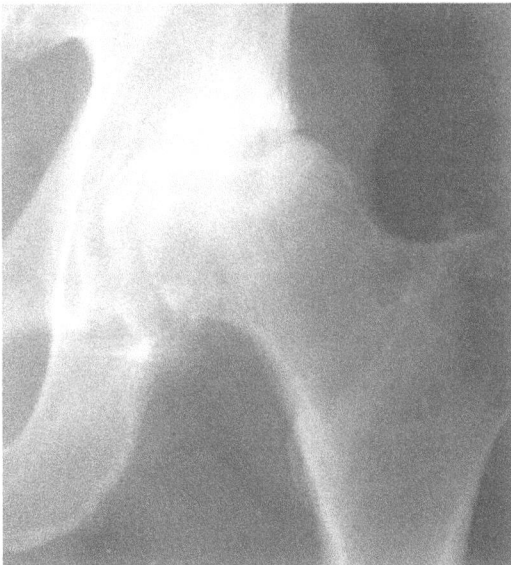

Figure 6.1
OA of the hip. There is loss of the superior hip joint space, subchondral sclerosis and cyst formation, and thickening of the medial neck of femur.

6.1.2 OA of the knee

- common site for OA, most common in females.

- almost all show medial joint space narrowing, with or without femoropatellar joint involvement (figure 6.2). In severe cases varus deformity of the knee may develop.

- lateral joint involvement is rare. If all compartments involved underlying rheumatoid arthritis must be considered.

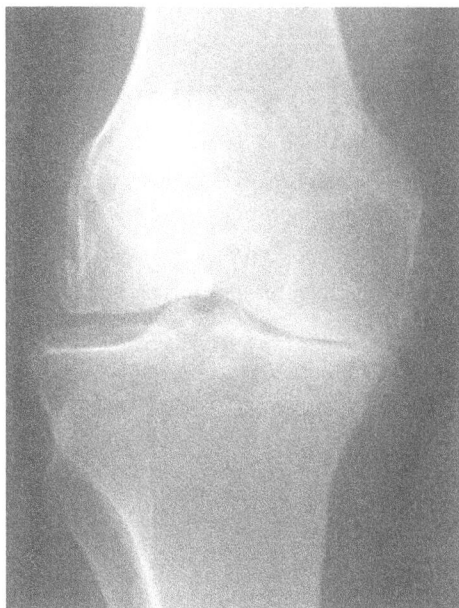

Figure 6.2
OA of the knee. There is loss of the medial joint space, subchondral sclerosis and marginal osteophyte formation.

6.1.3 OA of the ankle and foot

- typically involves the talonavicular and first metatarsophalangeal joints (hallux rigidus) (fig 6.3).

- if it involves intertarsal joints underlying neuropathy (e.g. diabetes) must be considered.

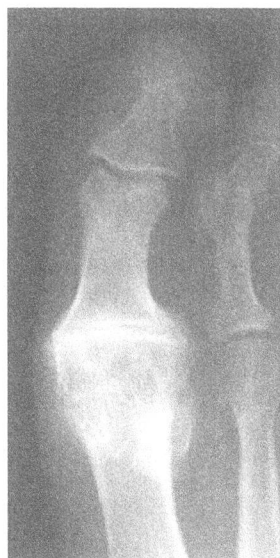

Figure 6.3
OA of the first MTP joint. There is joint space narrowing, subchondral sclerosis and osteophyte formation.

6.1.4 **OA of the shoulder**

- OA confined to the glenohumeral joint is uncommon.

- most frequently seen as the result of a longstanding rotator cuff defect.

6.1.5 **OA of the hand and wrist**

- involvement of the interphalangeal joints is common, particularly in middle-aged post-menopausal women. The first metacarpophalangeal joints are typically involved, usually bilaterally. This may be combined with OA of the scaphoid-trapezoid joint.

6.1.6 **OA of the spine**

- OA may affect the facet/apophyseal joints of the spine. In the lumbar spine, particularly at L4/5, facet joint OA may result in anterior slipping (degenerative spondylolisthesis) of the proximal segment with respect of the distal. If it is severe it can cause spinal canal and foraminal stenosis.

- patients with facet joint OA frequently also have degenerative disc disease (spondylosis deformans) which typically involves the lower cervical and lower lumbar discs.

6.2 **Rheumatoid Arthritis (RA)**

- *rheumatoid arthritis* is a common disease in some countries, rare in others. It is a generalized connective tissue disorder of unknown cause that can affect any synovial joint in the body.

- the radiographic signs of RA are;

      — soft tissue swelling
      — periarticular osteoporosis
      — diffuse joint space narrowing
      — marginal erosions
      — symmetric distribution of changes
      — fibrous or bony ankylosis in longstanding cases

- in early RA, synovial proliferation causes capsular distension and oedema of the surrounding tissues visible in the fingers as *fusiform soft tissue swelling*. Very early on the joint effusion may actually produce joint space widening before cartilage loss supervenes and causes joint space narrowing.

- the inflammatory hyperaemia causes localised demineralization seen as *periarticular osteoporosis*.

- the synovial proliferation causes *marginal erosions*. Early on these occur at the bare areas where the synovium is in direct contact with bone (fig 6.4).

- later on the erosive change destroys the articular cartilage with *joint space narrowing* (fig 6.5).

- Finally, joint deformity and rarely fibrous or *bony ankylosis* may develop.

6.2.1 **RA of the hand and wrist**

- earliest erosive findings are in the radial side of the metacarpal heads and bases of the proximal phalanges (fig 6.4). The distal interphalangeal joints are not affected early in the disease.

- early findings in the wrist are in the ulnar styloid, radial styloid, waist of scaphoid, triquetrum and pisiform.

- late findings in the hand include ulnar deviation/subluxation of the second to fifth metacarpophalangeal joints (fig 6.5).

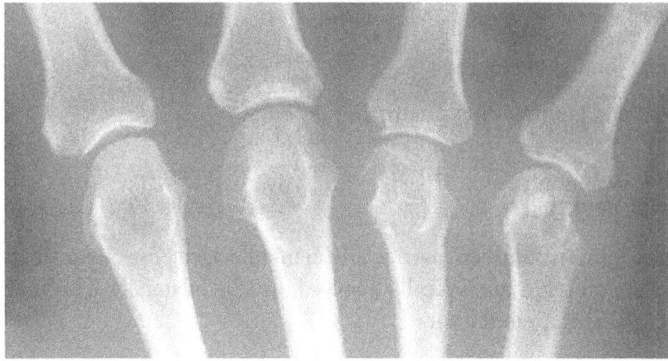

Figure 6.4
Early RA. There are marginal erosions affecting the 4th and 5th metatacarpal heads and the bases of the adjacent phalanges. The 2nd and 3rd metacarpophalangeal joints remain normal.

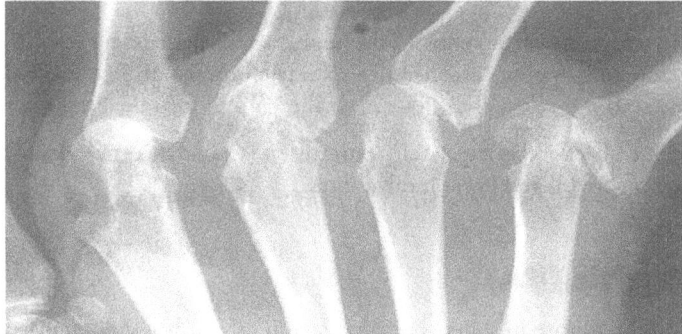

Figure 6.5
More advanced RA with large erosions, joint space narrowing and ulnar subluxations of the metacarpophalangeal joints.

6.2.2 RA of the foot

• earliest erosive findings are on the medial side of the metatarsal heads, particularly the fifth.

6.2.3 RA of the knee and hip

• uniform loss of joint space is typical (fig 6.6). In the hip concentric/axial narrowing of the joint occurs with a protrusion deformity in severe cases. Protrusio acetabuli refers to migration of the diseased hip into the pelvic cavity.

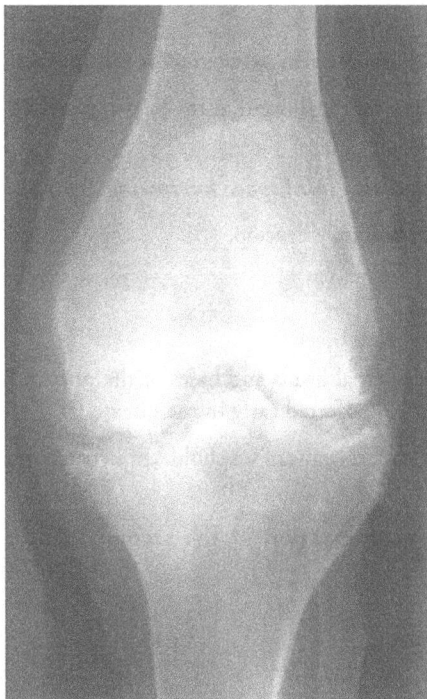

Figure 6.6
Chronic RA of the knee. Generalized reduced bone density. Uniform loss of joint space with erosions. Note that a similar appearance may be seen with a pyogenic arthritis (see Chapter 5).

- Osteophyte formation **not** seen in RA. However, with longstanding RA in weight bearing joints, degenerative joint disease may be superimposed. Then the degree of joint space narrowing is more severe than the sclerosis and osteophyte formation.

6.2.4 **RA of the spine**

- the cervical spine is more commonly involved than the thoracic or lumbar.

- atlantoaxial subluxation (anterior motion of C1 on C2) may occur due to transverse ligament instability. On the lateral radiograph an atlantoaxial distance greater than 2.5 mm indicates subluxation (figs 6.7 and 6.8). A lateral radiograph with the head flexed may be required to demonstrate the subluxation.

- impaction of the atlantoaxial joint is less common than atlantoaxial subluxation. There is then a cephalic (proximal) migration of the odontoid process relative to C1. This is as a result of rheumatoid disease of the C1/2 facet joint and is more often associated with neurologic symptoms (due to spinal cord compression) than atlantoaxial subluxation (fig 6.7).

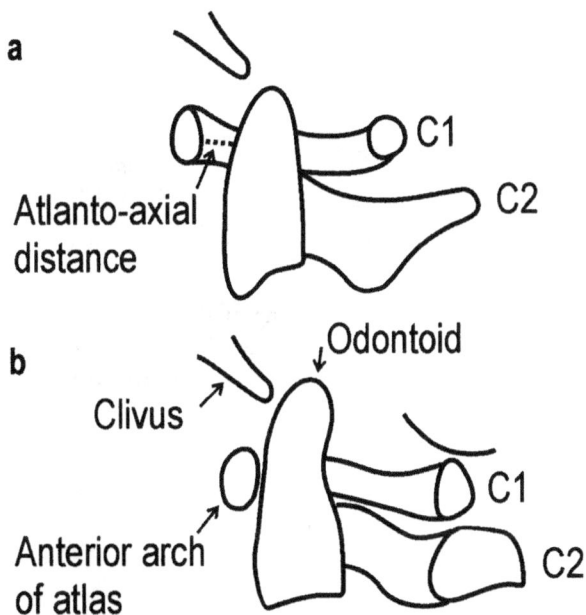

Figure 6.7
a) RA with atlantoaxial subluxation. The atlantoaxial distance exceeds 2.5 mm. b) RA with atlantoaxial impaction.

(modified from Manamaster, *Handbooks in Radiology: Skeletal Radiology*, Year Book Medical Publishers, Chicago, 1989).

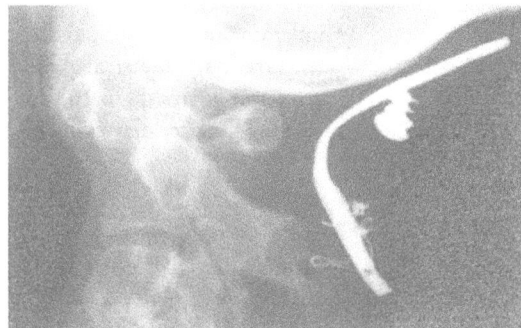

Figure 6.8
RA with severe atlantoaxial subluxation. The metal in the soft tissues behind the spine was an unsuccessful attempt at occipito-cervical fusion. Note the occipital screw has come loose.

6.3 **Seronegative Spondyloarthropathies**

- this group of conditions were formerly called "rheumatoid variants", and include a spectrum of arthritis and spinal complaints. They are all negative for rheumatoid factor autoantibodies.

- included are:
    - ankylosing spondylitis
    - psoriatic arthropathy
    - Reiter's syndrome
    - inflammatory bowel disease (ulcerative colitis and regional enteritis)

6.3.1 Ankylosing spondylitis (AS)

- a chronic inflammatory disease primarily affecting the spine. Commonest in young men.

- initial changes are a bilateral *sacroiliitis* (inflammation of the SI joints, fig 6.9). The stages of sacroiliitis are as follows;

    — initially affects lower and middle thirds of SI joint with the iliac side more severely affected than sacral
    — periarticular osteoporosis, erosions and subchondral sclerosis
    — further erosion leads to widening of joints
    — progresses to bony ankylosis

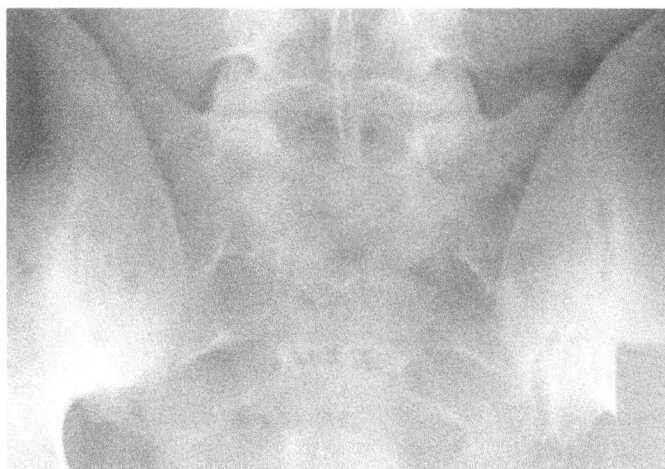

Figure 6.9
AS with early bilateral sacroiliitis. There is widening and irregularity of the SI joints with subchondral sclerosis.

- inflammatory changes at the discovertebral junction lead to squaring of the vertebral bodies (*osteitis*), symmetrical paravertebral ossification bridging the vertebral bodies (*marginal syndesmophytes*, fig 6.10) and in chronic cases discovertebral destruction (*pseudarthrosis*, fig 6.11). The latter may easily be mistaken for an infective discitis.

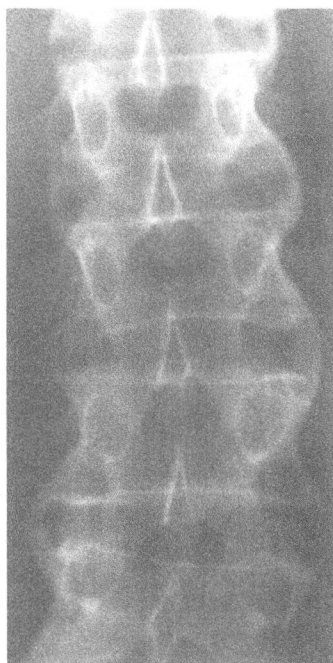

Figure 6.10
AS of the upper lumbar spine. Multiple level marginal syndesmophytes bridging the vertebral bodies.

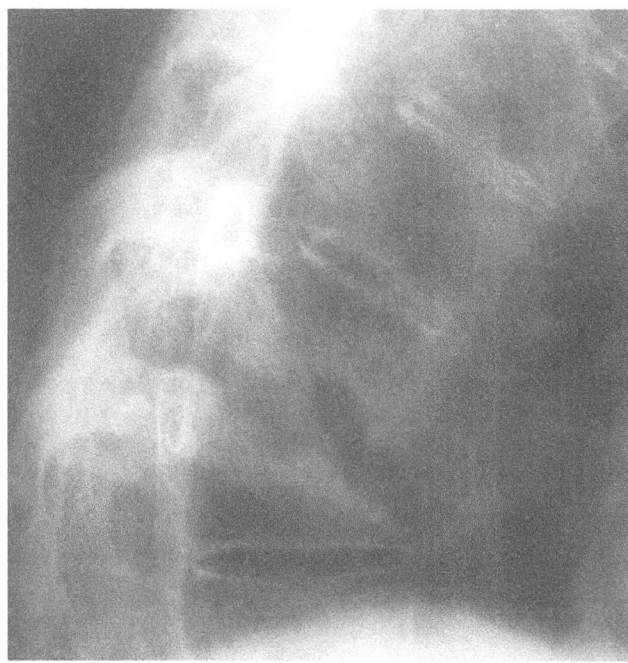

Figure 6.11
AS with discovertebral destruction (pseudarthrosis). The appearances mimic an infective discitis. Note the fusion above and below the pseudarthrosis.

- posteriorly in the spine, erosions, subchondral sclerosis and ankylosis affect the apophyseal joints, costotransverse joints, costovertebral joints and posterior ligaments. The end stage of AS is a fused spine (**bamboo spine**, fig 6.12).

- osteoporosis is a feature of longstanding disease. Because of the immobility and fragility of the spine, fractures following minor trauma are quite common. These fractures are frequently unstable because they involve all three columns of the fused spine (figs 4.70 and 6.13).

- involvement of the appendicular skeleton (i.e. the limbs) is eventually seen in about 50% of the patients. There is symmetric involvement of large joints with changes in the hands which are similar but less severe than RA.

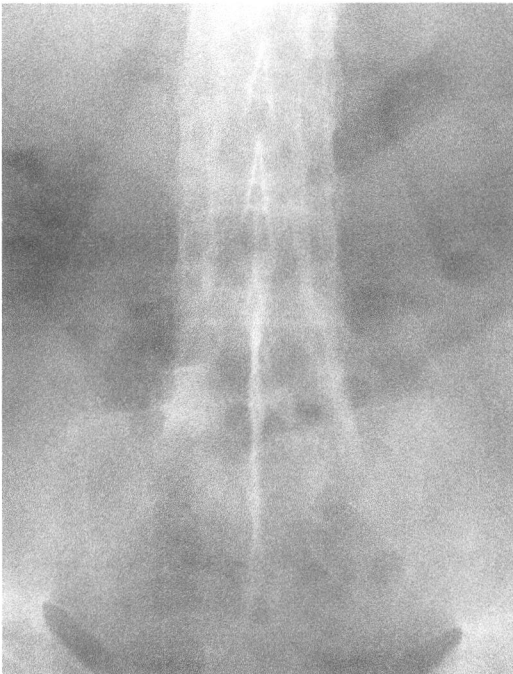

Figure 6.12
Chronic AS with a fused (bamboo) spine and fused SI joints.

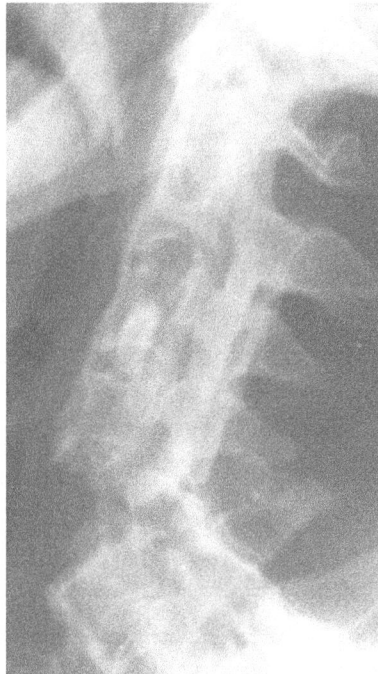

Figure 6.13
Chronic AS with a severe displaced unstable fracture of the cervical spine.

6.3.2 **Psoriatic arthropathy**

- psoriasis is a chronic skin condition in which an arthropathy may occur in a small number of the patients. Occasionally, the arthropathy may predate the skin changes.

- in the hands, the soft tissue swelling may be fusiform (as with RA) or more typically involve the entire digit. Bone density is generally normal (unlike RA). Erosions begin marginally (like RA) but progress to severe destruction with pencil-in-cup deformity (fig 6.14). The interphalangeal joints are involved more than the metacarpophalangeal joints. Productive changes produce small bony excrescence at and around joints. The distribution tends to be asymmetric (unlike RA).

- the SI joints may be involved in up to 30% cases. The sacroiliitis tends to be bilateral and symmetrical.

- in the spine, large bulky asymmetric osteophytes (non-marginal syndesmophytes) develop at the thoracolumbar junction. These tend to be more coarse than the marginal syndesmophytes seen in AS.

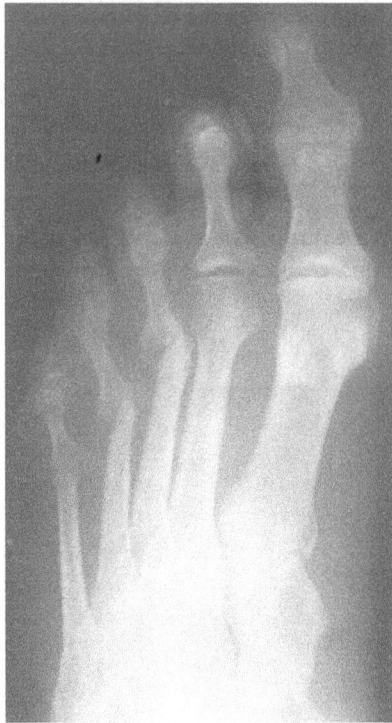

Figure 6.14
Psoriatic arthropathy with pencil-in-cup deformity affecting the 3rd to 5th metacarpophalangeal joints.

6.3.3 **Reiter's syndrome**

- this syndrome includes the triad of urethritis, conjunctivitis and arthritis occurring almost exclusively in males.

- there are two types: endemic, contracted by venereal exposure (sexually transmitted), and an epidemic type developing after dysentery.

- a distinctive feature is erosions with "fluffy" periosteal reaction at the metatarsal necks, proximal phalanges and calcaneus (fig 6.15).

- bilateral sacroiliitis, indistinguishable from AS and psoriatic arthropathy.

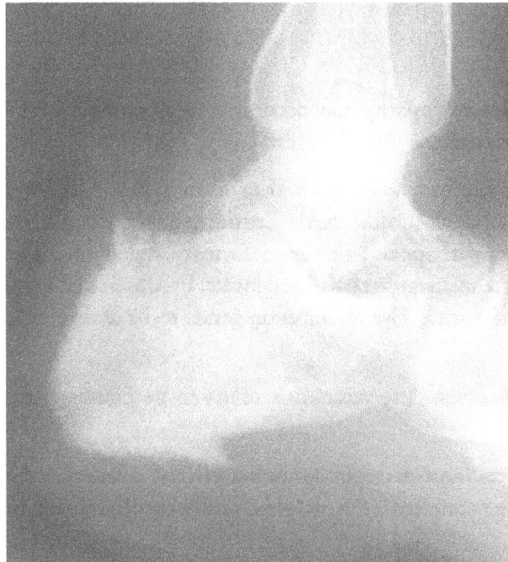

Figure 6.15
Reiter's syndrome. Combination of erosions and "fluffy" new bone formation at the insertion of the achilles tendon and origin of the plantar fascia.

6.4 Juvenile Chronic Arthritis (JCA)

- JCA consists of a heterogeneous group of joint diseases affecting children.

- most of the children have seronegative chronic arthritis, usually presenting before the age of 5 years.

- the early appearances are similar to RA, with soft tissue swelling and juxta-articular osteoporosis.

- because of hyperaemia the epiphyses show increased growth and appear large in relation to the diaphyses. The carpal bones appear irregular (fig 6.16).

- joint space narrowing and erosions are a late feature of the disease.

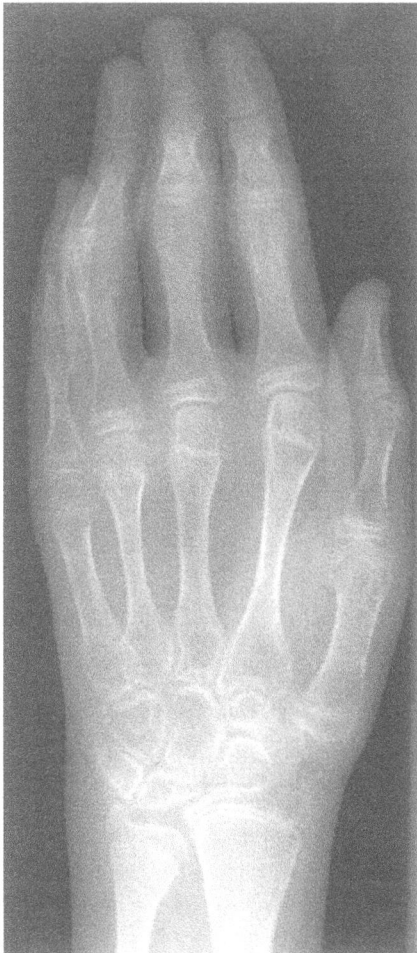

Figure 6.16
Juvenile chronic arthritis. There is generalized loss of bone density, with hypertrophy of the metacarpal epiphyses and squaring and irregularity of the carpal bones.

6.5 Crystal-induced Arthritis

- this is a heterogeneous group of arthropathies characterized by the deposition of different types of crystals in joints.

- the three common types are;
    — uric acid crystals (gout)
    — calcium pyrophosphate dihydrate deposition disease (CPPD)
    — calcium hydroxyapatite disease (CHD)

6.5.1 **Gout**

- there are 2 forms; *acute gout* and *chronic tophaceous gout*. In acute gout there is inflammatory capsular and soft tissue swelling in response to the precipitation of monosodium urate crystals in a synovial joint. 70% of the cases affect the 1st MTP joint.

- chronic tophaceous gout produces eccentric, asymmetrical nodular deposits of calcium urate (tophi) in the synovium, subchondral bone, soft tissues of the ear, hands, feet and around the elbow (figs 6.17 and 6.18). Calcification is an uncommon and late feature (fig 6.18). The joint space is relatively well preserved until late in the disease. Osteoporosis is **not** a feature of gout (unlike RA). The tophi produce large bone erosions which may be intra-articular, periarticular or well away from the joint (fig 6.17). An osteophyte-like overhanging lip to the erosions is characteristic of gout.

- when treatment is instituted early, radiographic bone changes are not seen.

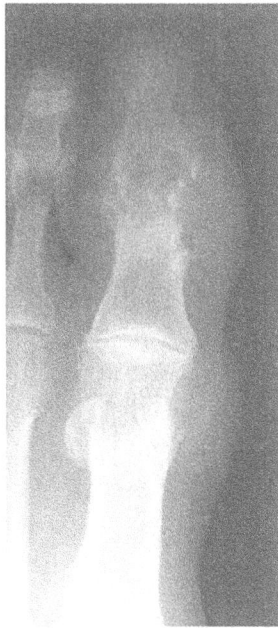

Figure 6.17
Chronic tophaceous gout involving the 1st MTP and IP joint of the great toe. Eccentric soft tissue swelling (tophi) with underlying relatively well defined erosions.

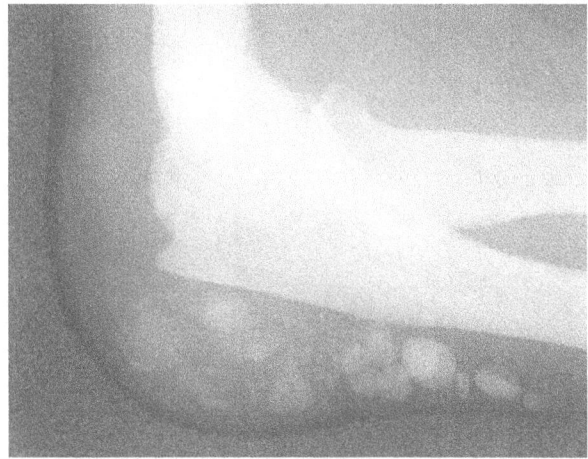

Figure 6.18
Chronic tophaceous gout with calcification of the tophi in the inflamed olecranon burrs.

6.5.2 **Calcium pyrophosphate dihydrate deposition disease (CPPD)**

- in CPPD crystals of calcium pyrophosphate become deposited in cartilage. The crystals become visible on radiographs as thin linear deposits of calcium in the articular hyaline cartilage and fibrocartilage (*chondrocalcinosis*) (fig 6.19). Longstanding CPPD is associated with degenerative joint disease.

- there is an acute synovitis if crystals are shed into the joint (*pseudogout*).

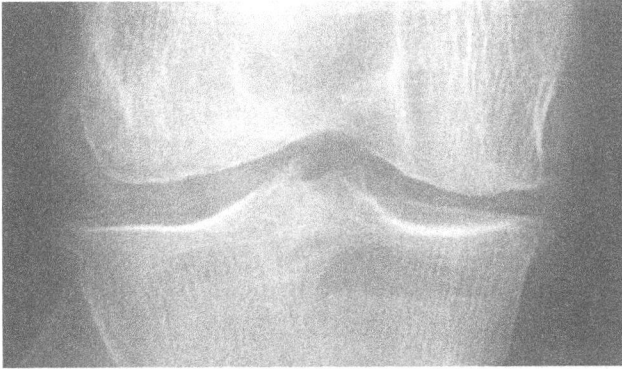

Figure 6.19
Chondrocalcinosis (cartilage calcification) due to CPPD.

6.5.3 Calcium hydroxyapatite disease (CHD)

- the typical appearance of CHD is an amorphous mineralized deposit in the rotator cuff or adjacent to the greater trochanter (fig 6.20).

- a localized inflammatory response is provoked if the crystals are shed into the adjacent bursa.

- CHD may also been seen in patients on renal dialysis, and in collagen vascular diseases such as scleroderma and dermatomyositis.

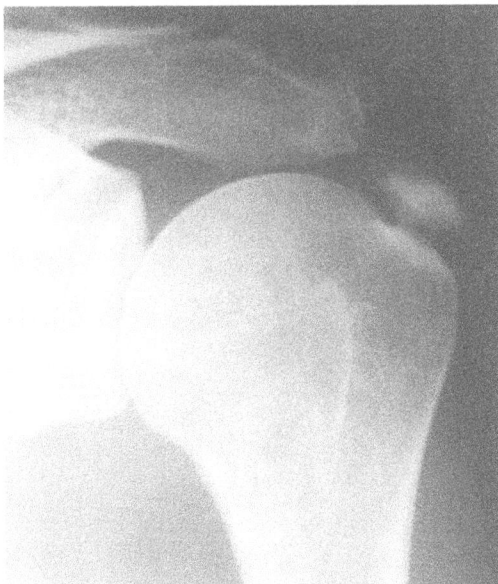

Figure 6.20
CHD deposition in the rotator cuff tendons.

6.6 Neuropathic Arthropathy (Charcot Joint)

- a severely destructive arthropathy, usually affecting a single joint, may develop in the presence of a neuropathy. Common causes include diabetes (in the foot), tabes dorsalis (tertiary syphilis) (in the hip and knee), and syringomyelia (i.e. cystic change in the spinal cord) and leprosy.

- typical features of the *hypertrophic form* of neuropathic arthropathy are (fig 6.21);

    — large joint effusion (seen as soft tissue swelling)
    — loss of joint space
    — bony debris/fragmentation
    — subluxation/dislocation of joint
    — normal or increased bone density

- approximately one third of neuropathic joints are the **atrophic form** with a sharp cut-off and resorption of the articular ends of the bone (fig 6.22).

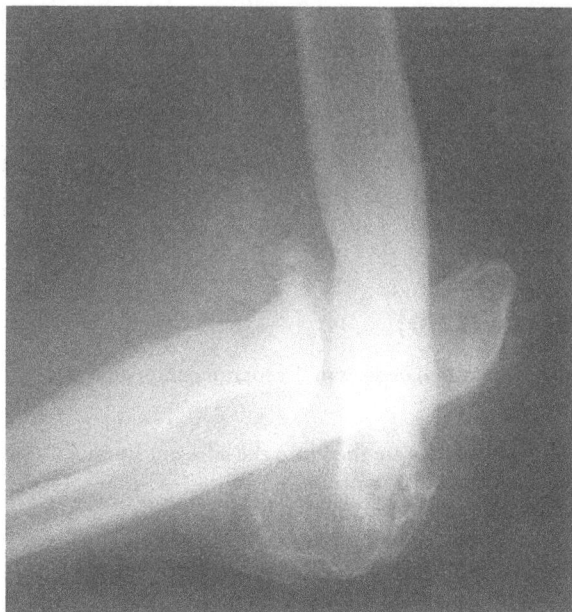

Figure 6.21
Hypertrophic form of neuropathic arthropathy affecting the elbow. There is increased bone density, dislocation, loss of joint space and bony debris/fragmentation.

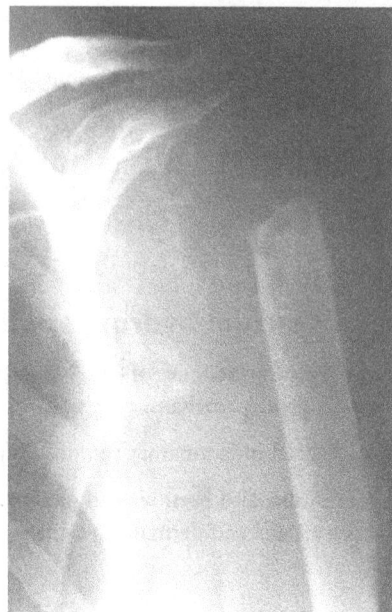

Figure 6.22
Atrophic form of neuropathic arthropathy affecting the shoulder in a patient with syringomyelia.

6.7 **Infective Arthritis**

- see Chapters 5.3 and 5.4.1

CHAPTER 7

Metabolic, Endocrine and Toxic Disorders

7.1 Metabolic Disturbances

7.1.1 Osteoporosis

- **osteoporosis** is the most common metabolic bone disease and is causing a decrease in bone mass. The microstructure of bone is normal, but the quantity of bone is reduced.

- the loss of bone density increases the risk of fractures, particularly the neck of femur, spine (wedge compression fractures, fig 4.141), and distal radius.

- there are numerous causes of osteoporosis including;

  — deficiency states and malnutrition
  — steroid therapy and Cushing's disease
  — chronic liver disease

- the radiographic features of osteoporosis are:

  — reduced bone density (at least 40–50% reduction must occur before it can be recognized on the radiograph)
  — loss of trabeculae (remaining trabeculae appear more prominent)
  — cortical thinning
  — fractures (vertebral wedge compression fractures)

- osteoporosis is a specific term referring to loss of bone mass and is not synonymous with osteopenia or de-ossification. Osteopenia and demineralization are general descriptive terms referring to reduced bone density, irrespective of the cause.

7.1.2 Rickets and osteomalacia

- **rickets and osteomalacia** are the same condition, occurring in children and adults respectively. There is lack of mineralization of normal osteoid.

- caused by **vitamin D deficiency** which may be due to;

  — dietary deficiency
  — gastrointestinal malabsorption
  — liver disease
  — anticonvulsant therapy
  — renal osteodystrophy
    (combination of osteomalacia and secondary hyperparathyroidism)
  — lack of sunlight (ultraviolet light)

- radiographic features common to both rickets and osteomalacia include;

  — generalized loss of bone density (osteopenia)
  — loss of corticomedullar differentiation
    (cortex and medulla of bone no longer seen as separate structures)
  — in severe cases bone softening with development of deformity

- the radiographic features of rickets are as above plus (figs 7.1);

  — splayed frayed metaphyses with widening of the growth plate
  — in less severe cases lucent metaphyseal band will be seen

- radiographic features of osteomalacia as above plus **pseudofractures** (demineralized zones) (fig 7.2);

  — a narrow lucent zone running perpendicular to cortex
  — this is due to insufficiency stress fractures repaired by non-ossified osteoid
  — frequently bilateral and symmetrical
  — common sites include pubic rami, proximal femur, scapula, ribs and ulna
  — uncommon in rickets

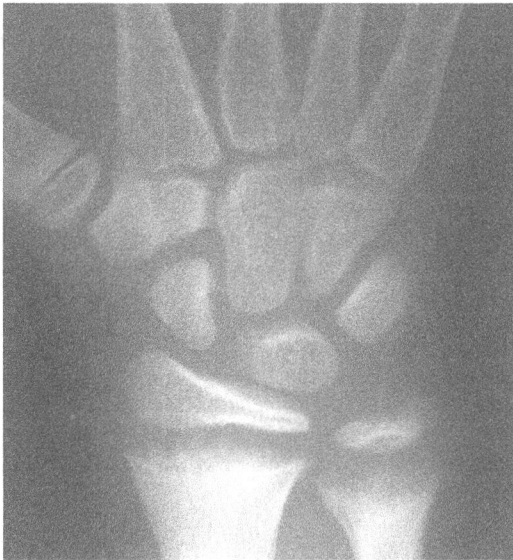

(a)

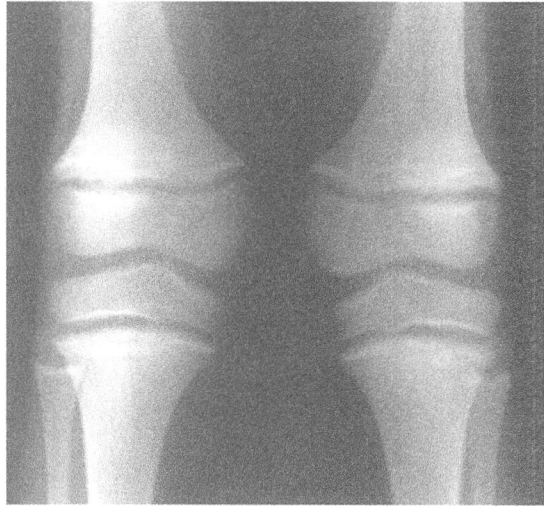

(b)

Figure 7.1
PA of the wrist (a) and knees (b) in a child with dietary rickets. There is generalized reduced bone density with widening of the growth plates and splaying of the metaphyses.

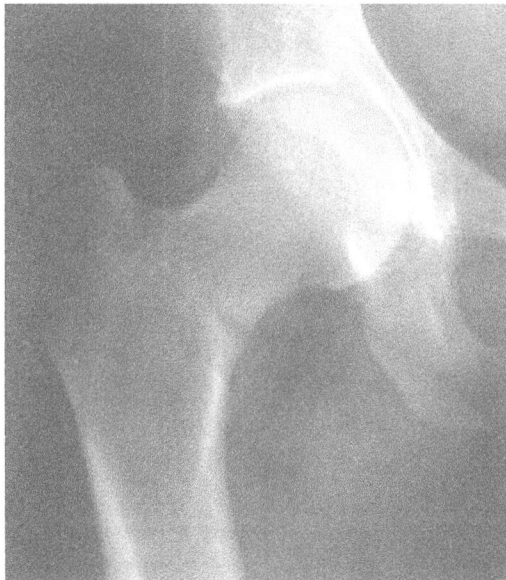

Figure 7.2
AP of the hip of an adult with osteomalacia. There is generalized reduced bone density and loss of corticomedullary differentiation of the femoral head. The lucent line traversing the medial cortex of the femoral neck is the typical appearance and site for a pseudofracture.

7.1.3 **Scurvy**

- *scurvy* is due to *vitamin C deficiency* resulting in abnormal collagen formation.

- the radiographic abnormalities in adults are nonspecific generalized loss of bone density (osteopenia).

- scurvy is rare under 6 months of age

- the radiographic features in children include (fig 7.3):

    — generalized loss of bone density (osteopenia)
    — subperiosteal haemorrhage leading to subperiosteal new bone formation
    — small sharply marginated epiphyses
    — dense metaphyseal line
    — metaphyseal corner fractures

- the radiographic findings of scurvy must be distinguished from those caused by child abuse (the battered child syndrome) which in some communities is more common than scurvy.

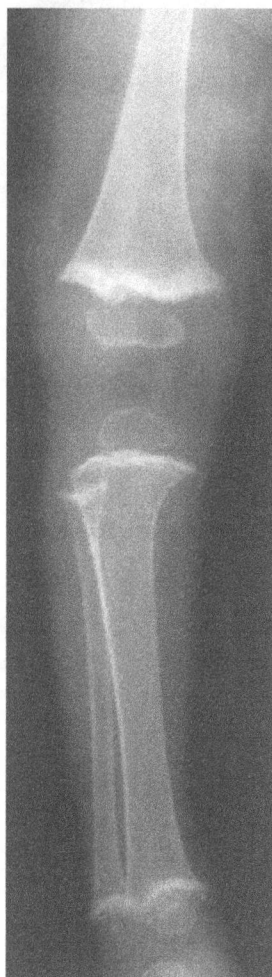

Figure 7.3
Lower leg in a child with scurvy. There is generalized reduced bone density, sharply defined epiphyses with sclerotic metaphyseal margins.

7.2 Endocrine Disturbances

7.2.1 Acromegaly

- skeletal overgrowth is known as *gigantism* in the immature skeleton, and *acromegaly* in the adult. Both result from excessive growth hormone production by a pituitary gland adenoma.

- the radiographic features include:

    — skull: pituitary fossa enlargement
                    frontal bossing (thickening of the frontal bones)
                    enlarged paranasal sinuses
    — spine: enlarged vertebral bodies
                    posterior scalloping (concave edges)
    — hand: large hands with spade-like terminal phalanges (fig 7.4)
                    widening of joint space due to thick cartilage
                    prominent bony projections at tendon attachments

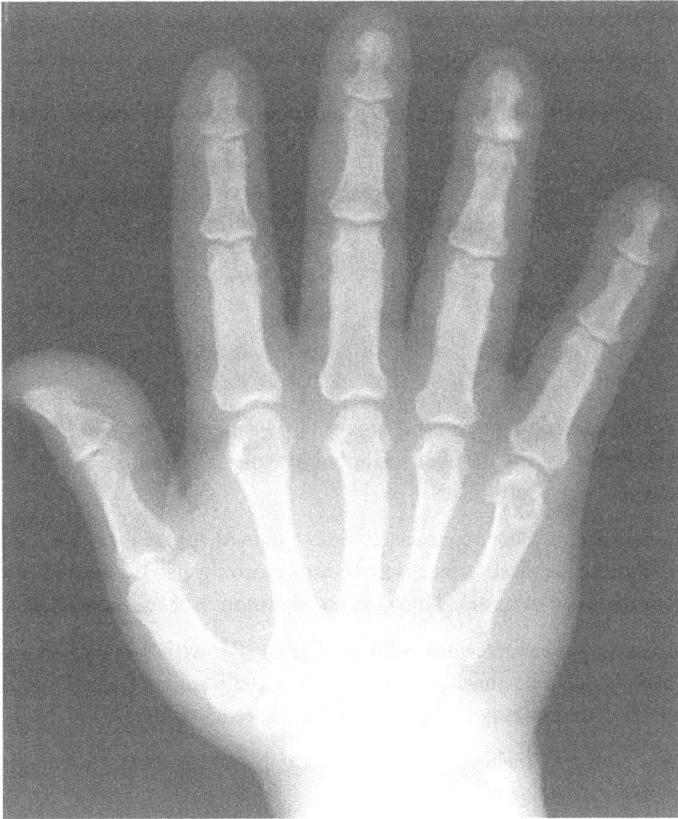

Figure 7.4
Acromegaly. Overall
enlargement of the hand with
spade-like terminal phalanges,
wide joint spaces and hook-like
appearance to the distal
metacarpals.

7.2.2 **Hypothyroidism**

- it is due to insufficient production of thyroxine.

- in children (cretinism) there is delayed skeletal maturation and growth retardation. The epiphyses, particularly the proximal femur, appear irregular and fragmented (fig 7.5).

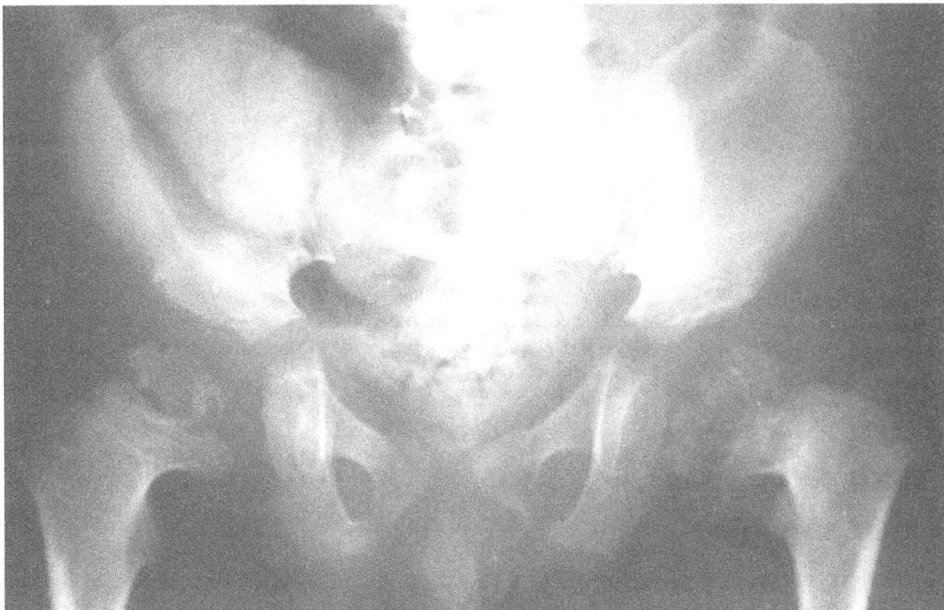

Figure 7.5
AP of the pelvis in a child with hypothyroidism (cretinism). There is irregular fragmentation of the *proximal femoral epiphyses mimicking a congenital* epiphyseal dysplasia. Note the severe constipation which is another feature of this condition.

7.2.3 **Hyperparathyroidism (HPT)**

- there are three forms of HPT; primary, secondary and tertiary.

  Primary HPT is due to excessive production of parathormone as a result of parathyroid adenoma (75%), hyperplasia or carcinoma.

  Secondary HPT is due to parathyroid hyperplasia in response to persistent hypocalcaemia (low blood calcium) and is seen in rickets, osteomalacia and chronic renal failure.

  Tertiary HPT applies to cases of secondary HPT which gives rise to autonomous HPT (i.e. HPT exists irrespective of the initial low blood calcium).

- the radiographic appearances of HPT are due to bone resorption which results in loss of bone density (osteopenia) and include (figs 7.6 and 7.7);

  — subperiosteal erosion (particularly along the radial aspect of phalanges in the hand)
  — subchondral resorption (erosions of the distal clavicle, pubic symphysis and SI joints)
  — Brown tumours (see below)

- ***Brown tumours***, called brown because of their macroscopic blood stained appearance, are lytic expansive lesions resulting from intense localized osteoclastic (bone-resorbing cells) activity. They are quite well defined and can mimic true tumours. They are less common in secondary HPT.

- in secondary HPT, the radiographic appearances are as in primary HPT with features of the underlying cause i.e. rickets, osteomalacia or chronic renal failure. Calcification of arteries and soft tissues occurs in secondary HPT particularly in cases with chronic renal failure.

- ***renal osteodystrophy*** is the term applied to the bone changes associated with chronic renal failure. These include secondary HPT, osteomalacia and osteosclerosis.

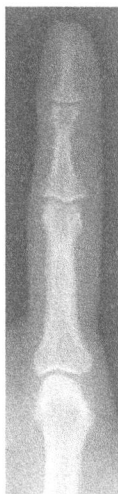

Figure 7.6
Primary hyperparathyroidism. Generalised osteopenia, terminal phalangeal and subperiosteal resorption.

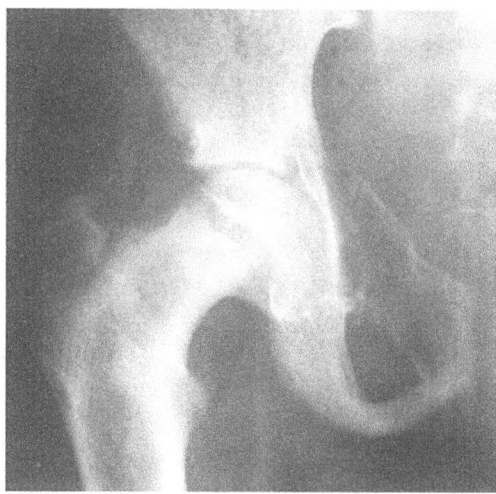

Figure 7.7
Secondary hyperparathyroidism due to chronic renal failure. There is a Brown tumour in the pubis and evidence of rickets with widening of the proximal femoral growth plate.

7.3 **Toxic Reactions**

7.3.1 **Lead poisoning**

- lead poisoning occurs in children who ingest lead-containing paints or water delivered by lead pipes. The typical radiographic appearance is a transverse band of metaphyseal sclerosis (fig 7.8).

- a similar appearance may be seen with Bismuth poisoning.

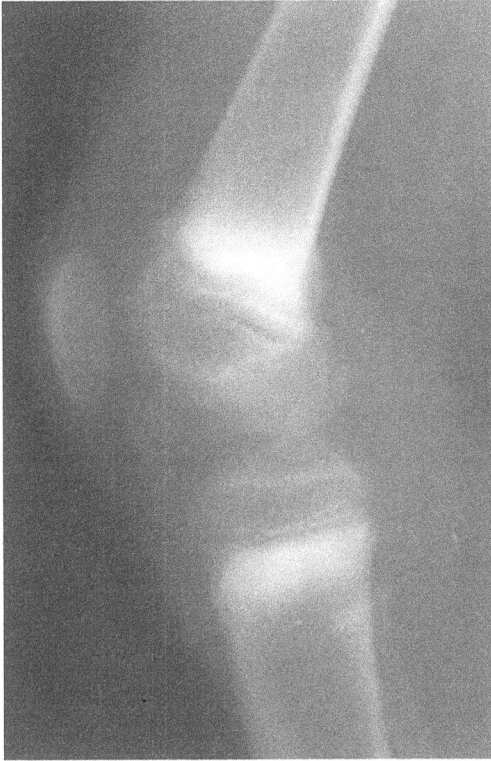

Figure 7.8
Child with lead poisoning. The diagnosis is indicated by the presence of a sclerotic metaphyseal bands.

7.3.2 **Fluorosis**

- fluorosis occurs due to chronic fluoride poisoning. It is endemic in some parts of the world.

- there is a generalized increase in bone density with prominence of ligamentous and musculotendinous attachments. It needs to be distinguished from other causes of diffuse increased bone density such as prostatic metastases and myelofibrosis.

CHAPTER 8

Haemopoietic and Lymphoreticular Disorders

8.1 Diseases Affecting Red Blood Cells

- these diseases, known as haemoglobinopathies, affect red bone marrow producing chronic haemolytic anaemia. The striking skeletal abnormalities result from severe marrow hyperplasia. Most are congenital and hereditary in origin.

8.1.1 Thalassaemia

- also known as Cooley's anaemia and Mediterranean anaemia. It is due to an inherited failure to produce sufficient globin.

- most common in the countries bordering the Mediterranean sea but also extending through Asia and West Africa.

- 2 forms – the most severe form, inherited from both parents and the less severe form, Thalassaemia Minor, inherited from one parent only. Thalassaemia Major presents during infancy or early childhood and affected patients often die in adolescence.

- the radiographic changes are secondary to the marrow hyperplasia and include (fig 8.1 and 8.2);

  — generalized osteopenia due to trabecular loss
  — expansion of long bones with thinning of the cortices
  — expansion of the diploic space (marrow between inner and outer tables of skull) with a so-called "hair-on-end" appearance on radiographs
  — infarcts and avascular necrosis less common than in sickle cell disease (see Chapter 8.1.2)
  — obliteration of facial sinuses due to extensive increase of "hyperactive" red marrow
  — "hyperactive" red marrow may also occur outside skeleton (extramedullary haematopoiesis) thereby producing soft tissue masses which are often located along the thoracic spine.

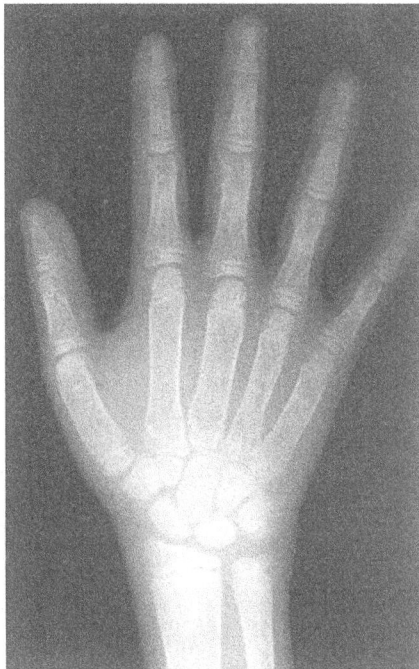

Figure 8.1
Thalassaemia showing generalised osteopenia, mild expansion of the tubular bones with thinning of the cortices.

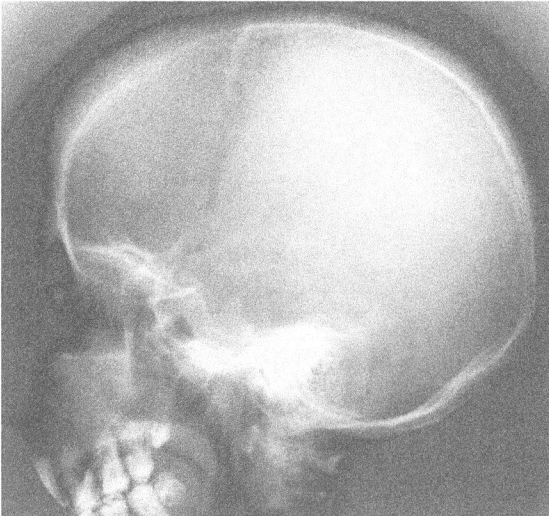

Figure 8.2
Thalassaemia with thickening of the skull vault and obliteration of the sinuses by the marrow hyperplasia.

8.1.2 **Sickle cell disease**

- an inherited disease causing production of abnormal haemoglobin.

- most frequently found in tropical African countries, but also in North and Central America and the Caribbean.

- 2 forms exist – the severe homozygous form and a less severe heterozygous form.

- clinically the severe form is characterized by severe anaemia and bone infarction often causing acute episodes of skeletal and abdomonal pain.

- the radiographic appearances, due to a combination of marrow hyperplasia and bone infarction, include (fig 8.3–8.5);

  — generalized osteopenia (less marked than in Thalassaemia)
  — deposition of new bone on inner surface of cortex (endosteal apposition) which may cause bone sclerosis and the so-called "bone-within-a bone"-appearance
  — bone infarction   acute (resembles osteomyelitis)
                                chronic (serpiginous calcification)
                                avascular necrosis (femoral and humeral heads)
                                vertebral endplates (central endplate depression)
  — osteomyelitis   there is an increased incidence of osteomyelitis usually associated with infarction. Staphylococcus is the most common organism but Salmonella osteomyelitis much more common in patients with sickle cell disease than the normal population.

- massive bone infarction in hands and feet (hand-foot syndrome) causes aseptic dactylitis (dactylitis = inflammation of the fingers or toes, fig 8.5). Radiographically this may be indistinguishable from osteomyelitis. In children the growth plates in the hands and feet may be damaged resulting in premature fusion and subsequent shortening of the affected limb or part of limb.

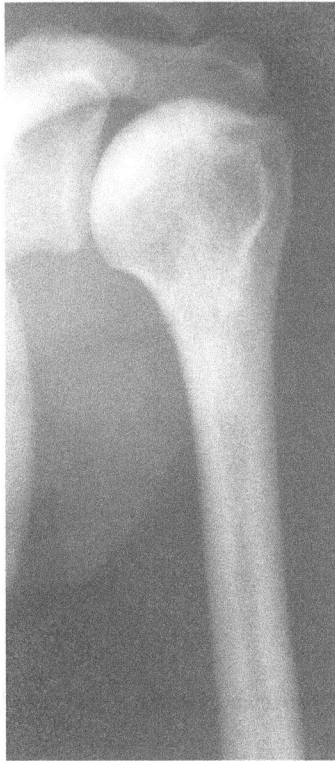

Figure 8.3
Sickle cell disease. There is
sclerosis in the humeral head
indicating chronic avascular
necrosis. There is also thickening
of the proximal humeral cortex
due to the endosteal apposition of
new bone.

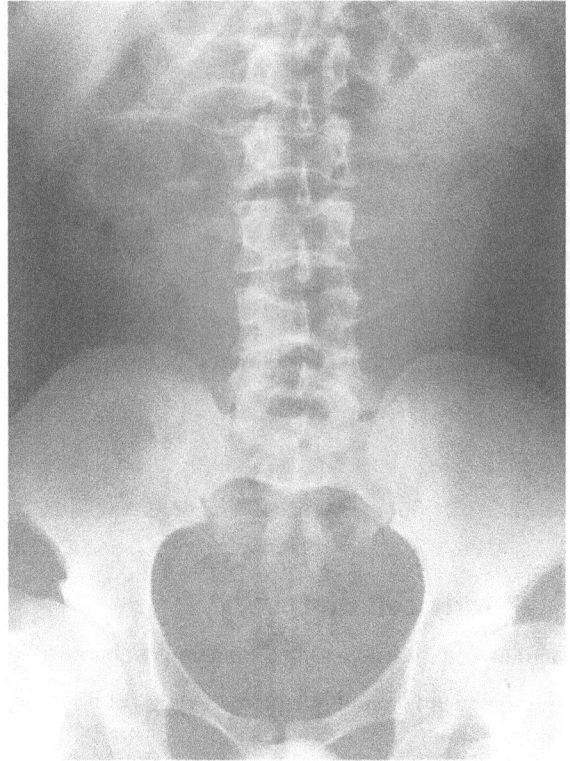

Figure 8.4
Chronic sickle cell disease. There are endplate depressions
affecting multiple lumbar vertebrae. The flattened dysplastic
hips are due to avascular necrosis in childhood.

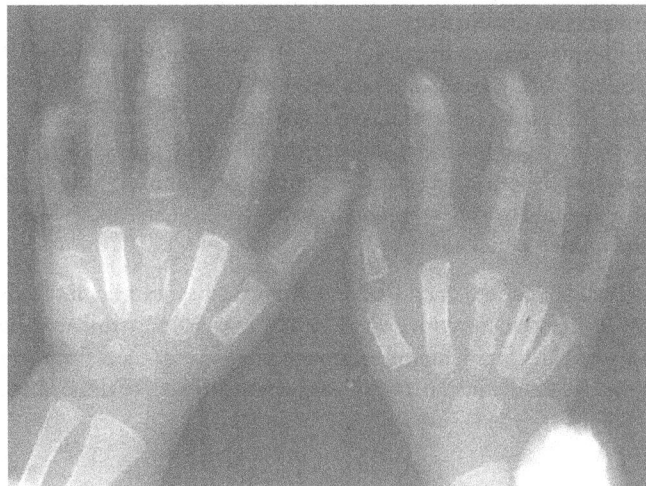

Figure 8.5
Acute sickle cell dactylitis affecting
the metacarpals bilaterally.

8.2 **Diseases Affecting White Blood Cells**

8.2.1 **Leukaemia**

- acute leukaemia is the most common type in children, whereas chronic forms dominate in adults. Radiographically acute and chronic types cannot be distinguished from each other.

- over 50% of children, and less than 10% of adults, will develop radiographic changes of the skeleton, including (fig 8.6);

    — generalized osteopenia (may result in vertebral collapse)
    — transverse metaphyseal lucencies
    — medial metaphyseal erosions especially in the humerus and tibia
    — lytic bone lesions which can mimic a primary sarcoma

- the incidence of leukaemia shows marked geographic and racial variation.

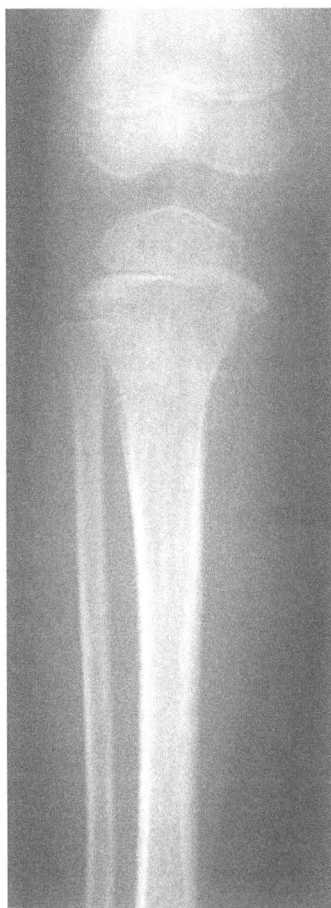

Figure 8.6
Acute leukaemia. There is loss of bone density with a destructive lesion in the proximal tibial metaphysis. Similar features may be seen in acute osteomyelitis and primary sarcoma of bone.

8.2.2 **Myelofibrosis**

- a disease seen in middle aged or elderly patients causing development of fibrous tissue from bone marrow cells. Also known as myeloid metaplasia and myelosclerosis.

- in later stages of disease the fibrous marrow is converted into bone, producing generalized bony sclerosis radiographically similar to some bone dysplasias (see Chapter 10) and diffuse sclerotic metastases (fig 8.7).

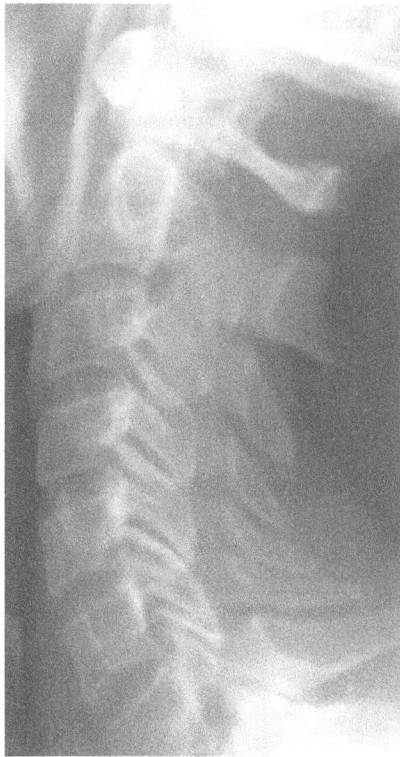
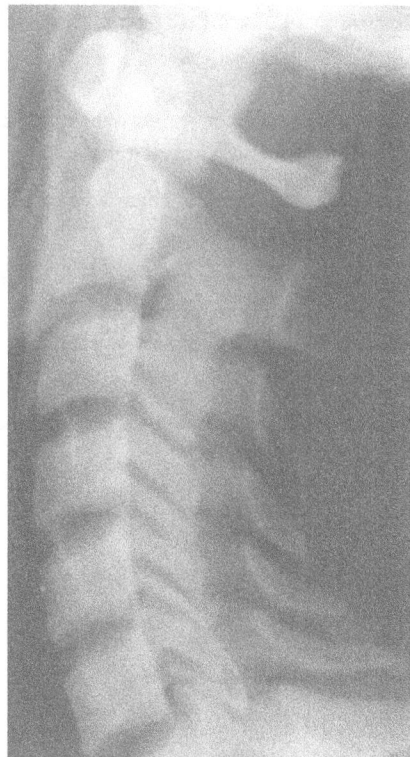

(a)   (b)

Figure 8.7
Middle aged woman with myelofibrosis. (a) At presentation the bone density is normal and the distinction between the cortex and marrow of the vertebral bodies preserved; (b) 5 years later there is now dense sclerosis affecting all the vertebrae.

8.3 **Disorders of the Lymphoreticular System**

8.3.1 **Lymphoma**

- malignant lymphomas can be divided into two groups

  1. Hodgkin's disease
  2. Non-Hodgkin's lymphoma

Hodgkin's disease

- primary Hodgkin's lymphoma of bone is rare. It is almost always secondary to primary lymph node disease.

- more than 75% of the cases involve the axial skeleton, particularly the spine.

- 25% of the lesions are lytic, 15% sclerotic and 60% mixed. In the spine sclerotic changes (so-called ivory vertebra) are typical (fig 8.8). A similar appearance may be seen with tuberculosis, Paget's disease and sclerotic metastases. Enlarged abdominal lymph nodes may produce pressure erosion of the anterior aspects of lumbar vertebrae (anterior scalloping).

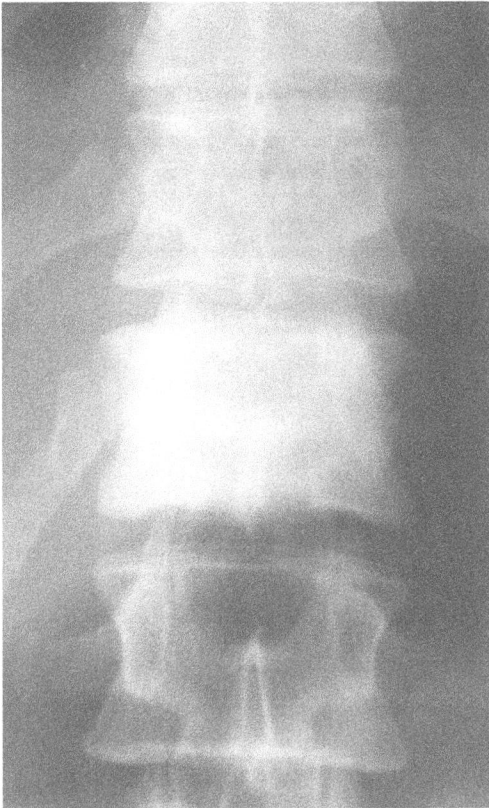

Figure 8.8
Ivory (uniformly dense) vertebra due to Hodgkin's lymphoma.

Non-Hodgkin's lymphoma

- the bone lesions are predominantly lytic with a large soft tissue component. Permeative bone destruction with a wide zone of transition may resemble a primary sarcoma or metastasis.

Burkitt's lymphoma

- this is a disease which occurs predominantly in children in the tropical zones of Africa, and South America. In parts of Africa it accounts for over 50% of all malignant tumours of childhood. It is associated with the Epstein-Barr virus.

- the disease is almost always multifocal at presentation and large destructive lesions in the mandible and maxilla are often seen as bone lesions are lytic. In addition ovarian and other soft tissue masses are common.

8.3.2 **Mastocytosis**

- a rare indolent condition comprising skin lesions (urticaria pigmentosa), hepatosplenomegaly and lymphadenopathy.

- in approximately one third of the cases, bone sclerosis develops. This may be focal or generalized. If generalized it can mimic myelofibrosis, diffuse sclerotic metastases and sclerosing bone dysplasias.

8.3.3 **Myeloma**

- neoplastic proliferation of plasma cells producing either a local tumour (plasmocytoma) or disseminated disease (multiple myeloma).

Plasmocytoma

- solitary tumour arising in adults over the age of 40, and causing lytic bone lesions. The vertebral bodies are the commonest site followed by pelvis, femur and humerus.

- located in bone the tumours appear lytic, coarsely trabeculated and mildly expansile with a thin zone of transition (fig 8.9). It can mimic expansile metastases (from renal or thyroid primaries) and, if at the end of a long bone, a giant cell tumour.

- after a latent period of 5–10 years most cases undergo transition to multiple myeloma.

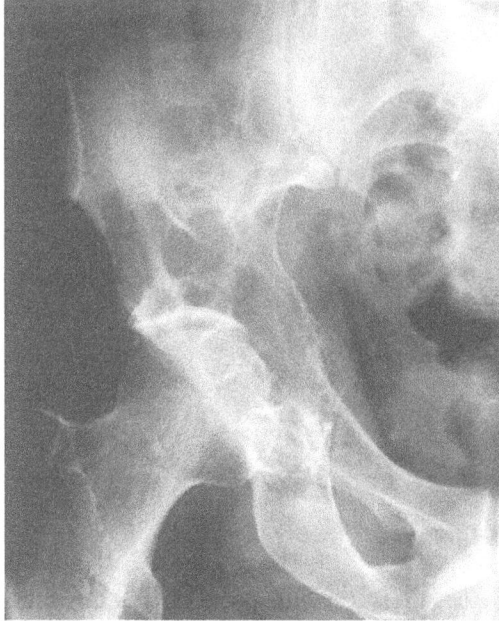

Figure 8.9
Plasmocytoma. Typical lytic, expansile, trabeculated lesion.

Multiple Myeloma

- disseminated form of plasma-cell infiltration. May be preceded by a solitary plasmocytoma.

- radiographic features include;

    — diffuse osteopenia which may result in vertebral collapse.
    — multiple, widespread punched-out (i.e. well-defined) lytic lesions. Sometimes called raindrop lesions in the skull vault (fig 8.10 and 8.11).
    — mimics multiple lytic metastases. Mandibular involvement is commoner in multiple myeloma than metastases.

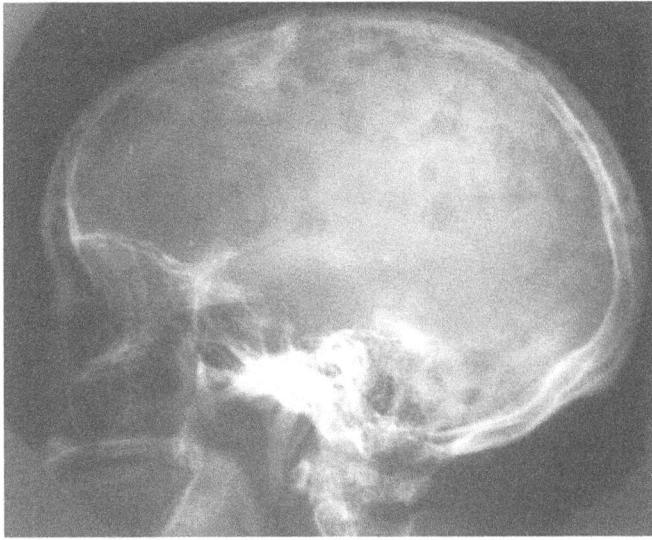

Figure 8.10
Multiple myeloma. Numerous raindrop lesions affecting the skull vault.

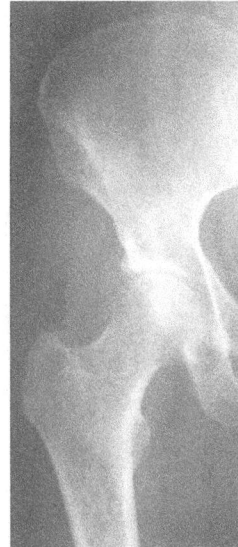

Figure 8.11
Multiple myeloma. Generalised widespread tiny lytic deposits.

8.3.4 Langerhans Cell Histiocytosis (LCH)

- a spectrum of diseases with histiocytic infiltration in bone marrow, spleen, liver, lymphatic glands and lungs.

Eosinophilic Granuloma (EG)

- the commonest (60–80%) and mildest form of LCH. Usually solitary, affects the skull vault (50%), axial skeleton (30%) and long bones (20%). Affects children more often than adolescents and adults.

- radiographic features include;

skull	— sharply defined, rounded lytic lesion
vertebral body	— collapse with flattening (vertebra plana)
long bone	— ill-defined diaphyseal lesion with lamellar periosteal new bone (fig 8.12)

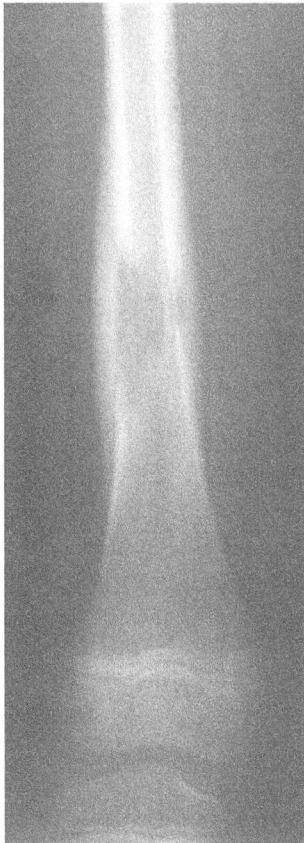

Figure 8.12
Langerhans cell histiocytosis. Eosinophilic granuloma showing a lytic lesion in the shaft of the femur with a lamellar periosteal reaction.

Hand-Christian-Schüller disease

- chronic disseminated form of LCH occurring in children under 10 years of age.

- bone lesions resemble EG but are much more numerous (fig 8.13). In the skull the lesions coalesce to produce large defects.

- 10% mortality usually associated with pulmonary infiltration.

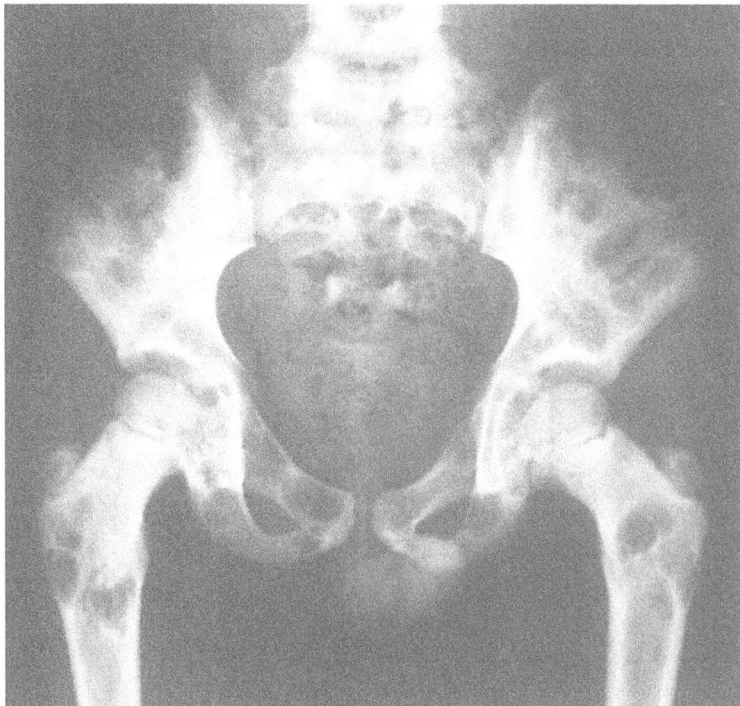

Figure 8.13
Langerhans cell histiocytosis. Hand-Christian-Schüller disease with multiple well defined lytic lesions.

Letterer-Siwe disease

- acute disseminated form of LCH occurring in infants below 2 years of age. Comprises less than 10% of LCH. Most cases prove fatal.

- bone lesions tend to be diffuse resembling leukaemia and metastatic neuroblastoma (fig 8.14).

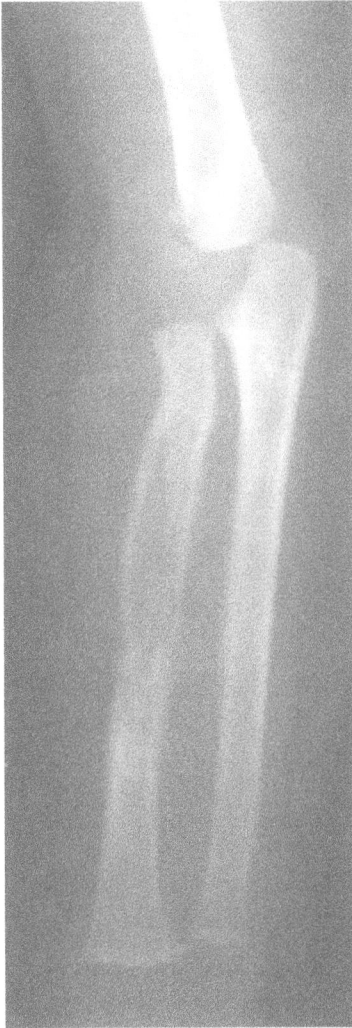

Figure 8.14
Langerhans cell histiocytosis. Letterer-Siwe disease with an infiltrative lesion of the radius. Similar features may be seen with acute osteomyelitis and a sarcoma.

8.3.5 Storage disorders

- there are a number of disorders of the lymphoreticular system due to the abnormal deposition of lipoproteins, usually as a result of inborn errors of metabolism. The commonest of these rare disorders are Gaucher's disease and Niemann-Pick disease.

Gaucher's disease

- an inherited disorder. Presents in childhood or early adulthood.

- radiographic features include (fig 8.15);

  — diffuse osteopenia
  — modelling deformity at the end of long bones ("Erlenmeyer flask"-appearence)
  — bone infarction
  — hip in children resembles Perthes disease
  — vertebral endplate depression
  — long bones sclerosis and bone-within-a-bone appearance (*similar to sickle cell disease*)

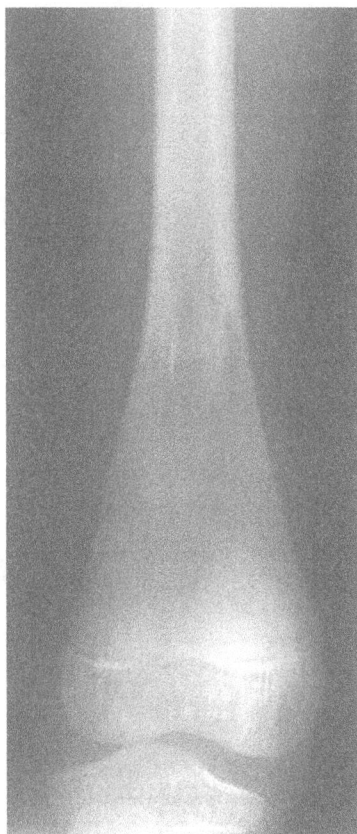

Figure 8.15
Gaucher's disease. There is loss of bone density and a modelling deformity of the distal femur (Erlenmeyer flask deformity).

8.4 **Disorders of Coagulation**

- the commonest disorder of coagulation is *haemophilia* due to a deficiency of factor VIII (haemophilia A) or IX (haemophilia B). It is a hereditary X-linked recessive disorder and is therefore only seen in males.

- the radiographic features are due to uncontrolled bleeding and include (fig 8.16 and 8.17):
    - dense joint effusions due to intra-articular deposition of haemosiderin
    - juxta-articular osteoporosis and overgrowth of epiphyses due hyperaemia
    - in the knee enlargement of the epiphyses and widening of the intercondylar notch
    - cartilage degeneration and premature degenerative joint disease
    - intraosseous and subperiosteal bleeding may produce large lytic lesions (haemophiliac pseudotumour) mimicking a neoplastic process.

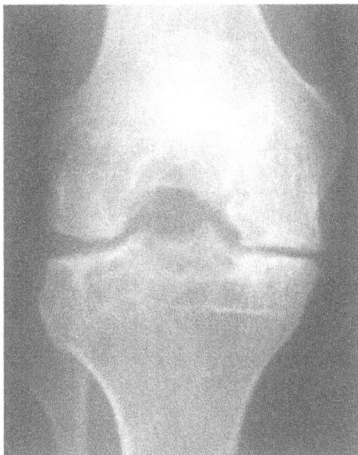

Figure 8.16
Haemophiliac arthropathy. There is enlargement of the epiphyses, widening of the intercondylar notch and premature degenerative joint disease.

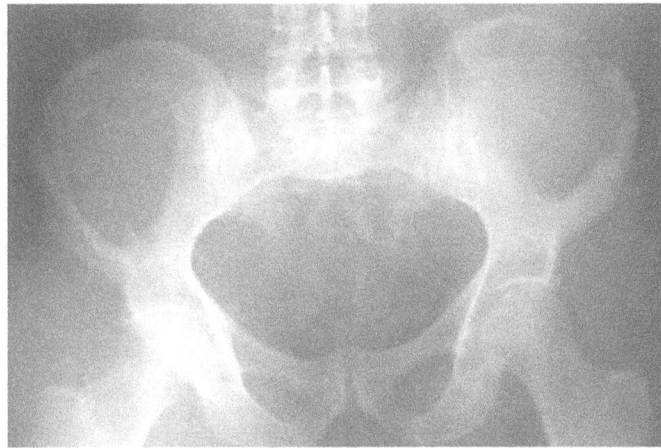

Figure 8.17
Haemophiliac pseudotumours. Well defined lytic lesions involving both iliac bones due to chronic pressure erosion from poorly controlled bleeding.

Tumours

Definitions

- the term **tumour** generally means mass; in common medical parlance it is usually synonymous with the term neoplasm.

- tumours can be subdivided into 2 groups

    1. *Benign tumours*
    2. *Malignant tumours*

- by definition, a neoplasm demonstrates autonomous growth (i.e. can enlarge). If in addition it produces remote spread (metastases) it is defined as a malignant tumour/neoplasm. Malignant tumours can be further classified as;

    1. *Primary*
    2. *Secondary*

- a primary tumour is the original tumour located in the tissue where it started growing. Secondary tumours (metastases) occur due to spread from a primary malignant tumour elsewhere. Tumours and metastases referred to in this chapter are those developing in and/or related to bony structures.

- occasionally the term secondary tumour is used to refer to a bone tumour developing within a pre-existing bone lesion e.g. osteosarcoma arising in Paget's disease.

- bone tumours can be further classified according to their tissue of origin including;

    — bone-forming (osteogenic)   e.g. osteosarcoma
    — cartilage-forming (chondrogenic)   e.g. chondrosarcoma
    — fibrous (fibrogenic)   e.g. fibrosarcoma
    — vascular   e.g. angiosarcoma

- although the aetiology of a number of conditions remains uncertain and some are not strictly neoplastic, they are usually included in discussion of tumours because they display radiographic appearances almost indistinguishable from true neoplasms. The most common of these are simple bone cysts (SBC) and aneurysmal bone cysts (ABC).

- the role of imaging in the management of a patient with a suspected bone tumour can be broadly subdivided as follows;

    1. detection
    2. diagnosis
    3. surgical staging
    4. follow-up

9.1 **Detection**

- despite the introduction of more sensitive techniques, such as bone scintigraphy and MR imaging, **conventional radiography** is the method by which the vast majority of bone tumours are first detected.

- it is important to remember that radiographs of trabecular bones have a relatively low sensitivity, and that pathological processes may be well established even if the radiographs are completely normal. At least 40–50% of the trabecular (marrow) bone must be destroyed before a discrete area of lucency can be demonstrated. Erosion or destruction of cortex are far more easily seen. Furthermore small tumours located in anatomically complex areas such as the spine and pelvis (fig 9.1) may be very difficult to detect

- early, **non-specific** signs of a bone tumour include (fig 9.2);

  — areas of ill-defined lysis or sclerosis
  — cortical erosion or destruction
  — periosteal new bone formation
  — soft tissue swelling

- one should be aware that primary bone tumours are very rare (less than 12 per million of the population per year), and when not suspected, such a diagnosis is easily missed.

- in the presence of a normal radiograph, referred pain from another site needs to be considered. In such situations further radiographs are required. In a child it is well recognized that hip joint pathology often presents with referred pain to the knee, and that neck pathology in adults may cause referred pain in the shoulders.

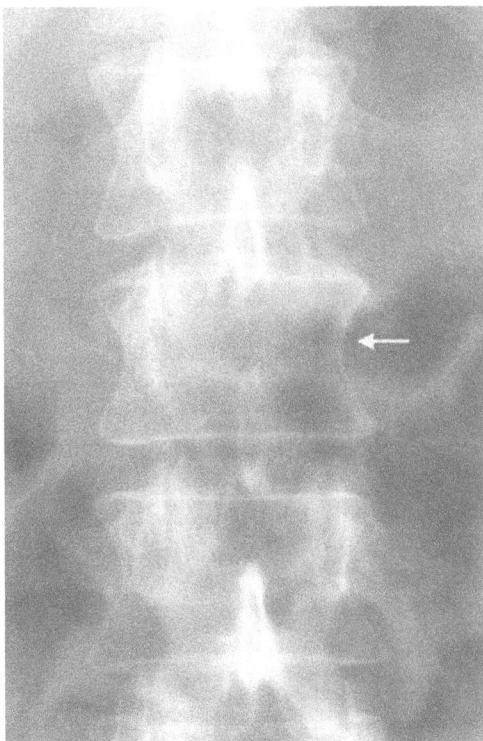

Figure 9.1
Breast cancer metastasis. The only abnormal feature on this AP view is absence of a left pedicle of one of the lumbar vertebrae (arrow).

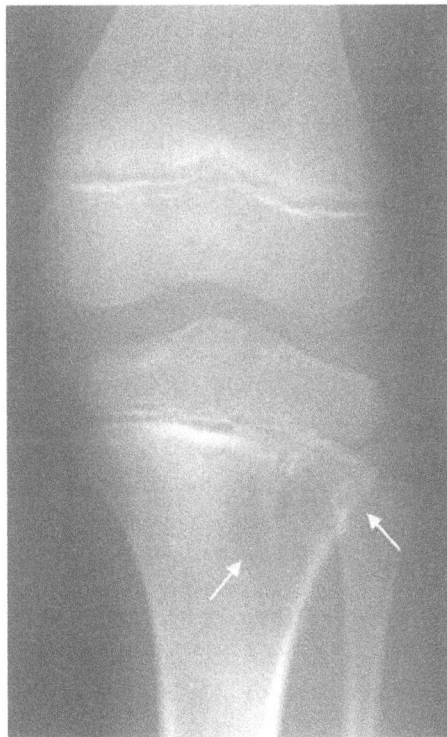

Figure 9.2
Child with an early osteosarcoma of the proximal tibial metaphysis. There is subtle bone destruction and thinning of the cortex (arrows).

9.2 Diagnosis of Bone Tumours

- when a bone tumour is suspected on a radiograph, it is important to consider all possible differential diagnoses, while examining **radiographic findings** in view of **clinical history and examination.**

9.2.1 Clinical history

Age

- the age of the patient is the most useful part of anamnestic information to be considered (Tables 9.1 and 9.2). Many tumours have a peak incidence at different ages. For a malignant bone-forming tumour, an osteosarcoma, this is between 10 and 30 years of age. Therefore, an osteosarcoma is unlikely to occur in a middle-aged or elderly patient. In a patient over 40 years of age, however, metastases and myelomas should always be considered first when a bone lesion is identified (fig 9.1). Similarly, metastatic neuroblastoma should be a differential diagnosis in children younger than 5 years, whereas a tumour arising in adolescence or early adulthood is unlikely to be of metastatic origin.

Table 9.1 **Age of incidence of benign bone tumours**

Tumour	Age (years)
Eosinophilic granuloma (LCH)	2–25
Simple bone cyst	5–20
Non-ossifying fibroma	5–20
Osteoid osteoma	5–30
Osteoblastoma	5–30
Aneurysmal bone cyst	10–30
Chondroblastoma	10–20
Chondromyxoid fibroma	10–20
Giant cell tumour	20–45

Table 9.2 **Age of incidence of malignant bone tumours**

Tumour	Age (years)
Leukaemia	0–5
Neuroblastoma metastases	0–5
Ewing's sarcoma	5–25
Osteosarcoma	10–25 (60–80) *
Lymphoma of bone	25–40
Parosteal osteosarcoma	25–35
Fibrosarcoma/MFH	30–50
Metastases and Myeloma	40+

*a second peak in osteosarcoma occurs in those countries where Paget's disease is common

Ethnic/geographic origin

- the differential diagnosis for a particular radiographic appearance will vary depending on the geographic origin of the case. For example, in many countries hydatid disease of bone is rare and would not be included in most differential diagnoses of a bone lesion. In other areas, e.g. North Africa, the Middle East Eastern Europe and South America where hydatid disease is common it would not be unusual to include it in a differential diagnosis. Kaposi sarcoma is common wherever

AIDS is prevalent. Burkitt's lymphoma is particularly common in children in tropical Africa. Giant cell tumours of bone are more common in the tropics while Ewing's sarcoma is rarely seen in African and Caribbean countries. Some conditions which, on occasion, may mimic bone tumours have a distinct racial predilection. These include sickle cell and Gaucher's disease.

Family history

- there is little evidence of a familial predisposition to the formation of bone tumours. The exceptions are certain hereditary bone conditions which may be associated with malignant transformation e.g. diaphyseal aclasis (multiple exostoses/osteochondromas) and Ollier's disease (multiple enchondromas, fig 9.3), where lesions can transform into chondrosarcoma in adult life.

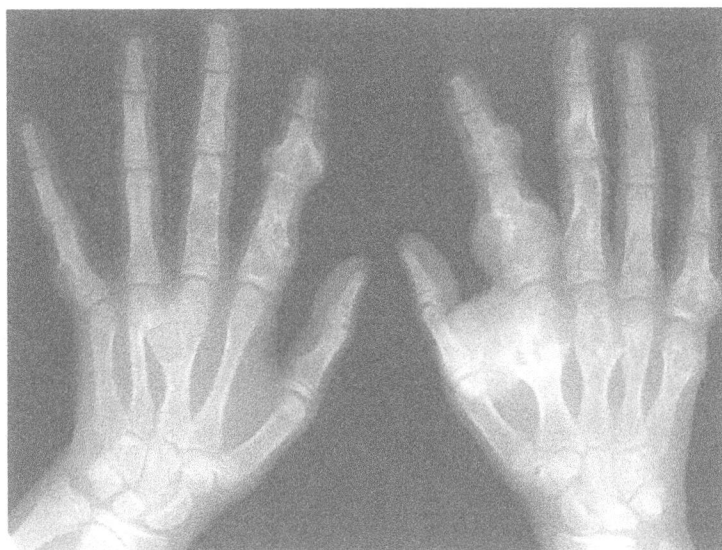

Figure 9.3
Child with multiple enchondromas (Ollier's disease) affecting the metacarpals and phalanges.

Previous medical history

- A history of prior malignancy, pre-existing bone disease or other medical details e.g. HIV status are always necessary to consider when trying to establish a diagnosis.

Multiplicity

- both from diagnostic and from therapeutic aspects it is important to know whether a lesion is solitary or multiple. Frequently this question can be answered only after obtaining radiographs from other parts of the body.

- all the factors mentioned above should be considered together. Multiple bone lesions in a child would suggest an inherited bone dysplasia (fig 9.3), Langerhans cell histiocytosis, leukaemia or metastatic neuroblastoma. In an adult, however, metastases and myeloma are the most likely diagnoses. If the patient is HIV positive or otherwise at risk for a Kaposi's sarcoma (see Chapter 5.12), the possibility for such a disease should be kept in mind.

9.2.2 Radiographic appearance

- having reduced the number of possible diagnoses by taking into account the above factors, it is time to analyse the radiographs in detail. When doing so, five questions should be answered;

    1. Which bone is affected?
    2. Where in that bone is the lesion (= suspected tumour) located?
    3. What is the tumour doing to the bone (pattern of bone destruction)?
    4. What form of periosteal reaction, if any, is present?
    5. What type of matrix mineralization, if any, is present?

Site in skeleton

- primary, malignant bone tumours often occur close to the knee joint. Cartilage tumours of the hands and feet, however, are almost invariably benign (fig 9.3 and 9.4). Chordoma characteristically arises from the clivus and sacrum, and Burkitt's lymphoma arises in the mandible and maxilla. Many tumours may develop in the spine but malignant tumours are found predominantly in the anterior part of the vertebra (the body), while benign lesions are characteristically found in the posterior elements (the neural arch).

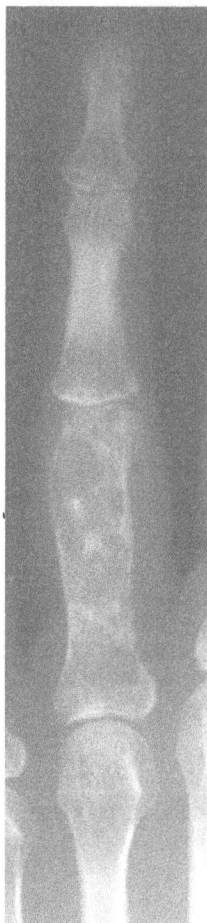

Figure 9.4
Typical enchondroma of a phalanx showing a lytic, mildly expansile lesion containing punctate cartilage calcification.

Location in bone

- the site of origin of a bone tumour can be an important parameter of diagnosis. Osteosarcoma usually arises in the metaphysis or metadiaphysis, whereas Ewing's sarcoma originates in the metaphysis or, more distinctively, in the diaphysis. In a child the differential diagnosis of a lesion arising in an epiphysis can be limited to a chondroblastoma (fig 9.5), epiphyseal abscess and rarely Langerhans cell histiocytosis. Following skeletal fusion, subarticular lesions, analogous in the adult to the epiphysis, include giant cell tumour, intraosseous ganglion and the rare clear cell chondrosarcoma. It is also helpful to identify the origin of the tumour with respect to the transverse plane of the bone. Is the tumour central, eccentric or cortically based? For example, a simple bone cyst, fibrous dysplasia and Ewing's sarcoma tend to be centrally located, whereas giant cell tumour, chondromyxoid fibroma and non-ossifying fibroma are typically eccentric. Lesions that usually arise in an eccentric position may appear central if the tumour is particularly large or the involved bone is of small calibre. There are numerous lesions that arise on the surface of bone. Most malignant surface lesions are the rarer forms of osteosarcoma e.g. parosteal osteosarcoma.

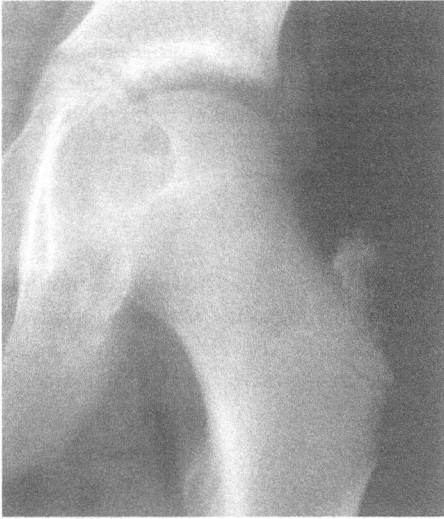

Figure 9.5
Child with a chondroblastoma of the proximal femoral epiphysis.

Pattern of bone destruction

- analysis of the interface between tumour and host bone is a good indicator of the rate of growth of the lesion. A well-defined, sharply marginated lesion indicates slower growth than an ill-defined, non-marginated lesion (fig 9.6). The faster the growth, the more aggressive the pattern of destruction and the wider the zone of transition between tumour and normal bone. As a rule, malignant lesions tend to grow faster than benign and therefore appear ill-defined. This aggressive pattern is called *permeative* or *moth-eaten* bone destruction. Destruction of the cortex with extension of the pathological process into the adjacent soft tissues is more suggestive of an aggressive (i.e. more likely malignant) process. Remember that acute osteomyelitis will also give an aggressive appearance with ill-defined bone destruction.

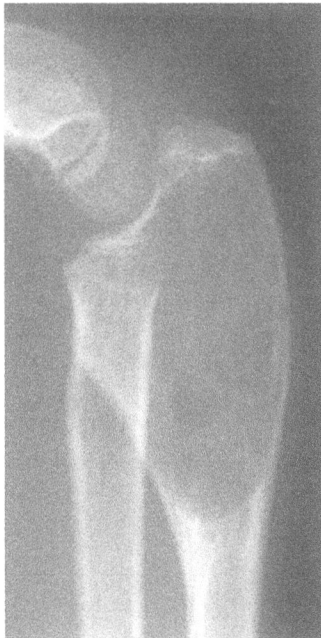

Figure 9.6
Child with an aneurysmal bone cyst of the proximal ulna. The tumour is lytic, expansile (only a shell left) and well defined.

Periosteal reaction

- the periosteum will mineralize/calcify in response to stimulation from tumour, blood and pus. The appearance and nature of this mineralization, known as periosteal reaction (or periosteal new bone formation) is frequently helpful in limiting the number of hypothetical diagnoses. The following patterns are recognised;

Shell

- expansion of the cortex gives the lesion a balloon-like appearance. In the young patient these lesions are usually benign e.g. simple bone cyst, aneurysmal bone cyst (fig 9.6) and chondromyxoid fibroma. In the adult this feature suggests expansile metastases from renal or thyroid primaries and plasmocytoma.

Lamellar

- denotes a thin sheet-like layer of mineralized periosteal new bone. It may be single or multiple (onion skin). A single lamella may be seen in many conditions including trauma. If relatively thick and generalized, hypertrophic osteoarthropathy should be considered (Table 9.3 and fig 9.7). Multiple lamellae/onion skin is a typical feature of Ewing's sarcoma and osteosarcoma (fig 9.8).

Interrupted

- if a periosteal reaction is interrupted (i.e. is discontinuous) it suggests an aggressive, rapidly evolving process. A triangular elevation of interrupted periosteal new bone is known as the Codman angle (named after the individual who first described it, fig 9.9). This pattern is suggestive, if not diagnostic, of bone malignancy as it may also be seen in osteomyelitis.

Combined/complex

- more than one pattern of periosteal reaction may be seen in the same case indicating varying rate of growth at different sites in the lesion. A divergent spiculated periosteal reaction, otherwise known as "sun-ray", is an example of the fastest growing complex pattern and is suggestive (but not diagnostic) of an osteosarcoma (fig 9.9).

Table 9.3 **Causes of hypertrophic osteoarthropathy**

Pulmonary
1. Carcinoma of bronchus
2. Abscess
3. Bronchiectasis/chronic chest infection

Pleural
1. Mesothelioma
2. Pleural fibroma

Cardiovascular
1. Cyanotic congenital heart disease

Gastrointestinal
1. Ulcerative colitis
2. Crohn's disease
3. Amoebic dysentery
4. Whipple's disease
5. Colic disease
6. Primary biliary cirrhosis
7. Nasopharyngeal carcinoma

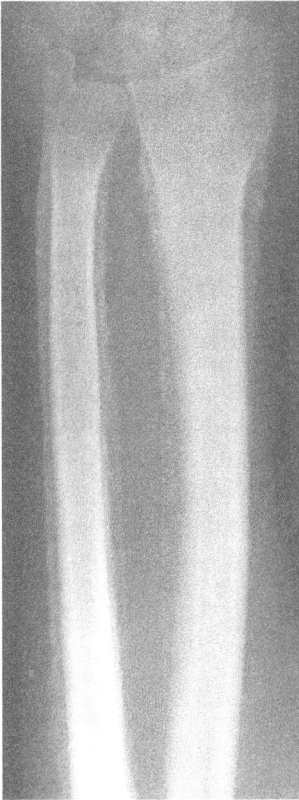

Figure 9.7
Hypertrophic osteoarthropathy of the forearm in a patient with lung cancer. The thick periosteal reaction is typical (see Table 9.3 for other causes).

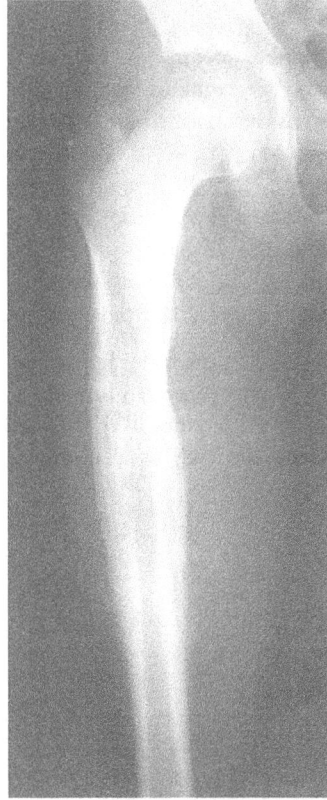

Figure 9.8
Child with a Ewing's sarcoma of the femoral metaphysis. There is permeative bone destruction, a lamellar (onion skin) periosteal reaction laterally and spiculated periosteal reaction medially.

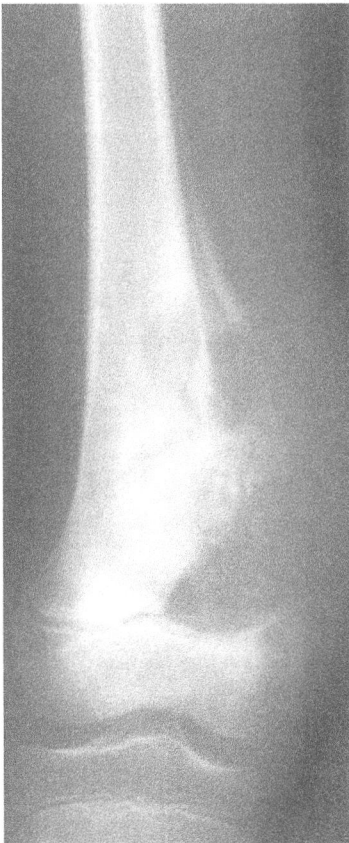

(a)

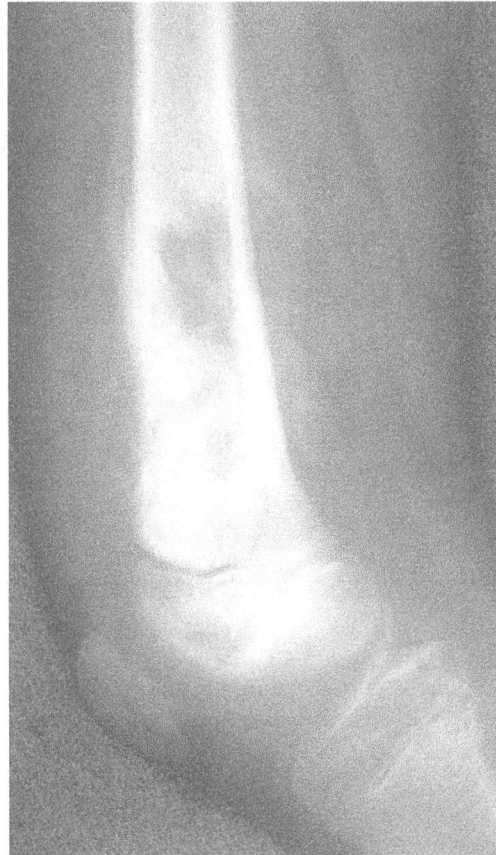

(b)

Figure 9.9
(a) AP and (b) lateral views of a high grade osteosarcoma in a child. There is ill-defined bone destruction, an interrupted lamellar periosteal reaction with Codman's angles, malignant osteoid mineralisation and soft tissue extension.

Matrix

- a number of tumours produce matrix, the intercellular substance that can calcify or ossify. Radiodense tumour matrix is either osteoid (bony) or chondroid (cartilaginous). The exception is fibrous dysplasia, where the collagenous matrix may be sufficiently dense to give a ground glass appearance (fig 9.10). Tumour osteoid is typified by solid (sharp-edged) or cloud to ivory-like patterns (fig 9.9). Tumour cartilage is variously described as stippled, flocculent, ring-and-arc and popcorn in appearance (fig 9.4). Identifying the pattern of matrix calcification will significantly reduce the differential diagnosis but has no influence as to whether the tumour is benign or malignant i.e. it can indicate that a tumour is of cartilaginous origin but does not differentiate a benign chondroma from a malignant chondrosarcoma.

- by analysing the features detailed above it should be possible in the majority of cases to indicate whether the suspected tumour is aggressive (i.e. more likely malignant) from those that appear indolent, i.e. more likely to be benign (fig 9.11). It should also be possible in some cases to indicate the likely tissue of origin thereby shortening the list of differential diagnoses.

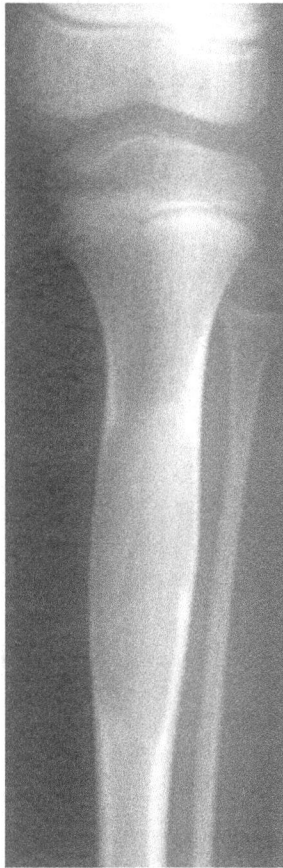

Figure 9.10
Fibrous dysplasia of the tibial shaft showing mild expansion of bone and the ground-glass matrix.

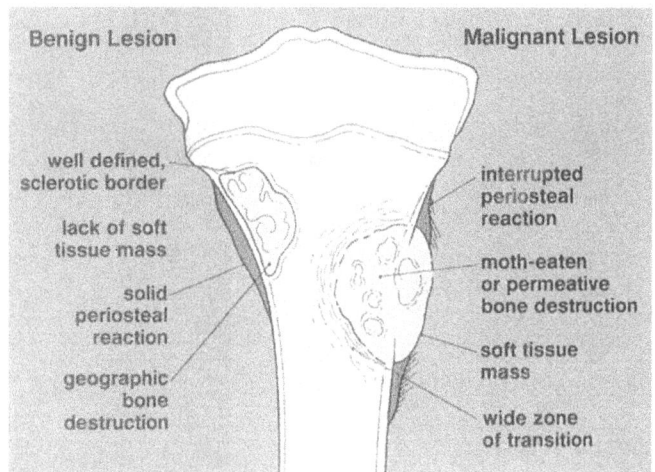

Figure 9.11
Schematic diagram of the radiographic features that can help differentiate benign from malignant bone lesions.

(from Greenspan A, *Orthopaedic Radiology*, 2nd edition, Raven Press, 1992, with permission)

9.3 Surgical staging

- when planning surgery, it is necessary to decide if the tumour is solitary or has already spread locally or elsewhere in the body. This procedure is called *surgical staging*.

- where possible, staging is best done by using CT or MR imaging, exclusion of other bony lesions with bone scintigraphy (radionuclide bone scanning) and pulmonary metastases with a CT scan of the thorax. Where these techniques are not available the primary tumour can be assessed with conventional radiographs, bony metastases with a radiographic skeletal survey and pulmonary metastases with a chest radiograph. Remember that, because of the permeative nature of many malignant bone tumours, radiographs will underestimate the full extent of involved bone.

- many primary sarcomas of bone will present late when the only surgical option will be amputation. It should be noted that long term survival in most of these high grade sarcomas is poor (<20% 5 year survival) unless treatment is early and combines surgery and chemotherapy.

9.4 Follow-up

- most sarcomas will spread to the lungs. Therefore, follow-up imaging is usually confined to routine chest radiographs.

- if limb-salvage surgery is the initial surgical treatment there is a risk of local recurrence at the operated site. Local recurrence is only likely to be detectable on radiographs if it is large enough to distort intermuscular fat planes or if there is tumour mineralization as might be seen with recurrent osteosarcoma.

9.5 Radiographic Diagnosis of Soft Tissue Tumours

- the lack of contrast resolution in the soft tissues is a well recognised limitation of radiography. Therefore, many soft tissue tumours will not be detectable on radiographs. Ultrasonography may then be of great help.

- in a minority of cases, part or all of the tumour may have sufficiently different radiodensity compared to surrounding tissue to be visualized on a radiograph.

- lipomas, the most common of all soft tissue tumours, have low radiodensities, and its greytones on a radiograph are somewhere in between water/muscle (higher density) and air (lower density), (fig 9.12). For this reason, lipomas are often well demarcated from the surrounding soft tissues. It should be noted that some liposarcomas may contain variable amounts of lipomatous tissue, thereby showing various degrees of radiolucency.

- calcification and ossification are easily detected on radiographs and and may be seen in a large spectrum of disease including congenital, metabolic, endocrine, traumatic and parasitic infections, whereas calcifications in soft tissue tumours are less common. Analysis of the pattern of calcification/ossification within a soft tissue mass may often indicate type of tissue involved.

  For example;

    — phleboliths (small circular calcifications in veins with a central lucency) are typical of haemangiomas (fig 9.13)
    — ring-and-arc calcification is typical of a cartilage-based tumour. In the soft tissues this includes soft tissue chrondoma as well as chondrosarcoma and also synovial chondromatosis.
    — central calcification is a feature of mineralizing soft tissue sarcomas such as osteosarcoma and synovial sarcoma.
    — peripheral calcification/ossification is typical of myositis ossificans which is frequently mistaken for a sarcoma (fig 9.14).

- Kaposi's sarcoma is a multicentric vascular tumour thought to have a viral aetiology. It is particularly common in immunosuppressed patients (e.g. HIV). This is covered in more detail in Chapter 5.12.

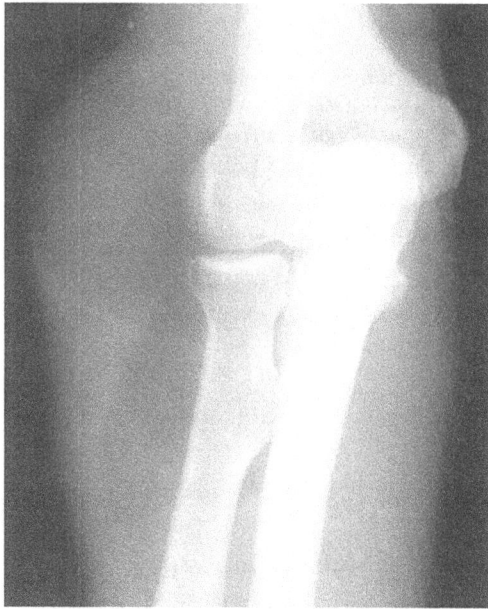

Figure 9.12
Low density lipoma within the soft tissues over the lateral aspect of the elbow.

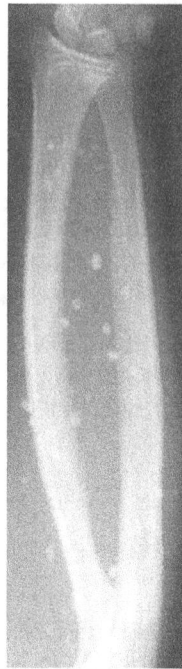

Figure 9.13
Soft tissue haemangioma of the forearm indicated by the multiple calcified phleboliths.

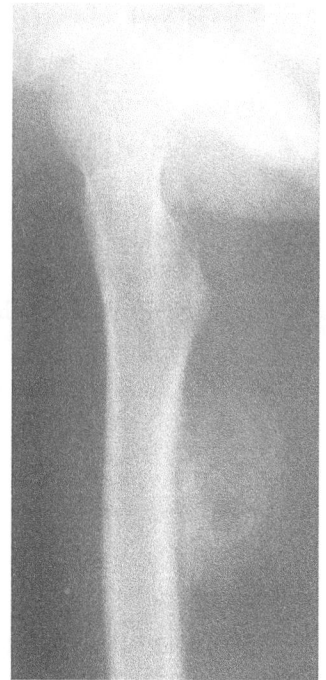

Figure 9.14
Post-traumatic myositis ossificans arising within the soft tissues of the posterior aspect of the femur in a child.

9.6 Specific Bone Tumours

- Although a discussion of the total range of bone tumours is out of the scope of this manual, a short presentation of the most common types and some of their characteristics are listed below.

9.6.1 Benign bone-forming tumours

Osteoma

- a benign dense/sclerotic focal tumour located on the surface of a bone. Common sites include the skull vault, paranasal sinuses and the mandible. Osteomas are usually found by chance. If they arise from the mandible, they may be combined with potentially malignant colonic polyps (Gardner syndrome).

Bone island/enostosis

- a benign focus of dense bone within a medullary cavity ranging from 2 mm to 2 cm in diameter. Usually an incidental finding of no clinical relevance. Multiple bone islands of no clinical importance are seen in bone dysplasia and osteopoikilosis.

Osteoid osteoma

- a small benign vascular tumour usually involving the cortex of long bones, and they are typically found in patients between 5 and 30 years of age. Typical radiographic appearances are of central lucencies ("nidus") which may, or may not contain calcification. Also varying amount of surrounding sclerotic new bone formation can be seen (fig 9.15). In the spine osteoma tends to involve the posterior elements (neural arch). The diagnosis should be considered in an adolescent presenting with a painful scoliosis. If the nidus is over 2 cm in size the tumour is called an *osteoblastoma*.

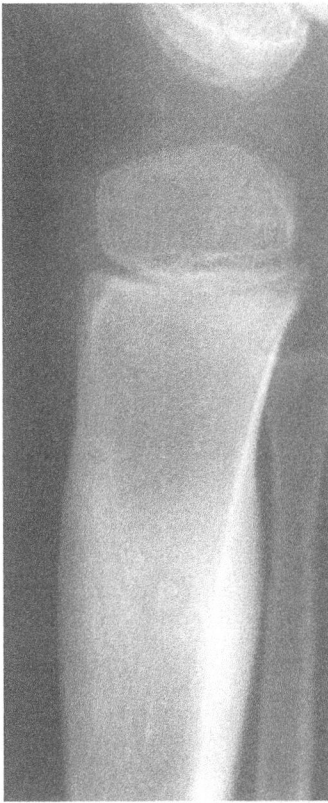

Figure 9.15
Child with an osteoid osteoma of the proximal tibia. Typical features include the rounded lucency containing a small focus of calcification (the nidus) and the adjacent cortical thickening.

9.6.2 Benign cartilage-forming tumours

Enchondroma

- benign tumour of mature cartilage arising within bone. It most commonly occurs in the tubular bones of the hands and feet. Typical radiographic appearances are well defined intramedullary lytic lesions containing variable amounts of cartilage calcification ("ring-and-arc", fig 9.4). Larger lesions, particularly in the hands and feet, may cause endosteal scalloping and mild bony expansion. Most are asymptomatic unless associated with a fracture. Malignant transformation of an enchondroma to a central chondrosarcoma is documented but rare. It occurs more frequently in the multiple form of the disease known as enchondromatosis or Ollier's disease.

Osteochondroma

- otherwise known as a cartilaginous exostosis, a benign bony protrusion covered by an outer cartilage cap. It is the most common of all bone tumours and tends to arise around the knee. It develops from the outer surface of the metaphysis and projects away from the adjacent joint. It may either have a relatively broad and flat base (sessile osteochondroma, fig 9.16a) or a stalk-like base (pedunculated osteochondroma, fig 9.16b). The cortical bone of the osteochondroma is continuos with the cortex of underlying bone, the cartilage cap may show variable amounts of calcification. If the cartilage cap appears particularly large (>2 cm thick) then a peripheral chondrosarcoma (the malignant counterpart of an osteochondroma) should be considered. Malignant transformation is more common, although still rare, in the multiple form of osteochondroma, the so-called diaphyseal aclasis.

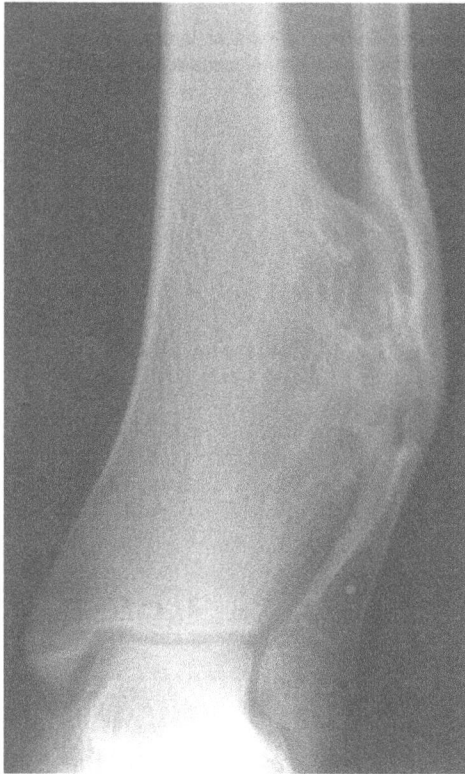
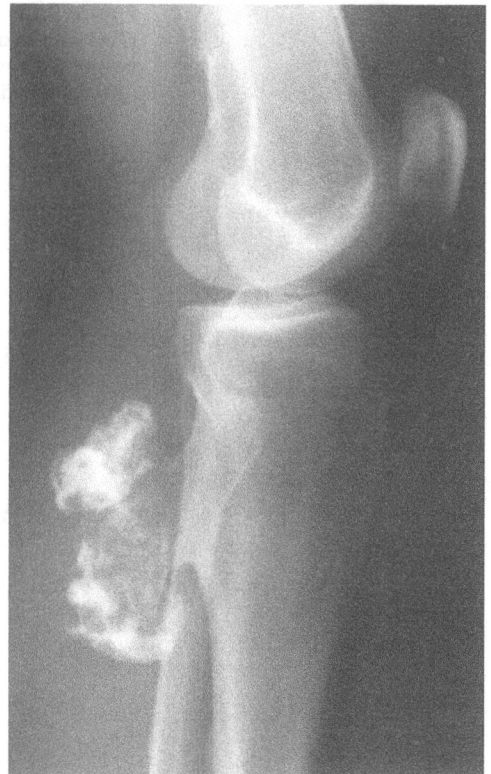

(a)   (b)

Figure 9.16
Osteochondroma (a) broad-based sessile type arising from distal tibia causing pressure deformity of the fibula;
(b) pedunculated type arising from the proximal tibia.

Chondroblastoma

- benign cartilage tumour arising within the epiphysis in children and adolescents. The main radiographic appearance is a well defined lytic lesion frequently containing faint calcifications (fig 9.5). Large lesions may eventually break through the growth plate.

Chondromyxoid fibroma

- a rare benign cartilage tumour typically arising eccentrically within the metaphyses around the knee.

9.6.3 Benign fibrous tumours

Fibrous cortical defect and non-ossifying fibroma

- common benign tumour usually seen close to the knee joint in children and adolescents. It appears as a well defined lytic lesion with a thin sclerotic border. Normally, it arises within the cortex and extends into the bone marrow cavity (fig 9.17). Small lesions are known as fibrous cortical defects. Large lesions which may appear trabeculated (septated), are known as non-ossifying fibromas. The majority are incidental findings in children X-rayed for other reasons, although large lesions may present with a pathological fracture (fig. 4.144).

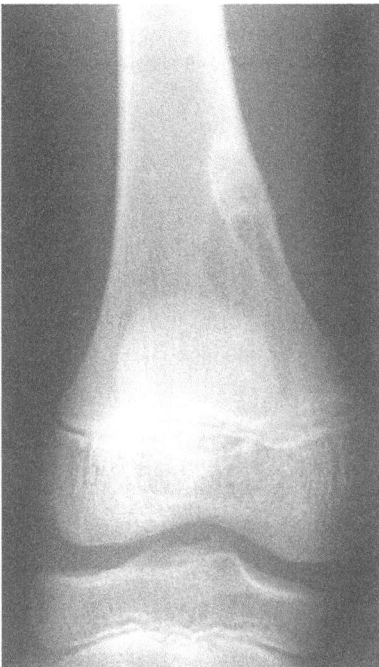

Figure 9.17
Well defined cortical based lytic lesion in an adolescent characteristic of a fibrous cortical defect.

Fibrous dysplasia

- benign lesion consisting of intramedullary fibrous tissue. Some 90% are solitary. The multiple form (polyostotic fibrous dysplasia) may be associated with skin pigmentation and precocious puberty in young females (Albright's syndrome). The radiographic appearance is a well defined lytic lesion within the medulla of long bones containing variable amounts of calcification. A usual feature is a so-called ground-glass appearance due to dense fibrous tissue (fig 9.10). Larger lesions may expand and weaken bone, leading to pathological fractures, and deformities may be seen after subsequent healing.

9.6.4 Benign vascular tumours

Haemangioma

- benign tumour of blood vessels occurring more commonly in soft tissues than in bone. When located in bone, they are mostly found within vertebral bodies appearing as lytic lesions with coarse vertically oriented trabeculae. The differential diagnosis includes Paget's disease, myeloma and metastases. Most are asymptomatic but vertebral collapse with spinal cord compression may occur, particularly during pregnancy.

Glomus tumour

- benign tumour arising in subcutaneous tissues of the tips of fingers causing well defined and often very painful erosion in terminal phalanges.

9.6.5 Benign tumours of unknown origin

Simple bone cyst

- is a benign non-neoplastic lesion otherwise known as a unicameral bone cyst. It is an intraosseous fluid filled cyst with a thin membrane lining. It occurs before skeletal fusion has finished most commonly in the proximal humeral metaphysis. The radiographic appearance is a well defined expansile lesion with thin sclerotic borders (fig 9.18). Sometimes a fragment of cortex may become displaced into the dependent portion of the cyst. This so-called "fallen-fragment sign" is highly suggestive of a simple bone cyst. Frequently a simple bone cyst presents with a pathological fracture.

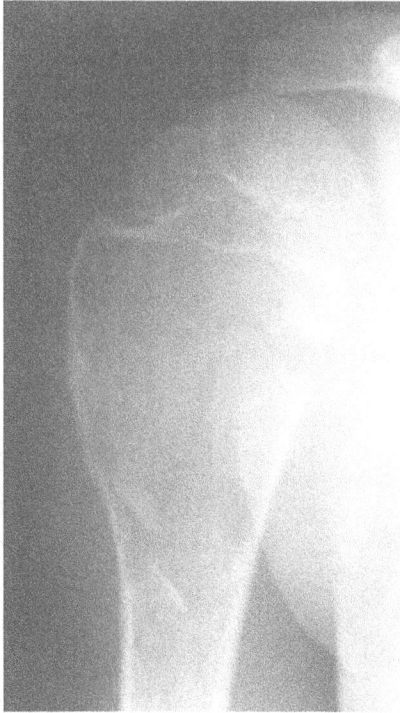

Figure 9.18
Simple bone cyst in a child. Typical features and site. Note the two fallen fragments of cortical bone in the lower portion of the lesion.

Aneurysmal bone cyst

- benign non-neoplastic lesion usually occurring before skeletal fusion and showing multiple intra-osseous cavities filled with blood. Approximately half of all cases occurs within long bones, whereas short tubular bones of the hands and feet, spine and pelvis are less frequently affected. The typical radiographic appearance is a well defined expansile lytic lesion. Larger lesions may appear septated (fig 9.19).

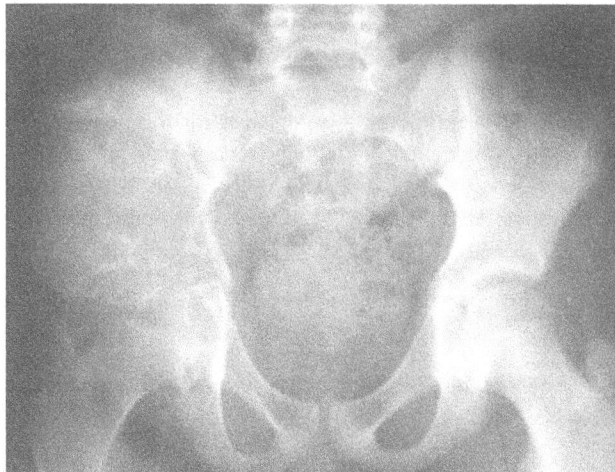

Figure 9.19
Large aneurysmal bone cyst of the ilium in a child. Larger lesions often have a septated appearance.

Giant cell tumour

- histologically benign but locally aggressive bone tumour occurring in the third and fourth decades of life. The most common sites are around the knee, proximal humerus, femur, and the distal radius. The radiographic appearance is a mildly expansile lytic lesion arising eccentrically within the subarticular bone (fig 9.20). The lesion may be well or ill defined. Curettage is usually the recommended treatment, but local recurrence occurs in up to 30% of the cases due to the locally aggressive nature of the tumour. Very rarely the tumour may cause metastases in the lungs.

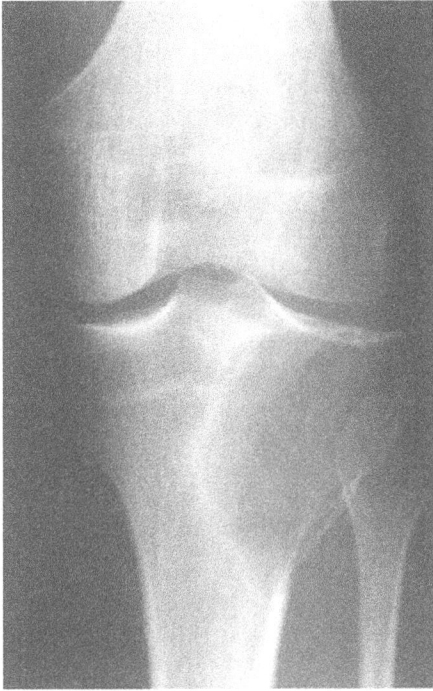

Figure 9.20
Adult with a giant cell tumour of the proximal tibia. The lesion is lytic, eccentrically located and subarticular.

9.6.6 Malignant bone-forming tumours

Osteosarcoma

- the most common primary malignant bone tumour being characterized by production of bone. The osteosarcomas can be divided into several subgroups depending on their site of origin.

High grade intraosseous osteosarcoma

- the most common type of osteosarcoma arising within the medulla of metaphyses or metadiaphyses of long bones particularly around the knee, and most often found in adolescents and young adults. It shows some or all the features of an aggressive malignant bone tumour, including permeative bone destruction, cortical destruction with soft tissue extension, a lamellated or spiculated periosteal reaction with Codman's angles (see Chapter 9.2.2) and malignant new bone formation (fig 9.9).

Parosteal osteosarcoma

• this is a low grade (= less malignant) tumour arising on the outer surface of bone. 50% arise on the posterior cortex of the distal femur. The radiographic appearance is a densely ossified mass closely adherent to the underlying bone (fig 9.21). Approximately one third of the cases shows early invasion of underlying bone, and over time many of them will transform into a highly malignant osteosarcoma.

Secondary osteosarcoma

• osteosarcomas may rarely arise in association with pre-existing bone lesions, but can be observed in patients with Paget's disease (Paget's sarcoma, fig. 5.44) or in bone structures previously exposed to high doses of ionizing radiation (radiotherapy) causing a so-called radiation osteosarcoma.

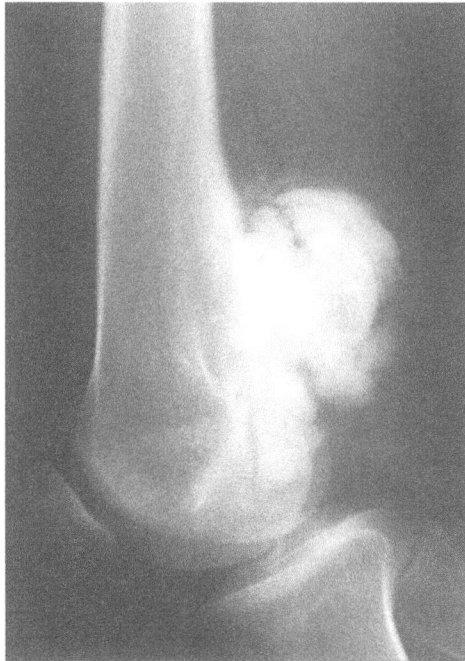

Figure 9.21
A parosteal osteosarcoma arising from the posterior metaphysis of the distal femur of an adult.

9.6.7 Malignant cartilage-forming tumours

Chondrosarcoma

• this malignant cartilage tumour may arise within a bone (central chondrosarcoma) or from the surface of a bone (peripheral chondrosarcoma), and is mainly seen in adults. The grade of malignancy varies from low to very high. Central lesions arise mainly in the metadiaphysis, are lytic, mildly expansile with cortical thickening, and contain cartilage calcifications (fig 9.22). If such a lesion exceeds 5 cm in length a chondrosarcoma is more likely than an enchondroma. Peripheral chondrosarcomas resemble osteochondromas but the cartilage cap is larger and calcifications are dispersed within a soft tissue mass (fig 9.23). In the presence of more aggressive features, a more malignant lesion such as a osteosarcoma or a malignant fibro histiocytoma should be considered.

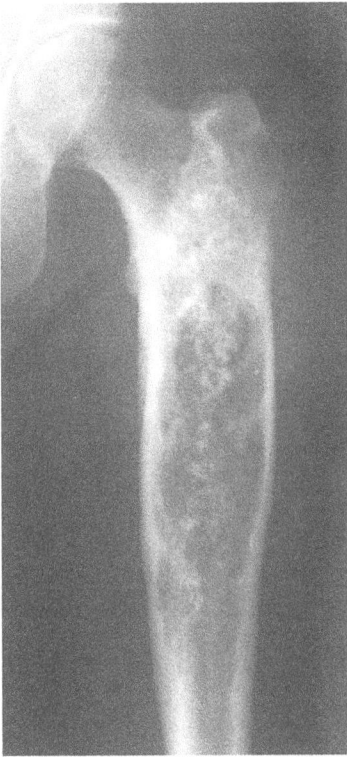

Figure 9.22
Adult with a large central chondrosarcoma of the proximal femoral shaft. There is a lytic lesion, with mild bony expansion, cortical thickening and multiple foci of cartilage mineralisation.

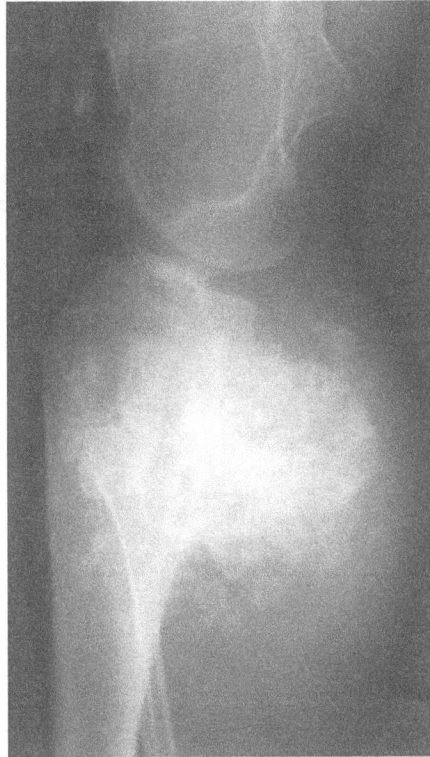

Figure 9.23
Adult with a peripheral chondrosarcoma arising from the posterior aspect of the proximal tibia. Compare the extensive calcifications with the benign osteochondroma in figure 9.16b. The abnormality of the distal femur is the result of osteochondromas indicating that this patient has diaphyseal aclasis. This is therefore a malignant transformation of an osteochondroma in a patient with diaphyseal aclasis.

9.6.8 Malignant fibrous tumours

Malignant fibrous histiocytoma

- the terminology of primary malignant bone tumours of fibrous origin has altered as histologists have reclassified these lesions. In the past many of these tumours were called fibrosarcomas, then malignant fibrous histiocytoma was preferred, and now many are simply called spindle cell sarcomas or classified as leiomyosarcomas of bone. Whichever terminology is applied, the radiographic appearances are the same.

- an aggressive bone tumour with cortical destruction, soft tissue extension, only minor periosteal new bone formation and no matrix mineralisation (fig 9.24). These tumours occur in the middle aged and elderly, and they may be indistinguishable from a bone metastasis.

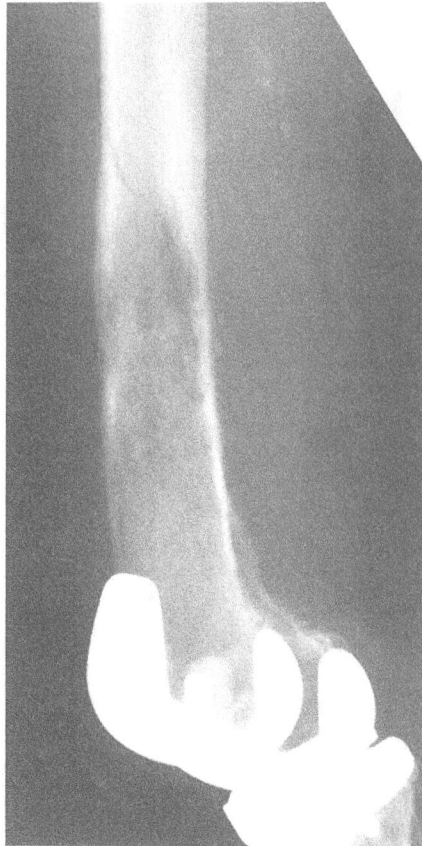

Figure 9.24
Malignant fibrous histiocytoma of the distal femoral shaft with a pathological fracture. Although there is evidence of a soft tissue mass there is no appreciable periosteal reaction.

The radiographic features are indistinguishable from a metastasis. The metal distally is a prosthetic knee replacement previously inserted.

9.6.9 Malignant tumours of marrow origin

Ewing's sarcoma

- there is a spectrum of malignant round cell tumours comprising Ewing's sarcoma and peripheral neuroectodermal tumours. They occur in the first and second decades slightly more often in long bones than in the flat ones. Ewing's sarcoma usually arises in the diaphysis of a long bone but frequently they are dia-metaphyseal in location. These are high grade tumours with typical aggressive/ malignant features on the radiographs. These include permeative bone destruction, lamellated (onion-skin) periosteal reaction with Codman's angles (see Chapter 9.2.2), cortical destruction and soft tissue extension (fig 9.8). Unlike osteosarcoma, there is no matrix mineralisation. The most important differential diagnosis to an early Ewing's sarcoma is acute osteomyelitis.

9.7 Bone Metastases

- metastases to bone are 25 times more common than primary bone tumours. Thus, the large majority of destructive bone lesions identified in patients over the age of 40 years will prove to be metastases or myeloma.

- 80% of bone metastases will originate from one of 5 primary sites

  — lung
  — breast
  — prostate
  — kidney
  — thyroid

- bone metastases are generally multiple (fig 9.25). Less than 10% are solitary, and when so, they are usually originating from a renal or a thyroid carcinoma.

- bone metastases develop mainly at sites of residual red marrow, such as the axial skeleton (ribs, vertebrae, skull vault, pelvis, fig 9.1 and 9.25) and the proximal humerus and femur (fig 9.26). Metastases distal (= more peripheral) to the elbows and knees are rare, and are usually secondaries from a lung carcinoma (fig 9.27).

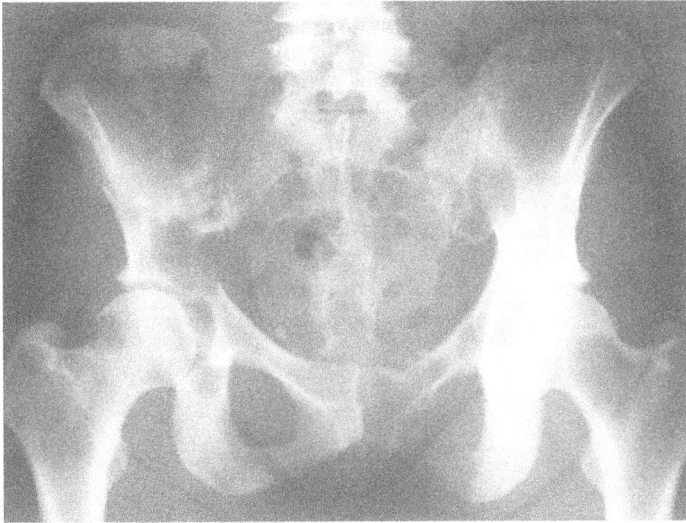

Figure 9.25
Multiple lytic metastases from breast carcinoma.

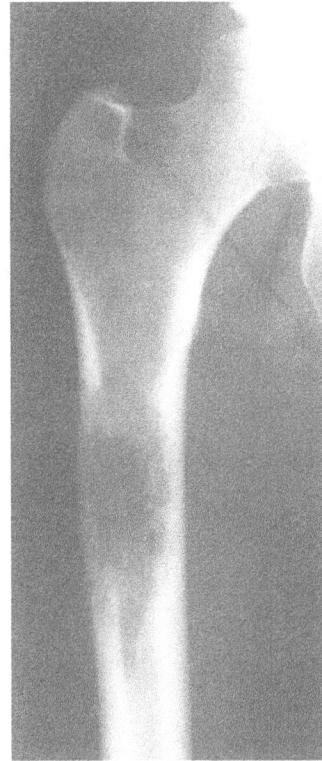

Figure 9.26
Lytic metastases from carcinoma of the lung.

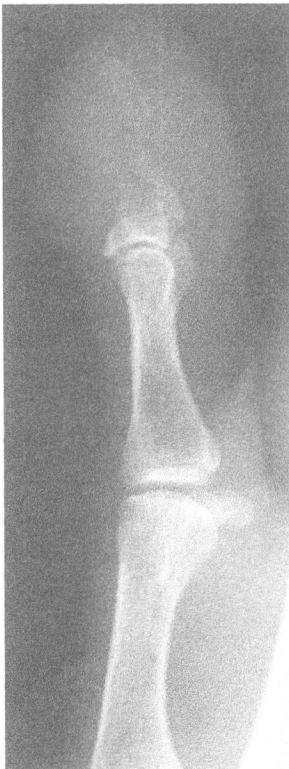

Figure 9.27
Lytic metastasis in the terminal phalanx from carcinoma of the lung.

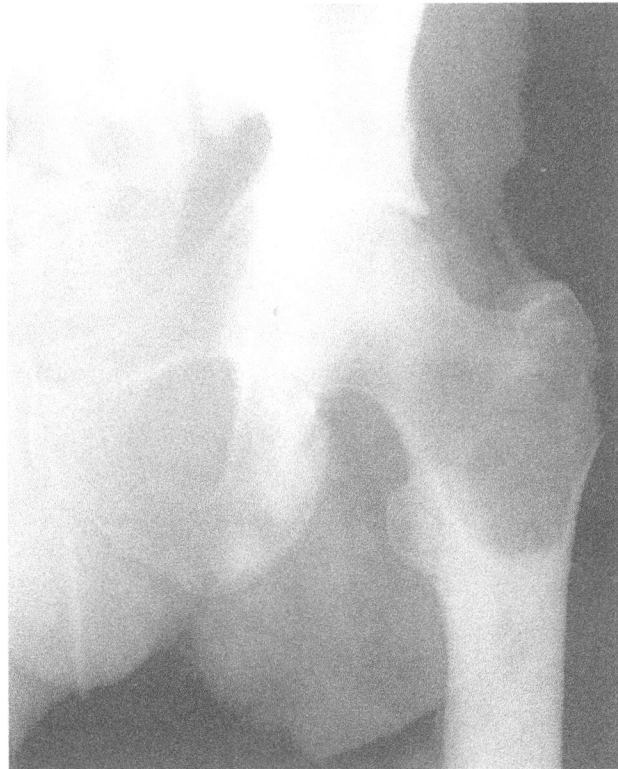

Figure 9.28
Multiple sclerotic metastases from carcinoma of the prostate. The apparent lucency in the intertrochanteric portion of the femur is the only area of normal bone.

- the radiographic appearances are those of an aggressive lesion with permeative bone destruction, cortical destruction and little or no periosteal reaction. Occasionally metastases may present as expansile masses, and these are usually originating from a renal or thyroid carcinoma. The density of metastases varies. Purely lytic metastases are mostly originating (in descending order) from carcinoma of the lung, the kidney, the breast or the thyroid gland (fig 9.25, 9.26 and 9.27). Mixed lytic and sclerotic metastases, however, mostly originate from primary malignancy of breast, lung, prostate or urinary bladder. Pure sclerotic metastases indicate prostate, breast, or gastrointestinal tract as site of origin (fig 9.28).

- radiographs useful in assessing possible risk for pathological fractures. If more than 50% of cortex in a weight bearing bone is destroyed, the risk for developing pathological fractures is relatively high, and prophylactic treatment should be considered.

CHAPTER 10

Congenital and Developmental Disorders

Definitions

- a full classification and discussion of congenital and developmental disorders are beyond the scope of this text.

- it is, however, important to distinguish between ***congenital abnormalities***, which may need treatment, and ***developmental variants*** of the normal, which will not require medical attention.

- when faced with a possible congenital abnormality the following questions should be answered:

    — is it an isolated/solitary lesion i.e. affects just one site?

    — is it an isolated but symmetrical lesion i.e. affects same site on both sides of body but no other site?

    — is it a generalised/multifocal condition?

10.1 **Isolated Conditions**

- such conditions can more precisely be classified by referring to anatomical location. Although referred to as *isolated* they may often be found together with other types of congenital/developmental changes.

10.1.1 **Shoulder girdle**

- "Sprengel's" shoulder refers to a congenital elevation of the scapula (fig 10.1). This can be unilateral or bilateral and is frequently associated with congenital abnormalities of the cervical and upper thoracic spine (Klippel-Feil syndrome).

- hypoplasia of glenoid due to growth disturbances is mostly found bilaterally. When unilateral only, it is often a result of birth trauma to the brachial nerve plexus. Unilateral it is often the result of birth trauma to the brachial plexus (causing palsy).

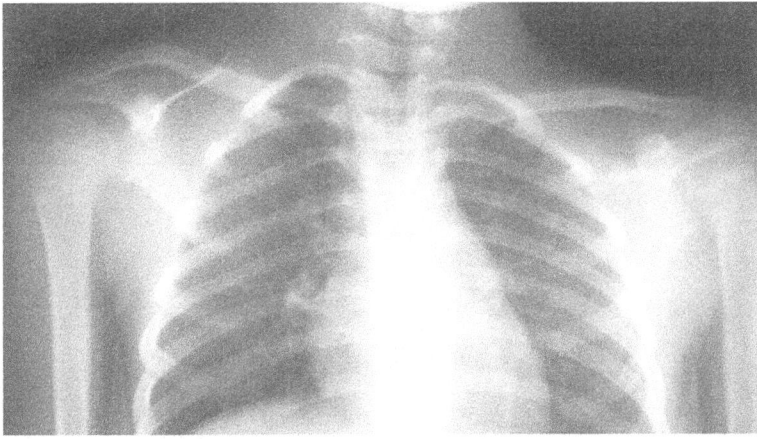

Figure 10.1
Unilateral elevation of the right scapula (Sprengel's shoulder).

10.1.2 **Madelung deformity (wrist maldevelopment)**

- growth disturbance of the medial aspect of the distal radial epiphysis causes a V-shaped deformity of the wrist (fig 10.2) usually found in females, and manifesting itself in adolescence. Such growth disturbances are assumed to be caused by localised trauma or infection leading to premature fusion of part of the growth plate. Sometimes they are accompanied by other bone dysplasias such as diaphyseal aclasis and enchondromatosis.

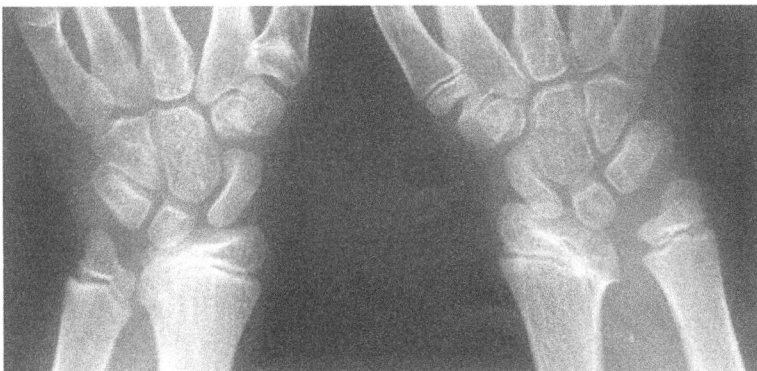

Figure 10.2
Bilateral Madelung's deformity.

10.1.3 **Duplication, hypoplasia and agenesis of upper limb bones**

- there is a wide spectrum of congenital upper limb abnormalities ranging from the clinically trivial to the very severe. Duplication of bones is one such manifestation (fig 10.3), hypoplasia and agenesis affecting the upper limb bones in a transverse or longitudinal manner are others (fig 10.4). Radial hypoplasia is found in some syndromes associated with congenital heart disease.

- congenital fusion of bones (synostosis) is well recognised in the wrist where it is mostly an incidental finding (fig 10.5, see also Chapter 4.4.6).

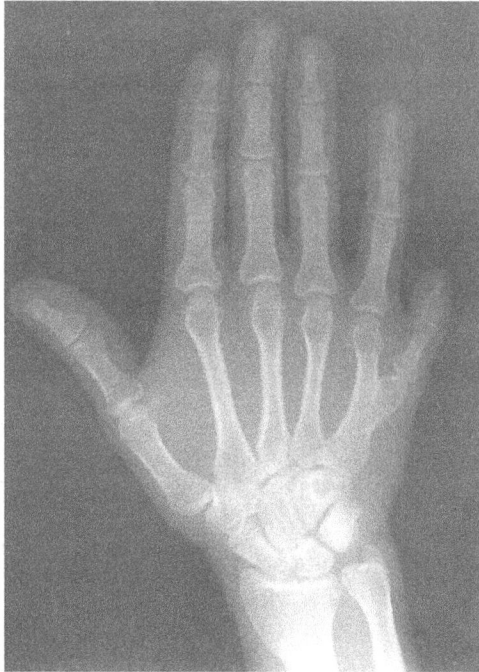

Figure 10.3
Congenital duplication with a 6th finger.

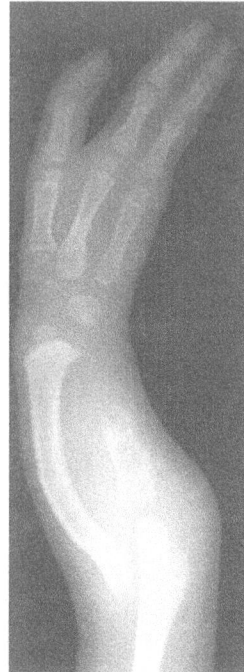

Figure 10.4
Longitudinal defect with a hypoplastic ulna and absence (agenesis) of the ulnar two rays of the hand.

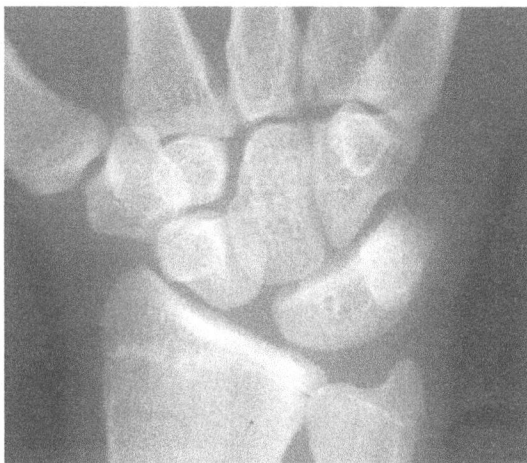

Figure 10.5
Incidental finding of congenital lunate-triquetral fusion.

10.1.4 Congenital dysplasia of the hip

- the hip joint is the most common site of congenital dislocations. The incidence is relatively high in the Caucasian population but very rare in China and parts of Africa. This may be explained by the way infants often are carried in those areas (on the mother's back with its hips flexed and abducted).

- imaging (most notably ultrasound) is used to detect abnormalities of the hip before true dislocation occurs i.e. prevention rather than cure.

- where ultrasound is not available, a combination of clinical testing and radiographs is required to establish the diagnosis (fig 10.6 to 10.8).

- the hip is a "ball-and-socket" joint. If the "ball" of the femoral head is not retained within the "socket" during growth, the acetabulum will fail to develop and will appear steep and shallow (fig 10.7).

- if congenital dislocation of the hip is inadequately treated, the femoral head will migrate upwards and develop a false acetabulum with the lateral ilium (fig 10.8).

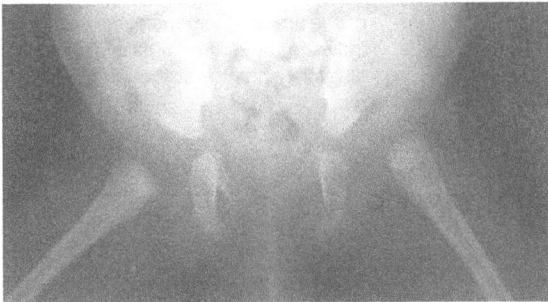

Figure 10.6
AP view with hips abducted of the pelvis in a newborn baby. A line drawn along the shaft of the right femur intersects the acetabulum. A similar line drawn on the left intersects the ilium indicating dislocation of the hip.

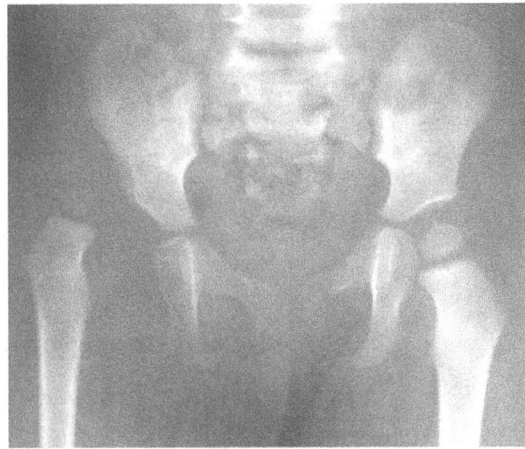

Figure 10.7
Child with congenital dislocation of the right hip. Note that, as a consequence, the right acetabulum is poorly developed.

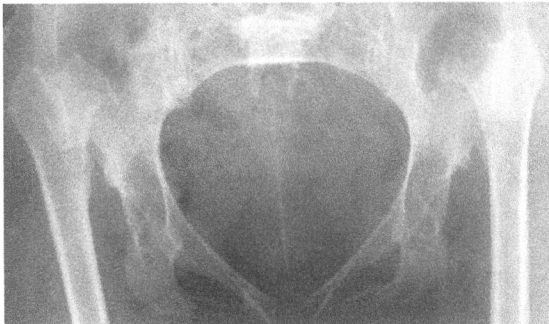

Figure 10.8
Adult with longstanding untreated congenital dislocation of the hip. The femoral heads have moved upwards and are articulating with the lateral aspect of the iliac bones. Both acetabulae are poorly developed.

10.1.5 Legg-Calvé-Perthes disease (coxa plana)

- usually known as Perthes disease, but also referred to as coxa plana. This condition is caused by osteonecrosis (ischaemic necrosis) of the proximal femoral epiphysis in children between the ages of 4 and 8 years. It is mostly affecting boys, and its occurrence differs from one geographical area to another.

- in approximately 10% of the cases the condition is bilateral but not starting at both sides at the same time. Therefore, the radiographic appearances are not symmetrical, and this is a useful diagnostic feature when trying to distinguish Perthes disease from other conditions with a fragmented proximal femoral epiphysis (e.g. epiphyseal dysplasias and cretinism).

- further progression of the disease includes increasing sclerosis, fragmentation, and flattening of the proximal femoral epiphysis (fig 10.9). In severe cases secondary growth disturbances of the acetabulum and irregularity of the proximal femoral metaphysis can be seen.

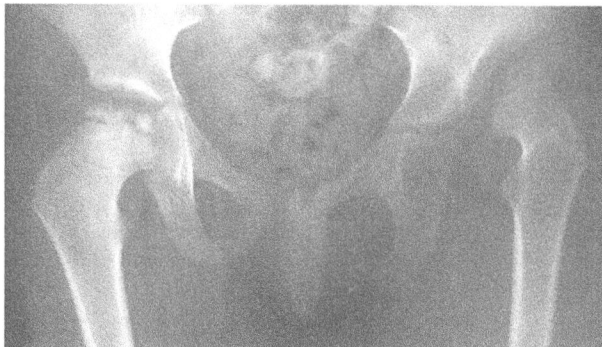

Figure 10.9
Child with sclerosis and fragmentation of the proximal femoral epiphysis indicative of Perthes disease. There is also congenital dislocation of the left hip.

10.1.6 Slipped upper femoral epiphysis

- see Chapter 4.7.1

10.1.7 Proximal focal femoral deficiency

- proximal focal femoral deficiency is a rare congenital abnormality characterized by varying degrees of hypoplasia (growth disturbances) of the proximal third of the femur (fig 10.10).

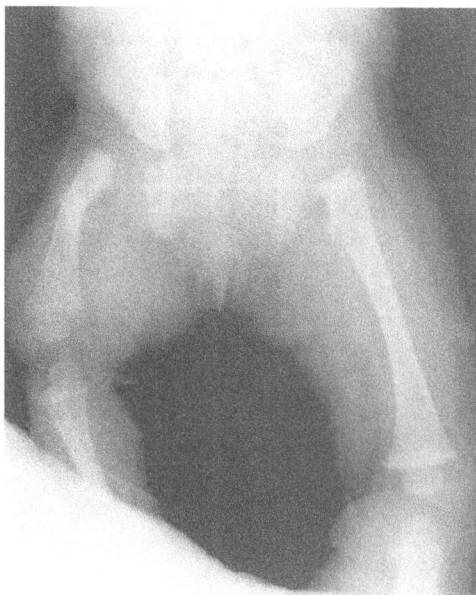

Figure 10.10
Proximal focal femoral deficiency with hypoplasia of the upper third of the right femur.

10.1.8 Congenital tibia vara (Blount's disease)

- Blount's disease, also known as congenital tibia vara, is a developmental condition principally affecting the medial portion of the proximal tibial growth plate. Two types the infantil (bilateral) type, and the adolescent (unilateral) type are known.

- when the medial tibial epiphysis and metaphysis do not grow properly, a progressive varus deformity of the knee will develop (fig 10.11).

- a similar deformity can be seen if there is premature fusion of the medial aspect of the proximal tibial growth plate due to inflammation (infectious or non-infectious) or trauma.

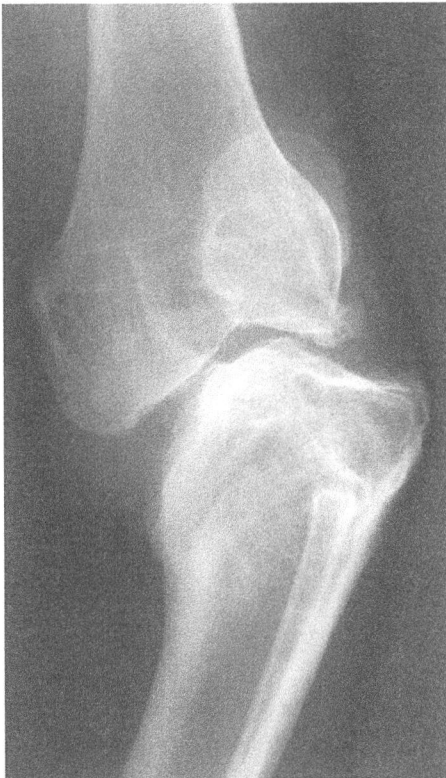

Figure 10.11
Adult with history of Blount's disease in childhood. There is depression of the medial tibial condyle with secondary degenerative changes and varus deformity of the knee joint.

10.1.9 "Ball-and-socket" ankle

- as the name implies the ankle joint develops into a "ball-and-socket" appearance (fig 10.12). The articular surface of the lower tibia and the upper talus are curved.

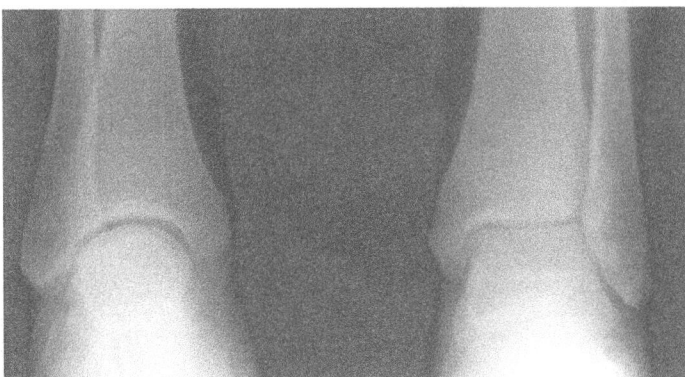

Figure 10.12
AP view showing a right ball-and-socket ankle. Compare with the normal left ankle.

10.1.10 **Talipes Equinovarus**

- also known as clubfoot. The incidence varies from area to area, and Talipes Equinovarus is in some communities observed as often as in one of 1000 births. The deformity includes (fig 10.13):

    — hindfoot equinus (plantar flexion of hindfoot causing a high arch)
    — hindfoot varus (bending inwards)
    — forefoot varus (bending inwards)

- a high arch (pes cavus) can also be seen in neuromuscular disorders.

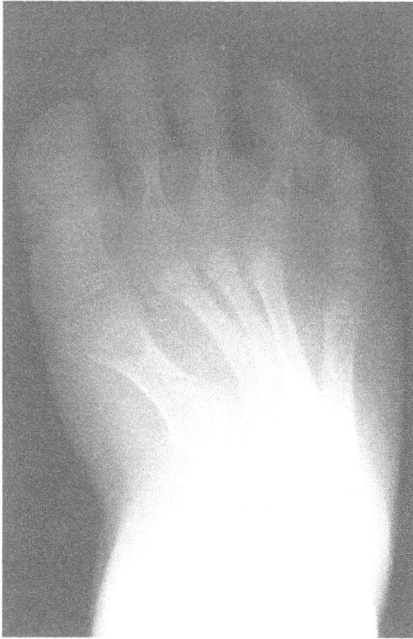

(a)

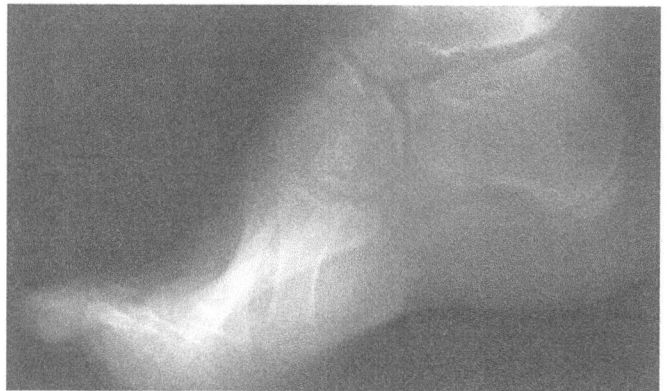

(b)

Figure 10.13
(a) AP and (b) lateral views of talipes equinovarus (clubfoot). Note the high arch (pes cavus) on the lateral view.

10.1.11 **Vertical talus**

- a congenital abnormality with extreme plantar flexion of the talus and dorsal dislocation of the navicular (fig 10.14). Results in a rigid flat foot.

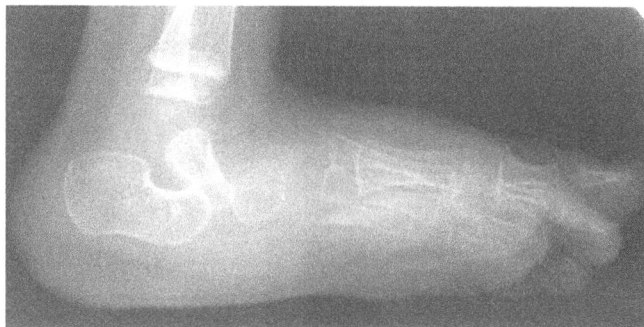

Figure 10.14
Congenital vertical talus with dislocation of the talonavicular joint.

10.1.12 **Tarsal coalition**

• tarsal coalition refers to the fusion of two or more tarsal bones forming a single structure. This fusion may be complete or incomplete, and the bridge may be fibrous, cartilaginous or osseous.

• despite being a congenital condition symptoms rarely develop before adolescence or early adulthood.

• multiple variations can occur (fig 10.15). The most common is fusion of the middle subtalar joint between the calcaneus and talus.

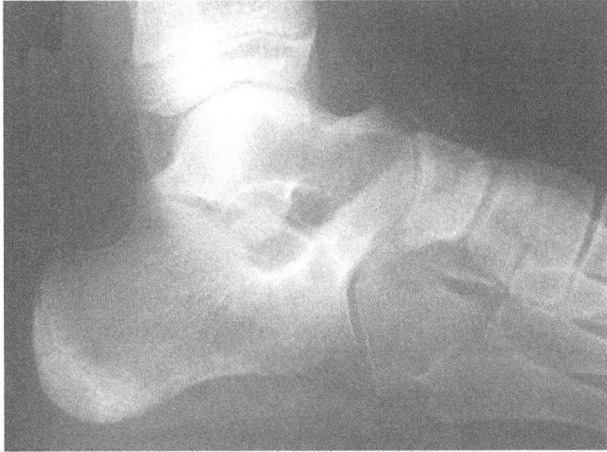
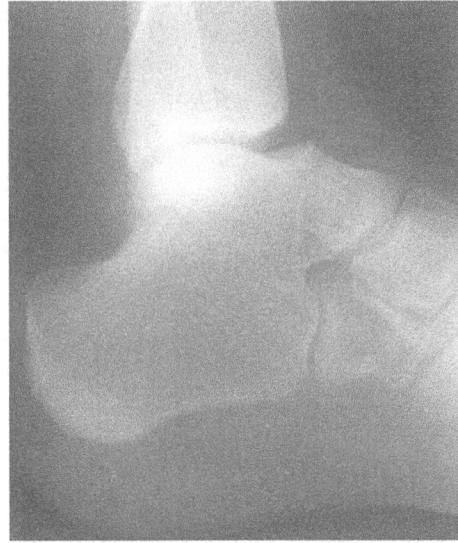

(a)   (b)

Figure 10.15
Two examples of congenital fusion (tarsal coalition): (a) Fusion between the anterosuperior process of the calcaneus and the navicular; (b) Fusion of the talus and calcaneus.

10.1.13 **Duplication, hypoplasia and agenesis of foot bones**

• as in the hand there is a wide spectrum of congenital abnormalities of the bones of the foot including duplication, hypoplasia and agenesis (fig 10.16).

• these tend to cause fewer problems than their counterparts in the upper limb as the functioning of the foot is less sophisticated and cosmetic deformities are usually hidden if shoes are worn.

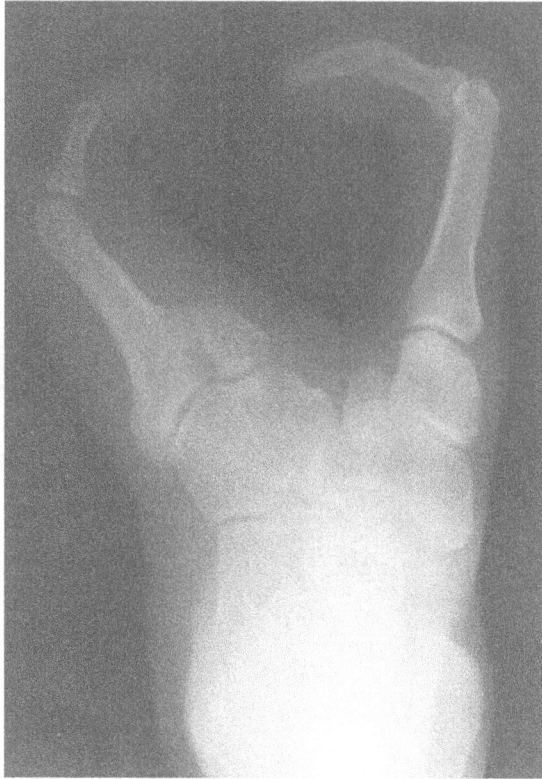

Figure 10.16
Congenital central defect of the foot (lobster-claw deformity).

10.2 Generalized Conditions

- there are numerous rare congenital conditions which can affect the skeleton to a greater or lesser extent. Most are remarkably rare and merit little mention. However, in many of these conditions radiographs are required to establish the correct diagnosis.

- these conditions are generally classified as "skeletal dysplasias", and most of these fall into one of the following broad categories;

    — dysplasia with predominantly **epiphyseal** involvement (with or without spinal involvement)
    — dysplasia with predominantly **metaphyseal** involvement (with or without spinal involvement)
    — dwarfisms
    — storage diseases
    — inherited metabolic disorders
    — dysplasia with reduced bone density
    — dysplasia with increased bone density
    — tumour-like dysplasia
    — malformation syndromes

- a few of the more common classic conditions are detailed below.

10.2.1 Multiple epiphyseal dysplasia

- symmetrical irregular growth of the epiphyses leads to premature degenerative change (fig 10.17).

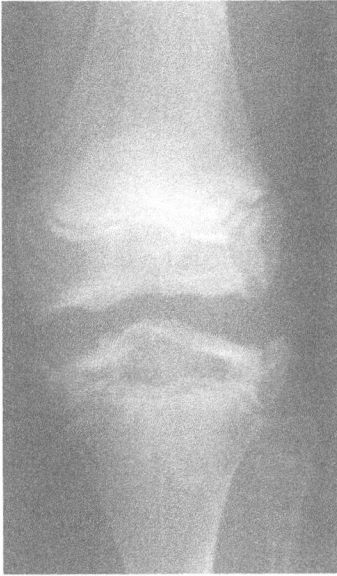

Figure 10.17
Knee joint in a child with multiple epiphyseal dysplasia. The epiphyses appear enlarged and irregular.

10.2.2 **Achondroplasia**

- achondroplasia is the most common type of short limbed dwarfism. The proximal limb segments (e.g. humerus and femur) are shorter than the distal (e.g. tibia, fibula, radius and ulna).

- the tubular (long) bones are shortened and thickened with flared metaphyses and normal epiphyses.

- the iliac bones appear squared with horizontal acetabular roofs (fig 10.18).

- the interpedicular distance decreases from the upper to lower lumbar spine (this distance increases in normal individuals, fig 10.18). As a result, adult achondroplastic dwarfs are prone to develop severe multiple level spinal canal stenoses causing nerve root irritation, paraparesis and paraplegia.

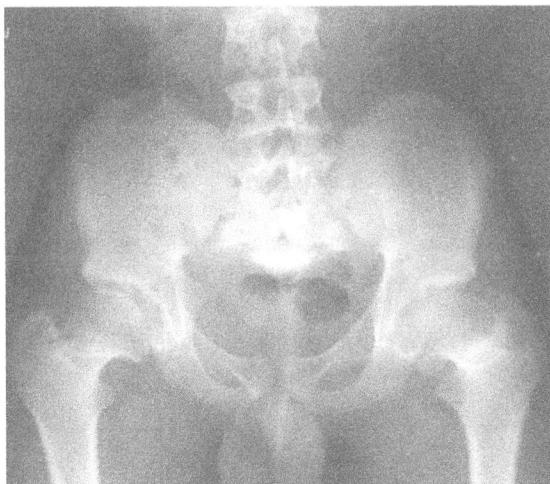

Figure 10.18
Achondroplasia with squared iliac bones, shallow roofs of the acetabuli and decreasing interpedicular distance in the lower lumbar spine.

10.2.3 **Osteogenesis imperfecta**

- a congenital connective tissue disorder causing severe reduction in bone density (osteopenia). This results in over-tubulation of the long bones (i.e. appear long and thin) and multiple fractures, which are slow to heal, and often leave marked residual deformity (fig 10.19).

- several different forms of the disease. Babies with the severest form (congenita) are usually stillborn or die in early infancy. Patients who survive infancy have a less severe form (tarda) although there is a wide spectrum of severity.

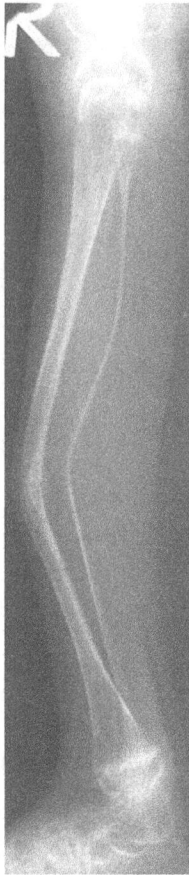

Figure 10.19
Child with osteogenesis imperfecta. The long bones are thinned, of reduced bone density and bowed. There is a healing fracture of the mid-shaft of the tibia.

10.2.4 **Sclerosing bone dysplasias**

- there is a number of bone dysplasias which can cause focal or generalised sclerosis of bone. These include;

  Osteopoikilosis – multiple small bone islands clustered at bone ends around the joints. Of no clinical significance.

  Melorheostosis – variable amounts of cortical and endosteal new bone formation likened to the pattern of dripping candle wax. Frequently affects only one limb (monomelic) or one side of the body (hemi-melic). Usually of little clinical significance but can be associated with joint contractures (fig 10.20).

  Osteopetrosis (marble bone disease) – generalized bone sclerosis resulting in brittle bones with an increased tendency to fracture (fig 10.21). The diffuse nature of the condition can simulate marrow infiltration from metastases or myelofibrosis.

  Mixed sclerosing bone dysplasia – often the distribution of bony sclerosis can exhibit a mixed pattern combining features from two or more different sclerosing dysplasias.

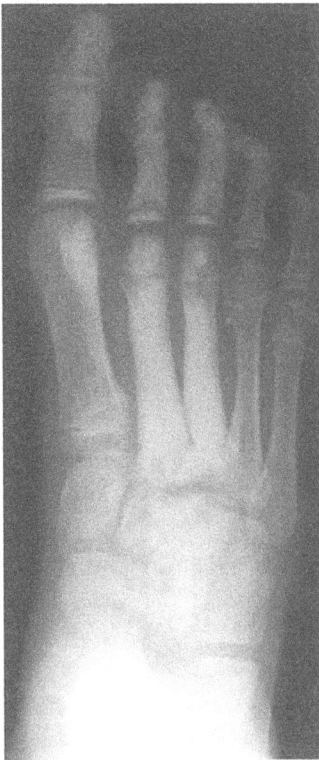

Figure 10.20
Child with the sclerosing
melorheostosis affecting the
medial three rays (digits and
metacarpals) of the foot.

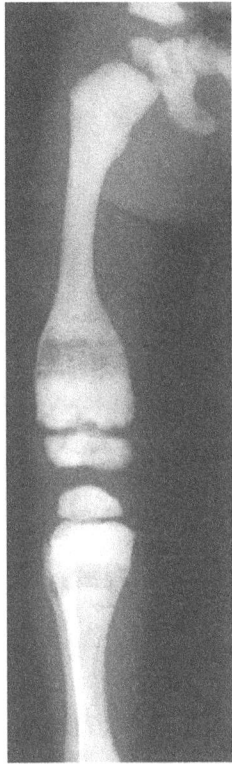

Figure 10.21
Child with osteopetrosis.
Generalised increase in
bone density with
modelling deformities of
the bone ends.

10.2.5 **Tumour-like dysplasias**

- this category includes;

  — multiple osteochondromas (diaphyseal aclasis, fig 10.22, see Chapter 9.6.2)
  — multiple enchondromas (Ollier's disease, fig 9.3 and 10.23, see Chapter 9.6.2)
  — polyostotic fibrous dysplasia (fig 10.24)

- individuals with diaphyseal aclasis and Ollier's disease have a small risk of malignant transformation of one of their lesions to a low grade chondrosarcoma (fig 9.22).

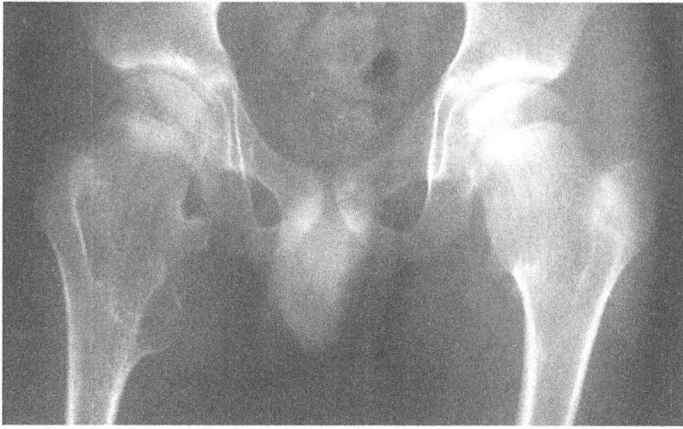

Figure 10.22
Child with diaphyseal aclasis. The circumferential nature of the osteochondromas arising from the proximal femurs results in the modelling deformities. (See Chapter 9.6.2.2)

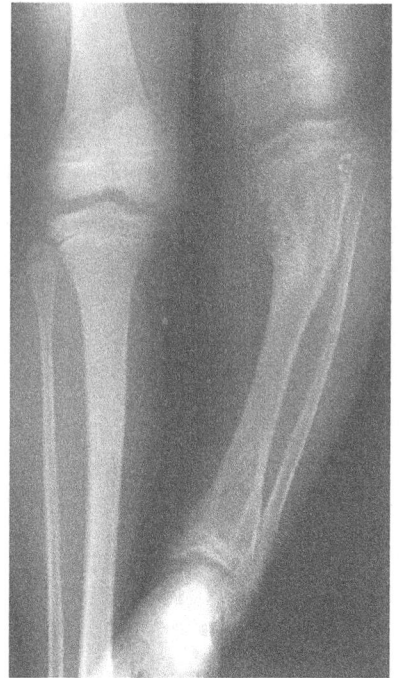

Figure 10.23
Multiple enchondromas (Ollier's disease) affecting the left lower limb.

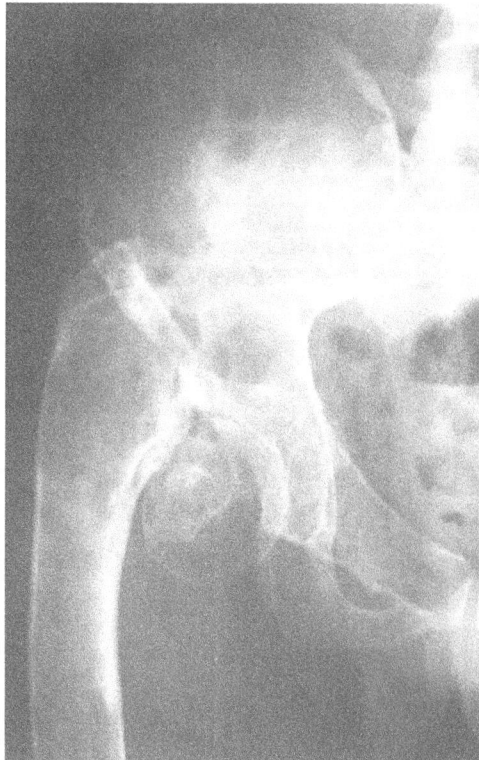

Figure 10.24
Multifocal (polyostotic) fibrous dysplasia. There is an ununited fracture of the femoral neck.

10.3 **Spinal Deformity**

10.3.1 **Scoliosis**

- scoliosis may be;

    — idiopathic
    — congenital
    — neuromuscular
    — other (including trauma, infection and tumours

Idiopathic scoliosis

- constitutes up to 70% of all cases of scoliosis

- 3 types depending on age of presentation – infantile, juvenile and adolescent.

- 85% are adolescent, more common in girls than in boys, usually involving the thoracolumbar spine with the convexity of the principle curve to the right.

Congenital scoliosis

- constitutes 10% of all cases of scoliosis.

- due to underlying congenital vertebral abnormalities. These include;

    — failure of formation e.g. hemivertebra, spina bifida (fig 10.25)
    — failure of segmentation e.g. fusion at one or multiple levels (fig 10.26)

- there is a recognized association of congenital scoliosis with other abnormalities such as tethering of the spinal cord and diastematomyelia (bony or fibrous bar across the spinal canal).

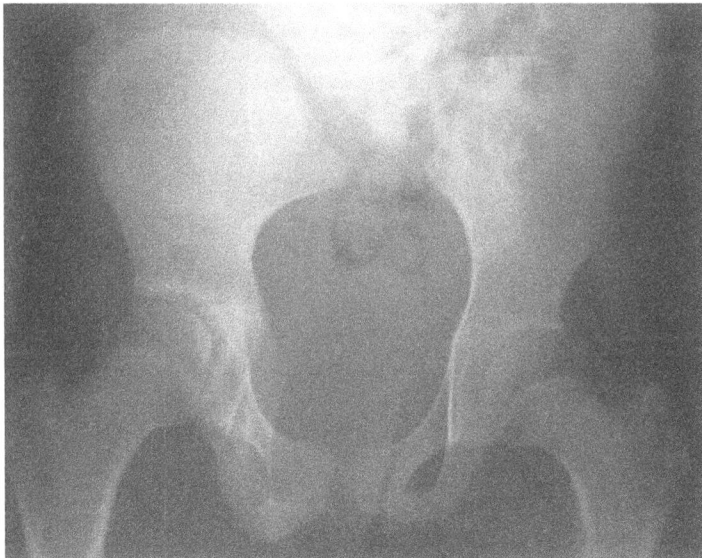

Figure 10.25
Child with absent sacrum (sacral agenesis). This condition is commoner in the children of diabetic mothers.

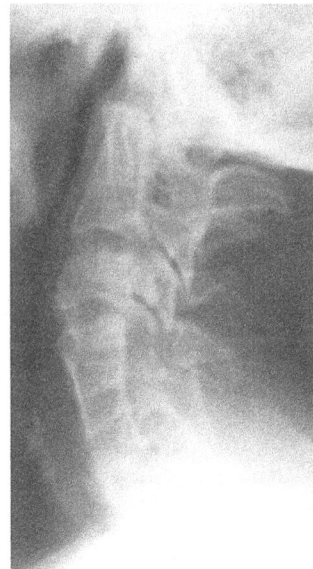

Figure 10.26
Multiple level congenital fusion in the cervical spine (Klippel Feil deformity).

Radiographs of scoliosis

- the initial radiographic examination should be an AP film to determine whether there are any underlying congenital vertebral abnormalities to indicate congenital cause. It can often be difficult to fully assess the extent of congenital vertebral abnormalities particularly if the deformity is severe. In this situation conventional tomography can be helpful (fig 10.27).

- follow-up films to assess the progress of the deformity should be performed PA to minimise radiation dose to the breast tissue.

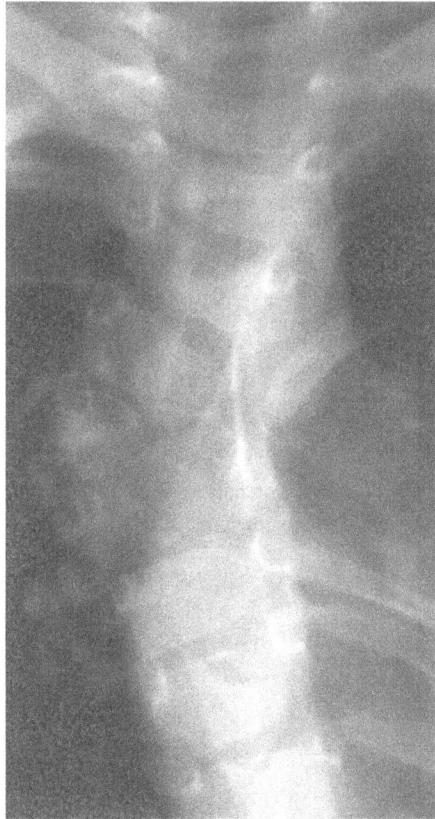

(a)

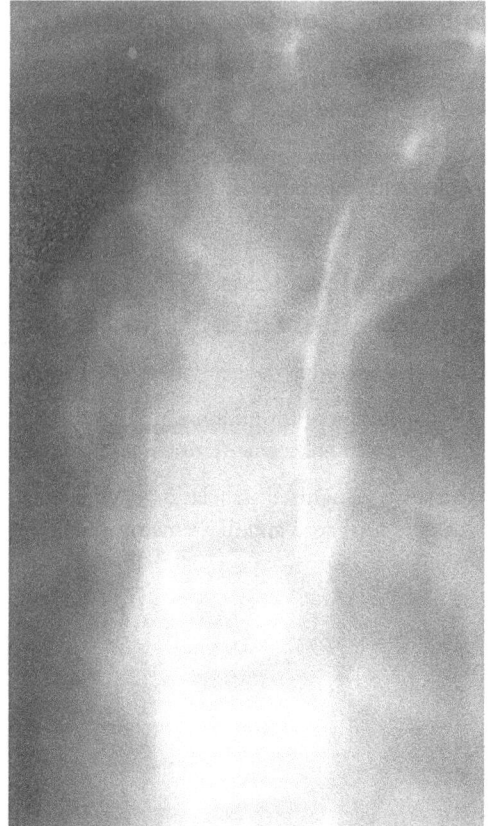

(b)

Figure 10.27
Congenital scoliosis. (a) the AP view shows a right sided hemivertebra; (b) the AP tomogram shows there is also a left sided posterior bar (fusion over several levels).

CHAPTER 11

Recommended Reading

• this manual is intended to be read and referred to by general practitioners, medical specialists, radiographers and radiologists working in small hospitals and institutions with little or no access to other radiological material. It is envisaged that the interested reader will wish to supplement her/his knowledge and seek out other sources of information. Continuing technological advances mean that in many fields textbooks rapidly become out-of-date. Fortunately, interpretation of conventional radiographs has changed little over the past years such that much of the subject matter in old textbooks remains as pertinent today as when the book was first published. Most textbooks published in the last few years concentrate on newer imaging techniques, not always available. Listed below are a few suggestions of useful texts.

Primers (basic texts)

Chapman S and Nakielny R. *Aids to Radiological Diagnosis*, Saunders

— *small book containing numerous useful lists.*

Manamaster BJ. *Handbooks in Radiology: Skeletal Radiology*, Year Book Medical Publishers

— *small book containing a lot of information in note form.*

Raby N, Berman L and de Lacey G. *Accident and Emergency Radiology: a survival guide*, Saunders

— *useful book detailing common fracture patterns and pitfalls.*

Thornton A and Gyll C. *Children's Fractures*, Saunders

— *short book concentrating on paediatric fractures*

Major textbooks

Keats TE. Atlas of Normal Roentgen *Variants that may Simulate Disease*, Year Book Medical Publishers

— *classic book showing literally thousands of normal variants.*

Schmidt H and Freyschmidt J. Köhler and Zimmer's *Borderlands of Normal and Early Pathologic Findings in Skeletal Radiography*, Thieme

— *covers much the same subject matter as Keat's Normal Variants but with more text and fewer illustrations.*

Rogers LF. *Radiology of Skeletal Trauma*, Churchill Livingstone

— *2 volume set. Arguably the most comprehensive book on the subject. The vast majority deals with conventional radiographs.*

Murray RO, Jacobson HG & Stoker DJ. *The Radiology of Skeletal Disorders*, Churchill Livingstone

— *classic 3 volume text on skeletal radiographs. Unfortunately, long out of print.*

Greenspan A. *Orthopedic Radiology: a practical approach*, Raven Press

— *a good general text concentrating on radiographs.*

Palmer PES & Reeder MM. *The Imaging of Tropical Diseases*, Springer

— *a comprehensive 2 volume book.*

www.ingramcontent.com/pod-product-compliance
Lightning Source LLC
Chambersburg PA
CBHW061104210326
41597CB00021B/3975